Thyroid Surgery

Thyroid Surgery
Principles and Practice

Edited by
Madan Laxman Kapre

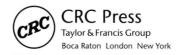

CRC Press
Taylor & Francis Group
Boca Raton London New York

CRC Press is an imprint of the
Taylor & Francis Group, an **informa** business

First edition published 2020
by CRC Press
6000 Broken Sound Parkway NW, Suite 300, Boca Raton, FL 33487-2742

and by CRC Press
2 Park Square, Milton Park, Abingdon, Oxon, OX14 4RN

First issued in paperback 2021

© 2020 Taylor & Francis Group, LLC
CRC Press is an imprint of Taylor & Francis Group, an Informa business

Library of Congress Cataloging-in-Publication Data

Names: Kapre, Madan, editor.
Title: Thyroid surgery : principles and practice / edited by Madan Kapre.
Other titles: Thyroid surgery (Kapre)
Description: First edition. | Boca Raton : CRC Press, 2020. | Includes bibliographical references and index. |
Summary: "This book will bridge a gap between the huge platform of literature available on the subject of thyroid surgery and the pratical working reality. The pearls in techniques and surgical procedures will be exhaustively detailed with authors' individual experience enriched with quality photographs"-- Provided by publisher.
Identifiers: LCCN 2020006268 (print) | LCCN 2020006269 (ebook) | ISBN 9781138483781 (hbk) | ISBN 9780429086076 (ebk)
Subjects: MESH: Thyroid Diseases--surgery | Thyroid Gland--surgery | Thyroid Neoplasms--surgery | Thyroidectomy
Classification: LCC RD599.5.T46 (print) | LCC RD599.5.T46 (ebook) | NLM WK 280 | DDC 617.5/39--dc23
LC record available at https://lccn.loc.gov/2020006268
LC ebook record available at https://lccn.loc.gov/2020006269

ISBN 13: 978-1-138-48378-1 (hbk)
ISBN 13: 978-1-03-224291-0 (pbk)

DOI: 10.1201/9780429086076

Typeset in Minion
by Nova Techset Private Limited, Bengaluru & Chennai, India

Publisher's Note
The publisher has gone to great lengths to ensure the quality of this reprint but points out that some imperfections in the original copies may be apparent.

CONTENTS

Preface   vii

Acknowledgments   ix

Editor   xi

Contributors   xiii

Introduction   xvii

CHAPTER 1 HISTORY AND EVOLUTION OF THYROID SURGERY   1

Cheerag Patel and Subhaschandra Shetty

CHAPTER 2 SURGICAL ANATOMY OF THE THYROID   7

Ashutosh Mangalgiri and Deven Mahore

CHAPTER 3 CLINICAL ASSESSMENT OF THE THYROID NODULE   15

Madan Laxman Kapre, Shripal Jani, and Priya Dubey

CHAPTER 4 IMAGING OF THE THYROID   21

Alka Ashmita Singhal

CHAPTER 5 PATHOLOGY OF THE THYROID   45

R. Ravi

CHAPTER 6 MEDICAL MANAGEMENT OF THYROID DISORDERS   51

Himanshu Patil and Shailesh Pitale

CHAPTER 7 ANESTHESIA FOR THYROID SURGERY   57

Vidula Kapre, Shubhada Deshmukh, Pratibha Deshmukh, Meghna Sarode, and Rajashree Chaudhary

CHAPTER 8 SAFE THYROIDECTOMY   67

Madan Laxman Kapre, Sankar Viswanath, Rajendra Deshmukh, and Neeti Kapre Gupta

CHAPTER 9 SURGERY FOR MULTINODULAR GOITER   75

Madan Laxman Kapre, Sanoop Elambassery, Neeti Kapre Gupta, M. Abdul Amjad Khan, and Gauri Kapre Vaidya

CHAPTER 10 MANAGEMENT OF RETROSTERNAL GOITER   79

Belayat Hossain Siddiquee

CHAPTER 11 REMOTE ACCESS ENDOSCOPIC AND ROBOTIC THYROIDECTOMY   83

Kyung Tae

CHAPTER 12 ROBOTIC THYROIDECTOMY   91

Neil S. Tolley and Christian Camenzuli

CHAPTER 13 INTRA-OPERATIVE NEURAL MONITORING   97

Rahul Modi

CHAPTER 14 SURGICAL MANAGEMENT OF DIFFERENTIATED THYROID CANCERS 105
Anil D'cruz and Richa Vaish

CHAPTER 15 MANAGEMENT OF NODAL METASTASIS IN THYROID CANCER 113
Neeti Kapre Gupta, Ashok Shaha, Madan Laxman Kapre, Nirmala Thakkar, and Harsh Karan Gupta

CHAPTER 16 COMPLICATIONS OF THYROID SURGERY 119
Gregory W. Randolph, Dipti Kamani, Cristian Slough, and Selen Soylu

CHAPTER 17 LOCALLY ADVANCED THYROID CANCER 127
Amit Agarwal and Roma Pradhan

CHAPTER 18 SURGICAL MANAGEMENT OF MEDULLARY THYROID CANCERS 135
Anuja Deshmukh and Anand Thomas

CHAPTER 19 SURGICAL MANAGEMENT OF ANAPLASTIC THYROID CANCERS 147
Deepa Nair and K.S. Rathan Shetty

CHAPTER 20 POST-TREATMENT SURVEILLANCE OF THYROID CANCER 151
Abhishek Vaidya

CHAPTER 21 APPLICATIONS OF RADIOISOTOPES IN THE DIAGNOSIS AND TREATMENT OF THYROID DISORDERS 161
Chandrasekhar Bal, Meghana Prabhu, Dhritiman Chakraborty, K. Sreenivasa Reddy, and Saurabh Arora

CHAPTER 22 SYSTEMIC THERAPY (TARGETED THERAPY AND IMMUNOTHERAPY) FOR THYROID CANCERS 173
Abhishek Vaidya and Amol Dongre

CHAPTER 23 SURGICAL MANAGEMENT OF PARATHYROID DISORDERS 179
Neeti Kapre Gupta, Gregory W. Randolph, and Dipti Kamani

CHAPTER 24 PEDIATRIC THYROID SURGERY 187
Rajendra Saoji

Index 191

PREFACE

The seeds of this book were sown by the students getting off the bus returning from their annual Thyroid Surgical Camp of Chikhaldara, Melghat. Armed with the art and craft of thyroid surgery, they wanted more insight into the science of it.

Our first book *Atlas of Thyroid Surgery* answered the question of "how?" but there were more questions, like "when?," "why?," and "how much?" that remained unanswered.

Thyroid surgery has undergone several paradigm shifts, from being a life-threatening exercise to a minimally invasive procedure. More than any other surgery, it highlights the need to respect tissues, nerves, and vessels. Skill, precision, and the fine line between aggression and conservatism in surgery is nowhere as important as it is in the management of thyroid disease. To do justice to all this was well beyond the scope of an atlas or a workshop.

It was then that, quite unexpectedly, Miss Shivangi from Taylor & Francis approached us and very kindly offered to take the thread of this new book forward.

I soon realized the magnitude of the task. Some unforeseen health issues almost stalled the process, and I am grateful to my publishers for graciously bearing with the delay.

With this book we have endeavored to bring forth a blend of surgical rationale, multidisciplinary decision-making, basic surgical principles, and techniques for both the novice and the expert alike.

We have tried to include authors from across the globe to present a holistic viewpoint on thyroid management.

Thyroid surgery can be performed with some grams of steel but needs nerves of steel.

ACKNOWLEDGMENTS

What worth is your knowledge if it does not dispel the darkness of ignorance? What worth is your skill if it does not make others skillful? What worth is a teacher's greatness if their students do not become greater than themselves?

I have been fortunate to find worthy colleagues, "Men and Women of Wisdom," and worthy publishers, CRC Press, Taylor & Francis Group, who came together to disseminate the wisdom, skill, and great clinical prowess in the field of thyroid surgery.

First, I wish to thank Miss Shivangi Pramanik and Miss Himani Dwivedi who had the faith and patience to bear with us, the authors and the editor. It was their disciplined approach that laid the foundation for this book, given to us by the publisher CRC Press, Taylor & Francis Group.

All my colleague authors who penned the chapters are the worthy men and women of wisdom. I am appreciative and conscious of how difficult it must have been for them to draw that extra ounce of energy and precious time to painstakingly write their chapters. I am grateful to all of them.

And I wish to express my gratitude to my colleagues in my own institute, fellows who worked with us, and the secretarial backup I received. Running the risk of missing a few names inadvertently and asking for their pardon, I am grateful to my fellows who have been burdened by tasks beyond their working hours. Dr. Neeti has been great in gathering bits and pieces provided by Amjad, Sankar, Sanoop, Shripal, and Priya. She has been my real support in compiling this book.

Finally, I am in great debt to my family, my wife Vidula, my daughters Neeti and Gauri, and my sons-in-law Abhishek and Harsh for their unconditional support and sufferings in the making of this book.

EDITOR

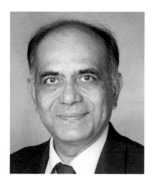

Dr. Madan Laxman Kapre is the Director at Neeti Clinics in Nagpur, India. He is the Founder and Governing Council Member of the Asia Pacific Thyroid Society, Seoul, South Korea; Advisory Committee of the Asia Pacific Society of Thyroid Surgery; and the Chairman of the Indian Subcontinent Symposium to 3rd WCTC, Boston, USA. He is the Founder and President of the Indian Society of Thyroid Surgeons, past President of the Foundation of Head & Neck Oncology in India, and the Founding President of the Vidarbha Society for Head and Neck Oncology. He has been President of the Laryngology and Voice Association of India and of the Maharashtra State ENT associations. For his work in tribal hills endemic for goiter, he has received lifetime achievement awards by two prestigious national organizations: Foundation of Head and Neck Oncology and Indian Academy of Otolaryngologist and Head and Neck Surgeons. His research work includes mandibular mucoperiosteal flap for closure of oral defects after surgery of oral cancers and intraoperative cytology for clearance of surgical margins. He is very active academically and has authored/edited many books including *Atlas of Thyroid Surgery* (Jaypee Brothers Medical Publishers, 2013), *Atlas on Surgery of Trismus of OSMF* (Springer Singapore, 2018), and *Essentials of Head and Neck Surgery* (Byword Books, December 2011).

CONTRIBUTORS

Amit Agarwal
Department of Endocrine Surgery
Sanjay Gandhi Post Graduate Institute
    of Medical Sciences (SGPGIMS)
Lucknow, India

Saurabh Arora
Department of Nuclear Medicine
All India Institute of Medical Sciences (AIIMS)
New Delhi, India

Chandrasekhar Bal
Department of Nuclear Medicine
All India Institute of Medical Sciences (AIIMS)
New Delhi, India

Christian Camenzuli
Hammersmith Hospital
Imperial College NHS Trust
London, United Kingdom

Dhritiman Chakraborty
Department of Nuclear Medicine
All India Institute of Medical Sciences (AIIMS)
New Delhi, India

Rajashree Chaudhary
Consultant Anesthesiologist
Neeti Clinics
Nagpur, India

Anil D'cruz
Consultant Head and Neck Surgeon
Apollo Hospitals
and
TATA Memorial Hospital
Mumbai, India

Anuja Deshmukh
Department of Head and Neck Surgery
TATA Memorial Centre
Mumbai, India

Pratibha Deshmukh
Department of Anesthesia
Indira Gandhi Medical College
Nagpur, India

Rajendra Deshmukh
Visiting Consultant ENT Surgeon
Neeti Clinics
Nagpur, India

Shubhada Deshmukh
Department of Anesthesia
Lata Mangeshkar Medical College
Nagpur, India

Amol Dongre
Consultant Medical Oncologist
Alexis Multispeciality Hospital
Nagpur, India

Priya Dubey
Association of Otorhinolaryngologists and
    Head and Neck Surgery (AOI-HNS)
Neeti Clinics
Nagpur, India

Sanoop Elambassery
ENT and Head and Neck Surgeon
Malabar Hospital
Kozhikode, India

Harsh Karan Gupta
Consultant ENT Surgeon
Neeti Clinics
and
Consultant ENT Surgeon
American Institute of Oncology
Nagpur, India

Neeti Kapre Gupta
Consultant Head and Neck Surgeon
Neeti Clinics
and
Consultant Head and Neck Surgeon
American Institute of Oncology
Nagpur, India

Shripal Jani
Foundation of Head and Neck Oncology (FHNO)
Neeti Clinics
Nagpur, India

Dipti Kamani
Division of Thyroid and Parathyroid Endocrine Surgery
Department of Otolaryngology – Head and Neck Surgery
Massachusetts Eye and Ear Infirmary
Harvard Medical School
Boston, Massachusetts

Madan Laxman Kapre
Neeti Clinics
and
Consultant Head and Neck Surgeon
American Institute of Oncology
and
R.S.T. Regional Cancer Institute
Nagpur, India

Vidula Kapre
Consultant Anesthesiologist
Neeti Clinics
Nagpur, India

M. Abdul Amjad Khan
Department of ENT and Head and Neck Surgery
Citizens Specialty Hospital
Hyderabad, India

Deven Mahore
Government Medical College
Gondia, India

Ashutosh Mangalgiri
Department of Anatomy
Chirayu Medical College
Bhopal, India

Rahul Modi
ENT – Head and Neck Surgery
Dr. L H Hiranandani Hospital
Mumbai, India

Deepa Nair
Head and Neck Oncosurgeon
Tata Memorial Hospital
Mumbai, India

Cheerag Patel
Department of Otorhinolaryngology,
    Head and Neck Surgery
Auckland District Health Board
Auckland, New Zealand

Himanshu Patil
Consultant Endocrinologist
Dew Hospital
Nagpur, India

Shailesh Pitale
Consultant Endocrinologist
Trinity Institute and Dew Hospital
Nagpur, India

Meghana Prabhu
Department of Nuclear Medicine
All India Institute of Medical Sciences (AIIMS)
New Delhi, India

Roma Pradhan
Department of Endocrine Surgery
DR Ram Manohar Lohia Institute of Medical Sciences
Lucknow, India

Gregory W. Randolph
The Claire and John Bertucci Endowed Chair
    in Thyroid Surgery Oncology
Harvard Medical School
and
Division of Thyroid and Parathyroid Endocrine Surgery
Department of Otolaryngology – Head and Neck Surgery
Massachusetts Eye and Ear Infirmary
Harvard Medical School
and
Department of Surgery, Endocrine Surgery Service
Massachusetts General Hospital
Boston, Massachusetts

R. Ravi
Institute of Surgical Pathology
Nagpur, India

K. Sreenivasa Reddy
Department of Nuclear Medicine
All India Institute of Medical Sciences (AIIMS)
New Delhi, India

Rajendra Saoji
Department of Pediatric Surgery
Government Medical College
Nagpur, India

Meghna Sarode
Consultant Anesthesiologist
Neeti Clinics
Nagpur, India

Ashok Shaha
Senior Consultant Head and Neck Surgery
Jatin P. Shah Chair in Head and Neck Surgery
Memorial Sloan Kettering Cancer Center
New York, New York

K.S. Rathan Shetty
Department of Head and Neck Oncology
Kidwai Memorial Institute of Oncology
Bangalore, India

Subhaschandra Shetty
ORL Head and Neck Surgery
Middlemore Hospital
Auckland, New Zealand

Belayat Hossain Siddiquee
Department of Otolaryngology
Bangabandhu Sheikh Mujib Medical
    University (BSMMU)
Dhaka, Bangladesh

Alka Ashmita Singhal
Senior Consultant Radiology
Medanta – The Medicity
New Delhi, India

Cristian Slough
Otolaryngology – Head and Neck Surgery
Willamette Valley Medical Center
McMinnville, Oregon

Selen Soylu
Department of General Surgery
Istanbul University
Cerrahpasa Medical Faculty
Istanbul, Turkey

Kyung Tae
Department of Otolaryngology – Head and
    Neck Surgery
College of Medicine
Hanyang University
Seoul, Korea

Nirmala Thakkar
Consultant ENT Surgeon
Neeti Clinics
Nagpur, India

Anand Thomas
Department of Surgical Oncology
Malabar Cancer Centre
Kerala, India

Neil S. Tolley
Senior ENT Consultant
ENT – Thyroid Surgeon
Hammersmith Hospital
Imperial College NHS Trust
London, United Kingdom

Abhishek Vaidya
Consultant
National Cancer Institute (NCI)
and
Visiting Consultant ENT and Head and Neck Surgeon
Neeti Clinics
Nagpur, India

Gauri Kapre Vaidya
Consultant ENT Surgeon
Neeti Clinics
and
Consultant ENT Surgeon
American Oncology Institute
Nagpur, India

Richa Vaish
Consultant
Head and Neck Oncosurgeon
TATA Memorial Hospital
Mumbai, India

Sankar Viswanath
Consultant ENT and Head and Neck Surgeon
Avitis Institute of Medical Sciences
Palakkad, India

INTRODUCTION

Madan Laxman Kapre

How common are thyroid nodules? The more you look for them, the more you find them. Their incidence is also directly proportional to the tools applied for their detection; clinical and radiological being the front-runners. Whether there is an absolute increase in the occurrence of thyroid nodules is debatable. Certainly, it is our observation that in central India, which is the author's work domain, the incidence in the urban population is almost on par with the rural population, which is quite a revelation given that it is thought to be endemic in the hilly areas of the Melghat district of central India. The prevalence of thyroid nodules detected by thyroid ultrasound at health check-ups was 34.2% [1]. Thyroid nodules were more prevalent in women and older age groups.

As most of the nodules are asymptomatic, and the incidence of thyroid carcinoma in them is quite low, about 1.2% [2], the clinician must be very judicious to select the patient for further evaluation. With increasing awareness and access to information on electronic media, not creating cancer phobia in patients is becoming a challenge. Preventing psychological stress to the patient and family while detecting early thyroid cancer that can be treated with less morbid surgery is becoming a tall task for surgeons.

It is very encouraging that even in developing countries, endocrinological, surgical, and medical services are growing at a rapid pace and are of high quality. As a result, there are several clinicians of varied backgrounds who are involved in initial diagnosis and subsequent surgical management. It is a matter of teamwork and evolving strategy to evaluate and manage thyroid nodules. Thyroid nodules are often diagnosed by endocrinologists while they are clinically small. Adding to this is the rising occurrence of "incidentaloma." Accurately diagnosing and evaluating a patient is a great clinical responsibility.

The incidence of thyroid nodules in the past was considered in a subset of patients in urban, rural, and hilly areas. It was also believed to be due to an iodine-deficient diet. However, the thyroid nodules pathogenesis has shifted away from the theory of iodine deficiency. Long study periods in large populations are needed, and this increases the likelihood of bias from changes in unmeasured risk factors other than iodine intake. There is also the additional uncertainty of the lag-time between changes in iodine exposure and changes in incidence of thyroid cancer; the lag-time between increasing iodine intake and the resolution of diffuse goiter and nodules in adult populations is several decades. Accurate dietary assessment of iodine intake is notoriously difficult [3].

WHICH THYROID NODULE NEEDS EVALUATION?

Symptomatic nodes are far easier to investigate, as the patient has shown willingness for further work-up. Asymptomatic nodules are the ones that require judicious examination in order to safeguard against a patient's anxiety and stress originating from investigating "tumorous" conditions.

For asymptomatic nodules detected either during a routine clinical examination by a general practitioner or by an observer, the patient requires sympathetic reassurance to prevent cancer psychosis, as these nodules are harmless and need not be subjected to further investigations.

The nodules detected by imaging and/or already being investigated by primary physician will merit its evaluation on the information presented by the imaging studies. Although more information on this topic shall be available to readers in relevant topics on imaging of the thyroid, it is rather relevant to make some basic observations. A small, <2 cm size solid nodule may be more ominous than a large cystic nodule.

THYROID FUNCTIONAL ASSESSMENT

Assessment of the functional status of the thyroid gland is vital for anesthetic assessment should the patient require surgical treatment. However, it will also help in assessing possible pathology. Hyperthyroid status is very rarely associated with malignancy, and such a situation will require a referral to an endocrinologist. Hypothyroidism indicates loss of functional thyroid parenchyma and suggests a disease accordingly.

CHANGING FRONTLINE INVESTIGATION

It is now fairly well accepted that ultrasonological assessment has overtaken fine needle aspiration cytology (FNAC) as the primary investigation method. Size, echogenicity, margins, loss of halo, and circularity will naturally give reasonable stratification of nodule. Similarly, the presence of occult lymph nodes in the neck away from the thyroid naturally indicates a papillary thyroid carcinoma. More details are available in relevant chapters.

FINE NEEDLE ASPIRATION CYTOLOGY (SCOPE AND LIMITATION)

FNAC was once a rare test; however, it has moved into second position after ultrasound in the current state of practice. It is a simple, painless office procedure, but it can be the beginning of stress and anxiety to the patient and family. Hence, we should be clear in our planning as to which of the thyroid nodules should be subjected to this test. It should be considered in situations where there is considerable evidence of clinical and radiological evaluation that a nodule under investigation has a considerable risk of being malignant.

NEWER ADVENTS OF RISK ASSESSMENT

Molecular/genetic mapping and the advent of elastography have added to our current risk assessment schemes. Genetic mutation guides our decision-making towards extents of surgery and in particular the clearance of nodal disease in the central compartment of neck level VI.

Elastography is another very helpful application of ultrasonography to characterize the compactness/hardness of thyroid nodules. It helps to differentiate thyroiditis of inflammatory origin from solid tumors which are likely to be malignant. Ultrasound elastography is a dynamic technique that estimates stiffness of tissues by measuring the degree of distortion under external pressure.

SUMMARY

The real reward of working through the maze of various tests and evaluating the results is the confidence of performing fewer surgical procedures, e.g., hemithyroidectomy, or less aggressive neck dissection particularly in the central compartment of neck level VI. This is the real progress over the decades where our patients are benefiting from fewer surgeries and have a better understanding of their condition.

We have tried to analyze and study the application of these procedures with their limitations of various risk evaluating tools in appropriate chapters. Beginning with history and clinical examination, one can start moving down the algorithm. Then by applying appropriate biochemical tests one can assess the functionality of the thyroid. Ultrasonography, FNAC, and more imaging such as contrast CT/MRI will map the disease more accurately.

Throughout the chapters of this book, we have envisaged a readership of learners and the learned. I, along with my colleague authors, hope this book will prove valuable for both.

REFERENCES

1. Moon JH et al. Prevalence of thyroid nodules and their associated clinical parameters: A large-scale, multicenter-based health checkup study. *Korean J Intern Med.* 2018;33:753–62.

2. Fernando JR, Raj SEK, Kumar AM, Anandan H. Clinical study of incidence of malignancy in solitary nodule of thyroid. *Int J Sci Stud.* 2017;5(4):232–6.

3. Zimmerman MB, Galetti V. Iodine intake as a risk factor for thyroid cancer: A comprehensive review of animal and human studies. *Thyroid Res.* 2015;8:8.

Chapter 1

HISTORY AND EVOLUTION OF THYROID SURGERY

Cheerag Patel and Subhaschandra Shetty

CONTENTS

Introduction 1
The History of Goiter 1
The History of the Thyroid and Parathyroid Hormones 2
The History of Surgery and of Surgical Instruments 3
The History of Thyroid Surgery 4
Future Directions 5
References 5

INTRODUCTION

It was Sir Winston Churchill who professed that:

"Those who fail to learn from history are doomed to repeat it."

This expression serves as an important reminder that as progress is made, it is of paramount importance that we acknowledge and appreciate the history that has brought us to the present. In modern day, thyroid surgery is commonly practiced throughout the world for a variety of pathological conditions. However, the history of thyroid surgery has been wrought with mortality, trepidation, and discouragement. In this first chapter, we explore this history in further detail so that we may duly appreciate the serendipitous discoveries, tenacious perseverance, and unfortunate mortalities that helped to pave the path to the operations that thyroid surgeons, all across the world, perform today.

THE HISTORY OF GOITER

The enlargement of the thyroid gland is a pathological phenomenon that has attracted physician and surgeon fascination throughout humanity's history.

As shown in Table 1.1, in around 2600 BC, the ancient Chinese were some of the first to describe thyroid enlargement and its treatment with seaweed [1]. Since this early reference, humanity's understanding of the thyroid gland in both its normal function and in disease has evolved constantly, with historic milestones marking groundbreaking discoveries and landmark achievements.

A review of the timeline of the treatment of goiter demonstrates a unifying theme that eventually culminated in a revolutionary discovery and subsequent treatment propositions. Seaweed, sponge, and eventually minced or ground thyroid extract feature heavily and repeatedly in the way we historically treated goiter [2]. In today's context, this makes resounding sense given the high concentrations of iodine that exist in all of these. However, it was not until 1820, in the last 200 years, that Swiss physician Jean-Francois Coindet understood and acknowledged the casual link between iodine deficiency (after Bernard Courtois' groundbreaking discovery of elemental iodine

in 1811) and goiter [1]. Since then, countless medical practitioners have prescribed iodine as an integral treatment for goiter—including French physician Jean Guillaume Auguste Lugol, after whom our commonly used *Lugol's Solution* (aqueous iodine) is named [2]—which features in the World Health Organization's *List of Essential Medicines* [3].

Equally as important as our understanding of goiter and the importance of iodine has been the evolution of our knowledge of the thyroid gland's anatomical structure and function.

Belgian physician and anatomist Andreas Vesalius was the first to provide the anatomical description of the thyroid gland in 1543 as "two glands…one on each side of the root of the larynx" [4]. Interestingly, he proposed that the function of the thyroid gland was to lubricate the tracheal lumen [2].

Adding to our anatomical understanding of the thyroid gland was the discovery of the *isthmus* in around the 1540s by Italian anatomist Bartholomew Eustachius—considered a founder of the modern discipline of human anatomy [1]. Humanity's appreciation and acknowledgment of thyroid enlargement is certainly evident in various pieces of artwork throughout our long history.

Perhaps one of the earliest artistic depictions of thyroid enlargement is the *Adena Pipe* (Figure 1.1), a pipe discovered in Ohio, USA in 1901, approximated by radiocarbon dating to be 2,000 years old [5].

Renaissance-era art from the 1400s–1700s in Europe demonstrates goiter in various pieces of artwork. One of the more iconic paintings that depicts thyroid enlargement is that of a boy "possessed by Satan" in the corner of *The Transfiguration* by Raffaello Sanzio (Figure 1.2) [6].

Though our understanding of the thyroid gland's anatomy was evolving significantly in the 16th century, it is evident that our understanding of its function(s) was still very much in its infancy. It seems that Vesalius's theory for the function of the thyroid gland persisted until the mid-18th century; from this point on in history, our understanding of its function underwent further evolution.

German anatomist C. H. T. Schreger (1768–1833) demonstrated an appreciation of the significant vascularity of the thyroid gland and attributed this to his proposed theory for the function of the thyroid gland—to act as a vascular shunt protecting against a sudden increase in blood flow to the brain [2].

German anatomist Herbert von Luschka (1820–1874) considered the thyroid gland to simply be a physical cushion against muscular pressure and trauma for the vital airway, phonatory, and neurovascular structures in the neck [2]. It was not until the late 18th century that our understanding of the thyroid gland's function

Table 1.1 A brief timeline of the history of goiter and our understanding of it

Time	Description
2600 BC	Goiter is known in China—treated with burnt sponge, seaweed, and animal thyroid.
1400 BC–400 AD	Ayurvedic (traditional Indian) medicine in India provides detailed descriptions of *galaganda* (goiter)
460 BC–375 BC	"…when glands of the neck become diseased themselves, they become tubercular and produce *struma*…" –*De Glandulis*, Hippocrates
23 BC–79 AD	"…Only men and swine are subject to swellings of the throat, which are mostly caused by the noxious quality of the water they drink…" –*Gaius Plinius Secundus of Pliny*
130–210 AD	Galen of Pergamon describes "mutism" and "semi-mutism" as complications of (thyroid) surgery by way of scraping with a fingernail, "tubercular" nodes.
340 AD	Ko-Hung, famous Chinese alchemist, recommends seaweed for treatment of goiter for people living in mountainous regions.
550 AD	Aëtius of Amida describes exophthalmic goiter and recognizes the importance of preservation of the *vocal nerves* (recurrent laryngeal nerve) for phonation.
~950–960 AD	Abu al-Qasim al-Zahrawi (Albucasis)—considered to be the greatest surgeon of the middle ages—first describes the thyroidectomy procedure and needle biopsies for goiter.
1170 AD	Roger of Palermo describes treatment of goiter with ashes of sponges and seaweed.
~1250 AD	*The Bamberg Surgery* (surgical textbook) provides a detailed description of surgical thyroidectomy.
1475 AD	Chinese physician Wang Hei describes treatment of goiter with minced/powdered animal thyroid.
1500 AD	Leonardo da Vinci first illustrates the thyroid gland.
~1540 AD	Bartholomew Eustachius first describes the *isthmus* of the thyroid gland.
1543 AD	Andreas Vesalius first provides anatomic description and illustration of the thyroid gland.
~1650 AD	Thomas Wharton provides the modern name, *thyroid*, after the shape of an ancient Greek shield.
1811 AD	Bernard Courtois discovers iodine.
1820 AD	Jean Francois Coindet describes iodine deficiency as the cause for goiter and begins treatment with iodine.
1829 AD	J. G. A. Lugol recommends aqueous iodine for the treatment of goiter.
1831 AD	Francisco Freire-Allemao (Brazil) proposes iodine prophylaxis to prevent goiter on a government administered, public health basis.
1835 AD	Robert Graves describes a syndrome of palpitations, goiter, and exophthalmos in three women.
1862 AD	Armand Trousseau introduces the term *Graves' disease*.
1883 AD	Emil Theodor Kocher describes myxedema as a complication of total thyroidectomy.
1909 AD	Emil Theodor Kocher—considered the father of modern thyroid surgery—receives the Nobel Prize for his work on thyroid surgery.

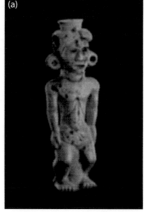
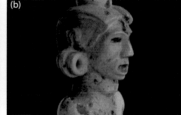

Figure 1.1 The Adena Pipe, Ohio Historical Society Archeology Collection, Columbus, Ohio, USA (a) Anterolateral view; (b) Closer view of neck region.

began to align with our current modern-day understanding. Swiss anatomist and physiologist Albrecht von Haller (1708–1788) proposed that the thyroid (along with thymus and spleen) was a ductless gland whose secretions directly entered the bloodstream [2].

THE HISTORY OF THE THYROID AND PARATHYROID HORMONES

As described earlier in this chapter, our understanding of the endocrine functions of the thyroid gland only seems to have begun emerging in the late 18th century. Punctuating the timeline of humanity's understanding of the thyroid gland and its disorders are the landmark endocrine discoveries of thyroid function: in 1914 by American chemist and Nobel Prize recipient Edward Calvin Kendall [7] and in 1952 by British biochemist Rosalind Pitt-Rivers and Canadian endocrinologist Jack Gross [8].

Edward C. Kendall was responsible (and famous) for the discovery of many hormones and biochemical compounds, which ultimately earned him the *Nobel Prize in Physiology or Medicine* (1950). One of his accomplishments was the isolation in 1914 of a crystalline, iodine-containing compound extracted from the thyroid gland that was responsible for the physiological effects of the thyroid function—a compound which he named *Thyroxine (T₄)* [7].

In 1950, Jack Gross joined Rosalind Pitt-Rivers at the National Institute for Medical Research (NIMR) in London to begin investigating an unknown iodine-labeled spot on paper chromatograms of human plasma extract [9]. In 1952 they published a scientific paper identifying a chemical compound that resembled Thyroxine but had a shorter half-life—*3,5,3′-Triiodothyronine (T₃)* [8].

Another important milestone in our understanding of thyroid endocrinology and a vital contribution to the field of thyroid-related clinical medicine was the synthesis of Thyroxine in 1927—thirteen years after its discovery and isolation—by Welsh chemist Charles Harington [10].

American physician John Thomas Potts is another important contributor to the field of endocrinology, his research interest focused on the endocrine control of calcium (and bone) metabolism [11]—though not a direct endocrine product of the thyroid gland, this is a crucial endocrine and physiological system to understand and appreciate as an important potential complication of thyroid

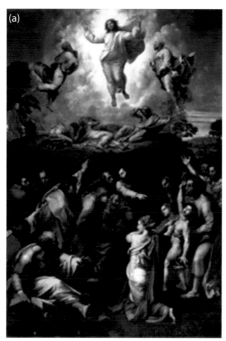
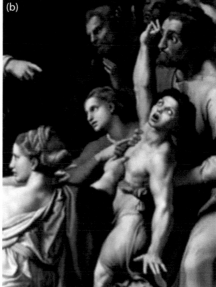

Figure 1.2   *The Transfiguration* by Raffaello Sanzio (Vatican Museum, Rome) (a) Complete painting; (b) View of *boy possessed by Satan.*

surgery. In 1972, J. T. Potts's laboratory at the National Institutes of Health (NIH) defined the amino acid sequence of the bovine *parathyroid hormone (PTH)*, followed shortly by the sequence for the human hormone [11]. This important milestone has allowed modern-day thyroid surgeons to specifically define the hormone deficiency that can result from thyroid surgery, where occasionally and certainly unintentionally—though sometimes intentionally— the neighboring parathyroid glands are removed or devascularized.

THE HISTORY OF SURGERY AND OF SURGICAL INSTRUMENTS

Surgery, a method of treatment for physical illness by means of bodily penetration and traumatic manipulation, has existed for many millennia. It has certainly evolved and been subject to its own share of adventurous discovery, refinement, and controversy over the course of human history.

Two procedures that are considered perhaps the oldest forms of surgery in humanity's history are male penile circumcision [12] and human skull *trephining* [13]. Though much debate still exists about the exact timing of circumcisions first being performed, there exist references to ancient Egyptian circumcisions around 450 BC as representations of socio-economic status amongst the upper class [12].

Trephining was the surgical procedure by which circular holes, often measuring approximately 4 cm in diameter, were made in the skull of the patient [13]. Again, the exact indication of this is unclear. It is hypothesized, however, that the procedure was perhaps a form of *decompressive craniotomy* for unremitting headaches. Evidence of this procedure dates back to at least the Neolithic period.

More recently, in the last two centuries, surgery has seen its most pronounced evolution, allowing it to cement its place in curative (and non-curative) treatment of physical illness. Without a doubt, the two most important advents that have permitted the explosion of the surgical specialty have been *anesthesia* and *asepsis*. Prior to the discovery of anesthesia in 1846, surgery was a limited practice

reserved for the more daring surgeons of the time, with pain being the single most important restricting factor. Evidence of this is the somewhat alarming fact that in pursuit of reducing operative pain, meticulousness and precision were often overwhelmingly substituted for "slashing speed" [14]. An above-knee amputation in London was once recorded as being completed in a mere 25 seconds from skin incision to wound closure (1846–1847) [14]. November 18, 1846 marked the date that American surgeon Henry Jacob Bigelow published his landmark paper titled "Insensibility during surgical operations produced by inhalation" [15]. Though initially met with a degree of skepticism, with some surgeons describing this newly discovered inhalational anesthesia as needless luxuries, it eventually became abundantly clear that the advent of this procedure afforded surgeons the time to be more precise in their surgical technique [14]. It also afforded them the opportunity to surgically venture into parts of the human anatomy that were previously restricted by unbearable pain and the echoing screams of the awake patient.

Though again initially met with resistance and skepticism by the surgical community, the works of Viennese obstetrician Ignaz Semmelweiss and British surgeon Joseph Lister were landmark milestones in the evolution of surgery [14]. In 1847, Ignaz Semmelweiss reported a significant reduction in puerperal sepsis simply by the adoption of rigorous handwashing by all medical staff involved in the delivery of each baby.

Joseph Lister is appropriately credited for his emphasis on the importance of aseptic technique and the use of his antimicrobial carbolic acid (phenol) system for surgical asepsis (Figure 1.3) [14].

Equally as important to the evolution of surgery was the growing breadth and sophistication of surgical instruments.

Considered to be the oldest surgical instrument to have been used by humans, evidence of the surgical knife in the form of a flint dagger dates, according to archeological analysis, as far back as 10000–8000 BC [16]. Since these prehistoric variants of the modern day scalpel, the knife has undergone multiple reincarnations with the use of copper in 3500 BC, and bronze and then iron in 1400 BC. The disposable scalpel that is so well known to today's surgeons was first introduced by American surgeon John Murphy after he adapted the disposable

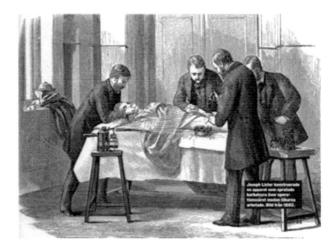

Figure 1.3   Joseph Lister demonstrates phenol system for surgical asepsis.

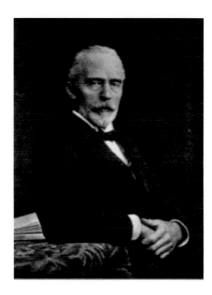

Figure 1.4   Emil Theodor Kocher.

safety razor produced by King Camp Gillette in 1901 (founder of the Gillette Safety Razor Company) [17]. John Murphy's disposable scalpel, however, was not technically satisfactory. In 1914, American engineer Morgan Parker adapted John Murphy's disposable three-piece scalpel to a significantly more technically intuitive two-piece scalpel—the same that is used in operating theatres across the world today [17].

The timeline for the evolution of surgical instruments is interspersed with certain milestone inventions.

Hungarian surgeon Aladar Petz is credited as being the inventor of modern-day surgical staplers after modifying a much more clunky mechanical suturing device invented by Hungarian surgeon Humer Hultl in 1909 [18]. He used his instrument for the very first time in 1920 on a young patient who underwent partial gastrectomy for gastric ulcer disease.

History reports that the thermal energy from heated stones was used as a means of cautery for hemostasis in prehistoric times and that surgeons had used electricity and cautery before the early 20th century [19]. However, the single most important figure in this particular sub-field of surgical technology is American inventor William T. Bovie who invented the first practical electrosurgical device, which was popularized by American surgeon Harvey Cushing (the father of modern day neurosurgery) [19]. Bovie's invention has gone on to be the basis for modern-day electrocautery devices so commonly used for cutting tissue and coagulating blood during surgery (including thyroid surgery).

American surgeon William Wayne Babcock is credited for many innovations in modern day surgery. One of the most recognized of these by modern-day thyroid surgeons is probably the invention of an atraumatic tissue holding forceps specifically designed to hold tubular organs—appropriately named after him: the *Babcock forceps* [20].

More recent advances in surgical technology that have added to the success of surgery include intraoperative neurophysiological monitoring; particularly its refinement at the turn of the new millennium that has added to the success of thyroid surgery (among other surgeries) by helping reduce the intraoperative complication of recurrent laryngeal nerve injury [21].

THE HISTORY OF THYROID SURGERY

As described earlier in this chapter, thyroid disease—particularly that characterized by goitrous enlargement—has been acknowledged, documented, and treated for at least the last four millennia.

The surgical management of thyroid disease, however, has been viewed with trepidation, as a rather daring undertaking, and has only really evolved to what it is today in just over the last century.

One of the earliest records of a successful thyroid surgery is from ~950–960 AD when Moorish physician/surgeon Albucasis removed a large goiter under opium sedation using simple ligatures and cautery irons to achieve adequate hemostasis [22]. Attempts and records in history of further thyroid surgery since then were somewhat sparse, particularly relative to the frequency with which they are performed today.

Famed American surgeon William Steward Halsted analyzed completed thyroid surgeries before the mid-19th century and reported 40% mortality [22]. Other important surgeons of the time such as Scottish surgeon Robert Liston and American surgeon Samuel David Gross emphasized the dangers of operating on the thyroid and discouraged it. Samuel D. Gross is quoted in his 1,000-page surgical textbook *A System of Surgery* as saying: "Can the thyroid in the state of enlargement be removed? Emphatically, experience answers no. Should the surgeon be so foolhardy to undertake it…every stroke of the knife will be followed by a torrent of blood and lucky it would be for him if his victim lived long enough for him to finish his horrid butchery…" [22]. It was not until esteemed Swiss surgeon Emil Theodor Kocher (Figure 1.4)—the first ever surgeon to receive the Nobel Prize in Physiology or Medicine (1909)—demonstrated his meticulous technique before and during thyroid surgery and reported his successes, that thyroid operations became more common [22]. He was a pupil of Austrian surgeon Theodor Bilroth, who himself first reported on 36 thyroidectomies with an over 40% mortality rate (16 died). Subsequently, as more advanced methods of antisepsis and hemostasis were emerging, Theodor Bilroth reported on a further 48 thyroidectomies between 1877 to 1881, this time with a dramatic decrease in mortality to 8.3% [22].

Theodor Kocher—considered the father of modern-day thyroid surgery—practiced with stringent aseptic technique both before and during surgery on the thyroid [22]. He also preached an astute focus on anatomy and carried out precise enucleation of the thyroid with an emphasis on hemostasis. He sought to achieve hemostasis by carefully dissecting and controlling vessels as they traversed from the thyroid gland's surrounding capsule to its substance. Towards the end of his surgical career, Kocher reported on more than 500 thyroidectomy cases at the Swiss Surgical Congress in 1917 with a mortality rate of 0.5% [22].

FUTURE DIRECTIONS

The likes of Henry Jacob Bigelow (anesthesia), Joseph Lister (antisepsis), Theodor Kocher (father of modern-day thyroid surgery techniques), and others described in this chapter have been vital in laying down the bedrock for what has become today's significantly safer thyroid surgery. Additional important technological advancements over the last few decades, particularly for thyroid surgery, have been those in improving hemostasis—achieving what has arguably been the biggest historical hurdle in thyroid surgery.

New technologies such as mechanical clip appliers (i.e., Ligaclip®, Surgiclip®), electrothermal bipolar-activated devices (i.e., Ligasure®), and ultrasonic vibration systems (i.e., Harmonic Focus®) have all contributed to this growing pool of vessel-ligating instruments in the pursuit of improved surgical hemostasis [23].

Considering the prevailing focus of current emerging technologies in thyroid surgery, it seems that a particular future direction (among others) will be the pursuit and refinement of minimalizing surgical access.

Robotic thyroidectomy surgeries appear to be the most significant advancement with respect to minimalizing access, particularly with their variety of approaches, including gasless transaxillary approach, axillo-breast approach (both unilateral and bilateral), and transoral approach [24].

Though it may be difficult to predict with certainty what the next century of thyroid surgeries will look like, one is inclined to say that the future of thyroid surgery looks to be as bright as its history has been colorful.

REFERENCES

1. Leoutsakos V. A short history of the thyroid gland. *Hormones (Athens).* 2004;3(4):268–71.

2. Clements FW et al. *Endemic goitre.* World Health Organization. monograph series; no. 44, 1960.

3. WHO Model List of Essential Medicines. 2017.

4. Thyroid History Timeline. 2019.

5. Bauduer F, Tankersley KB. Evidence of an ancient (2000 years ago) goiter attributed to iodine deficiency in North America. *Med Hypotheses.* 2018;118:6–8.

6. Sterpetti AV, Fiori E, De Cesare A. Goiter in the art of Renaissance Europe. *Am J Med.* 2016;129(8):892–5.

7. Kendall EC. Landmark article, June 19, 1915. The isolation in crystalline form of the compound containing iodine, which occurs in the thyroid. Its chemical nature and physiologic activity. By E.C. Kendall. *JAMA.* 1983;250(15):2045–6.

8. Gross J, Pitt-Rivers R. 3:5:3′-triiodothyronine. 1. Isolation from thyroid gland and synthesis. *Biochem J.* 1953;53(4):645–50.

9. Tata JR. Rosalind Pitt-Rivers and the discovery of T3. *Trends Biochem Sci.* 1990;15(7):282–4.

10. Harington CR, Barger G. Chemistry of Thyroxine: Constitution and synthesis of Thyroxine. *Biochem J.* 1927;21(1):169–83.

11. Marcus R. Present at the beginning: A personal reminiscence on the history of teriparatide. *Osteoporos Int.* 2011;22(8):2241–8.

12. Raveenthiran V. The evolutionary saga of circumcision from a religious perspective. *J Pediatr Surg.* 2018;53(7):1440–3.

13. Prehistoric Surgery January 1/8, 2019. *JAMA.* 2019;321(1):110.

14. Gawande A. Two hundred years of surgery. *N Engl J Med.* 2012;366(18):1716–23.

15. Bigelow HJ. Insensibility during surgical operations produced by inhalation. *Bost Med Surg J.* 1846;35(16):309–17.

16. Brill JB. The history of the scalpel: From flint to zirconium-coated steel. 2018.

17. Ochsner J. Surgical knife. *Tex Heart Inst J.* 2009;36(5):441–3.

18. Olah A. Aladar Petz, the inventor of the modern surgical staplers. *Surgery.* 2008;143(1):146–7.

19. O'Connor JL, Bloom DA. William T. Bovie and electrosurgery. *Surgery.* 1996;119(4):390–6.

20. Laios K. Professor William Wayne Babcock (1872–1963) and his innovations in surgery. *Surg Innov.* 2018;25(5):536–7.

21. Kim SM et al. Intraoperative neurophysiologic monitoring: Basic principles and recent update. *J Korean Med Sci.* 2013;28(9):1261–9.

22. Sarkar S et al. A Review on the history of 'thyroid surgery'. *Indian J Surg.* 2016;78(1):32–6.

23. Upadhyaya A et al. Harmonic versus LigaSure hemostasis technique in thyroid surgery: A meta-analysis. *Biomed Rep.* 2016;5(2):221–7.

24. Pan JH et al. Robotic thyroidectomy versus conventional open thyroidectomy for thyroid cancer: A systematic review and meta-analysis. *Surg Endosc.* 2017;31(10):3985–4001.

Chapter 2

SURGICAL ANATOMY OF THE THYROID

Ashutosh Mangalgiri and Deven Mahore

CONTENTS

Introduction 7
Embryology of the Thyroid Gland 7
Capsule of the Thyroid Gland 9
Blood Supply of the Thyroid Gland 10
Parathyroids 12
The Nerves 12
Ligament of Berry 13
Pyramidal Lobe 13
References 13

INTRODUCTION

The thyroid gland probably boasts of one of the most intricately arranged anatomical configurations and innumerable variations. Therefore, sound knowledge of anatomy is paramount for performance of successful and safe surgery. The following text will discuss the surgical anatomy of the thyroid in a manner akin to performing the steps of thyroidectomy. This would aid the readers in cadaveric dissection as well as live surgery. In a nutshell, the elevation of flaps should be sub-platysmal, you should retract or cut the strap muscles, identify the middle thyroid vein if present, address the superior pole, identify the recurrent laryngeal nerve, address the inferior pole, and finally the ligament of Berry. However, the skill of preserving the nerves and the parathyroids, especially respecting their vasculature, is what sets apart an accomplished surgeon.

"When you learn to treat the nerves and the parathyroids with respect and care during the performance of thyroid surgery, then you will be a man, my friend…."

EMBRYOLOGY OF THE THYROID GLAND

An endodermal diverticulum descends in the form of primordium of the thyroid gland. The thyroid diverticulum descends as the thyroglossal duct from the foramen cecum of the tongue. The thyroglossal duct follows a particular pathway during its descent. First, it passes through the tongue, then descends anterior to the hyoid, winding round the inferior border of the hyoid, until it reaches behind the hyoid. Finally, it descends in the neck. In the neck, the thyroglossal duct forms a bi-lobed structure, which finally attains a definitive shape of the thyroid gland. The fifth pharyngeal arch contributes as ultimobranchial body. C-cells of the thyroid gland are believed to be originating from neural crest cells. In the neck, the two lobes are connected by the isthmus. Many anomalous presentations have been described in the literature, like the absence of one of the lobes, the absence of the isthmus, two lobes connected from below, and the presence of a pyramidal lobe unilaterally or bilaterally. One of the rare forms is the presence of the isthmus above the cricoid cartilage [1].

SURGICAL ANATOMY
PLATYSMA MUSCLE

The platysma is classified under panniculus carnosus, a muscle present in the superficial fascia. The platysma is supplied by the cervical branch, one of the terminal branches of the facial nerve. The platysma of both sides runs upwards medially from the level of the second rib to the lower border of the mandible. Raise the flap in a sub-platysmal plane. The sub-platysmal plane is an avascular plane. We have to keep in mind that the platysma is absent in the midline, so we should identify it laterally (Figure 2.1).

ANTERIOR JUGULAR VEINS

Anterior jugular veins are paired veins running parallel upwards from the jugular venous arch. The midline avascular plane is

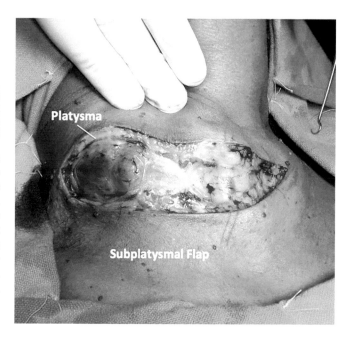

Figure 2.1   Intra-operative picture of the platysma muscle.

identified between these anterior jugular veins. Usually the anterior jugular veins are paired but you may get single or multiple veins also. The anterior jugular veins are now exposed.

STRAP MUSCLES

Now let us see the relation of the strap muscles. They are in two planes: superficial and deep. In the superficial plane we can identify the sternohyoid and the superior belly of the omohyoid.

So, the relation of the strap muscles from within outward is sternothyroid, sternohyoid, superior belly of omohyoid, and part of sternomastoid. If we want to know the lateral, anterior, and inferior relation, laterally is the sternothyroid, anteriorly are the sternohyoid and the superior belly of the omohyoid, and inferiorly is the sternomastoid.

Strap Muscles: These infrahyoid muscles are arranged in two planes: superficial and deep. The sternohyoid and the superior belly of the omohyoid are arranged in the superficial plane and the sternothyroid in the deep plane (Figures 2.2 through 2.4).

In large goiters, strap muscles are so thinned out that they appear as thin fascia. Strap muscles are to be preserved during surgery as far as possible.

If the need to cut the strap muscle arises, we should keep in mind that the nerve supply of the strap muscles should be preserved. The division of muscle should be above the nerve supply done by the ansa cervicalis.

ANSA CERVICALIS

The straps are innervated by a looped structure known as ansa cervicalis, embedded in the anterior wall of the carotid sheath. Ansa cervicalis has (1) anterior root, (2) posterior root, (3) loop of ansa (Figures 2.5 and 2.6).

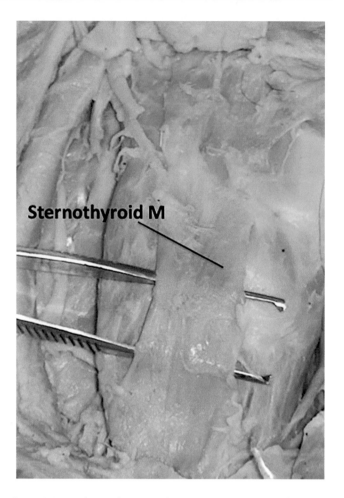

Sternothyroid M

Figure 2.3 Cadaveric dissection showing strap muscles and their nerve supply.

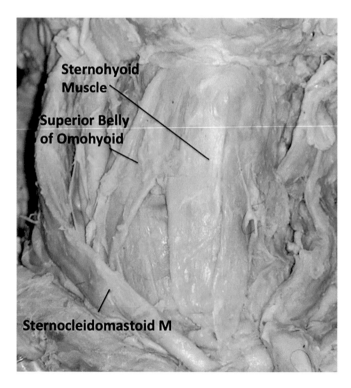

Sternohyoid Muscle

Superior Belly of Omohyoid

Sternocleidomastoid M

Figure 2.2 Cadaveric dissection showing strap muscles and their nerve supply.

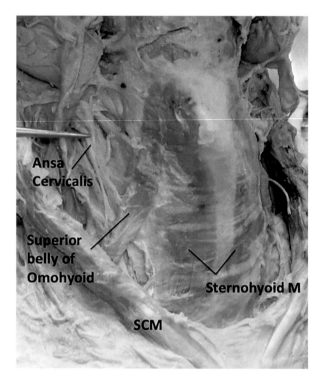

Ansa Cervicalis

Superior belly of Omohyoid

Sternohyoid M

SCM

Figure 2.4 Cadaveric dissection showing strap muscles and their nerve supply.

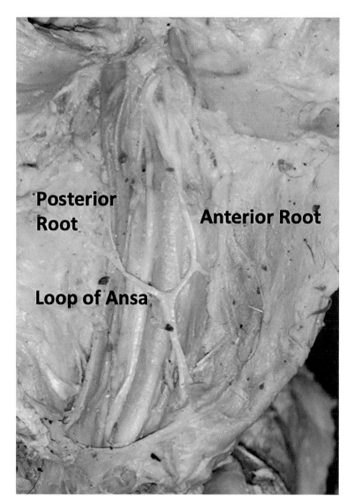

Figure 2.5 Anatomy of the ansa cervicalis.

CAPSULE OF THE THYROID GLAND

The thyroid is suspended by an investing layer of deep fascia, which forms the false capsule of thyroid and moves because of its attachment to the cricoid thyroid gland. A true capsule is formed by condensation of fascia surrounding the gland. The vascular plexus underlies the true capsule (Figure 2.7).

RELATIONS

Relations of the lobe of the thyroid gland:

- Each lobe has a medial, lateral, and posterior surface.
- The lateral surface is related outside inwards to the sternocleidomastoid, which covers the lower part of the thyroid lobe. The sternohyoid medially and the superior belly of the omohyoid laterally cover the gland in the superficial plane, and in the deeper plane the sternothyroid muscle covers the gland.
- The medial or the deeper surface of the gland is in relation with two tubes, i.e., the esophagus and the trachea; two nerves, i.e., the recurrent laryngeal nerve and the external branch of the superior laryngeal nerve; and two muscles, i.e., the inferior constrictor and the cricothyroid muscle.
- Posteriorly it is related to the carotid sheath and its contents (Figure 2.8).

RELATIONS OF THE ISTHMUS

The isthmus has two surfaces anterior and posterior and two borders superior and inferior. The isthmus may be absent at times. It may present above the cricoid cartilage in case the thyroid is an inverted U shape [1].

The anterior surface is related to the sternohyoid and sternothyroid muscles. The posterior surface is related to the 2nd to 4th rings of the trachea.

The upper border is related to the anastomosis between the anterior branches of the superior thyroid arteries and the pyramidal lobe when present. The inferior lobe is related to multiple inferior thyroid veins emerging at the inferior surface and the thyroid ima artery when present.

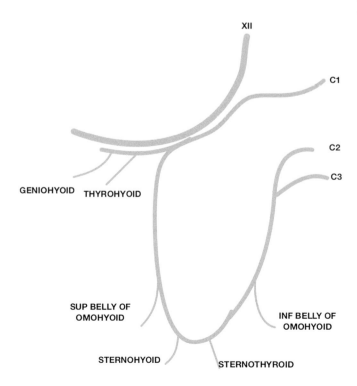

Figure 2.6 Anatomy of the ansa cervicalis.

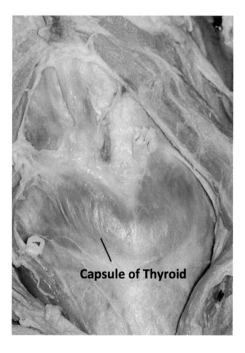

Figure 2.7 Capsule of the thyroid.

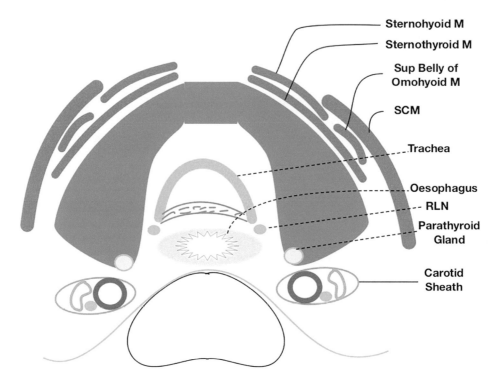

Figure 2.8   Relations of the thyroid gland.

BLOOD SUPPLY OF THE THYROID GLAND

The blood supply of the thyroid gland comes from the superior thyroid artery, the branch of the external carotid artery. This artery contributes in a major way to supply the thyroid gland. Another vessel supplying the thyroid gland is the inferior thyroid artery. The inferior thyroid artery provides a major contribution to the parathyroid gland.

The thyroid gland receives blood mainly through the superior and inferior thyroid arteries (Figure 2.9).

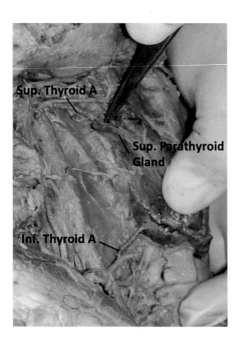

Figure 2.9   Blood supply of the thyroid gland.

SUPERIOR THYROID ARTERY

The superior thyroid artery lies at the upper pole along with the superior laryngeal nerve. The superior thyroid artery divides at the upper pole of the thyroid into anterior and posterior branches. The anterior division runs over the anterior border and then at the upper border of the isthmus to the anastomosis with its fellow from the other side. It is important to remember this branch as it may serve as a major bleeder. The posterior division descends over the posterior border and forms the anastomotic channel with the ascending branch from the inferior thyroid artery.

INFERIOR THYROID ARTERY

The inferior thyroid artery branches off from the thyrocervical trunk, ascends behind the carotid sheath, and then descends at the lower pole. At the lower pole, the inferior thyroid artery divides into multiple branches to supply the thyroid gland. It also provides a separate branch to the inferior parathyroid gland.

The ascending branch from the inferior thyroid artery supplies the superior parathyroid gland through the anastomotic channel. Thus, the inferior thyroid artery supplies both the parathyroid glands and should be regarded as the parathyroid artery.

THYROID IMA ARTERY

An additional branch from the innominate or right common carotid or from the arch of the aorta may arise to supply the thyroid gland. If present, it ascends in front of the trachea and terminates into the isthmus; this may be the reason for severe bleeding during tracheostomy.

PYRAMIDAL ARTERY

The pyramidal artery was described recently by Mangalgiri et al. [2] in a study on cadavers and during live surgeries. The pyramidal artery was present in those cases in which the pyramidal lobe was well developed. The pyramidal artery branches off from the superior thyroid artery just before its division. The pyramidal artery runs medially and then upwards along with the pyramidal lobe. If the pyramidal lobe runs along the right side of the artery, it will arise

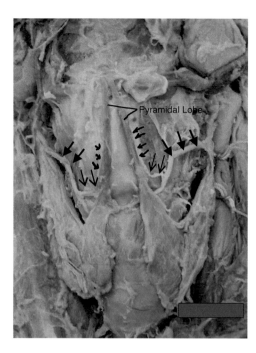

Figure 2.10   Pyramidal lobe artery.

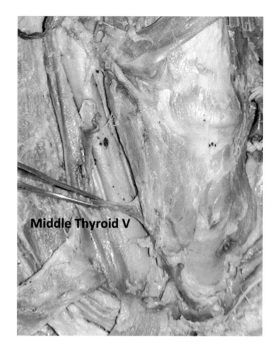

Figure 2.12   The short and stumpy middle thyroid vein.

from the right superior thyroid artery (STA), and if the pyramidal lobe runs along the left side, it will arise from the left STA. If the pyramidal lobe arises from the isthmus, then the artery may arise from the left or right STA (Figure 2.10).

THYROID VEINS

Usually, the thyroid gland is drained by the superior thyroid vein, the middle thyroid vein, and the inferior thyroid vein. The superior thyroid vein and the middle thyroid vein drain into the internal jugular vein. The inferior thyroid vein drains into the brachiocephalic vein. Often, a fourth vein is seen between the middle thyroid artery and the inferior thyroid vein. If it drains into the internal jugular vein, then it is called the fourth vein of Kocher (Figure 2.11).

IMPORTANT STEP TO AVOID DISASTER

The middle thyroid vein is of utmost importance. It is to be identified and secured. It is not really in the middle but a little towards the inferior pole. It is a stout and short vein but may look thinner if it is stretched by traction and countertraction of the thyroid lobe (Figure 2.12).

NERVE SUPPLY OF THE THYROID GLAND

The nerve supply of the thyroid gland comes from the parasympathetic and the sympathetic nerves; from the vagus nerve and the superior, middle, and inferior ganglia of the sympathetic trunk respectively (Figure 2.13).

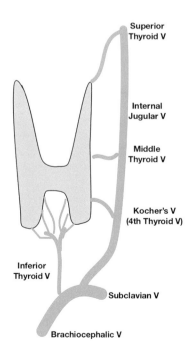

Figure 2.11   Venous drainage of the thyroid gland.

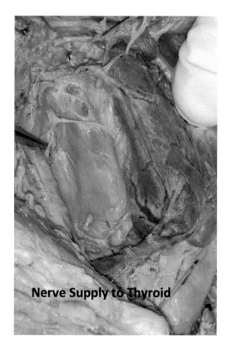

Figure 2.13   Nerve supply of the thyroid.

The lymphatic drainage of the gland is categorized in two groups: (1) the upper one into the prelaryngeal and jugulo digastric lymph node (JDLN) (III) and (2) the lower one into the pretracheal and level 4, 5, 6.

PARATHYROIDS

DEVELOPMENT
The parathyroid (PT) glands have variable positions. The position of the superior PT gland is almost constant. The paired superior glands arise from the IV branchial pouch. They are situated at the junction of the upper and middle thirds of the posterior border of the thyroid, one on each side and embedded in the capsule of the gland.

The paired inferior parathyroid glands arise from the III branchial pouch. They may have ectopic locations such as the intrathyroid, anterior mediastinum, posterior mediastinum, or central compartment of the neck. The inferior parathyroids are known for their variable location and number.

The inferior parathyroid glands are commonly found in relation to the inferior thyroid artery, and the ligation of this vessel should be done after preserving the blood supply of the parathyroid.

LYMPHATIC DRAINAGE
The lymphatic of the parathyroid follows the blood vessels and drains into pre- and paratracheal lymph node (LN), the deep cervical LN, and the mediastinal LN.

The nerve supply of the parathyroid comes from non-myelinated nerves derived from the superior or middle sympathetic ganglion or directly from the plexus on the fascia on the posterior surface of the lateral lobe of the thyroid gland.

THE NERVES

Two nerves which lie in close proximity to the thyroid gland are the external branch of the superior laryngeal nerve (EBSLN) and the recurrent laryngeal nerve (RLN). Both are to be identified and preserved. Still, many surgeons ignore the EBSLN or rather do not try to identify it. Identifying this nerve should be of high importance as it is the tenor of the vocal cord, and damage to it will definitely effect singers and professional voice users. The most feared nerve for beginners is the RLN. We now discuss the surgical anatomy of these two nerves.

EXTERNAL BRANCH OF THE SUPERIOR LARYNGEAL NERVE
Joll's triangle and Reeves's space are the accepted landmarks for identifying the EBSLN. Before describing the landmarks, let us understand the Cernia et al. classification of EBSLN. According to Cernia et al. [3], there are three variations of the EBSLN position:

Type 1 crosses the superior thyroid artery more than 1 cm away from the superior pole of the thyroid.

Type 2a crosses the superior thyroid artery less than 1 cm from the superior pole of the thyroid.

Type 2b crosses the superior thyroid artery under cover of the superior pole of the thyroid.

Joll's triangle is bounded laterally by the part of the superior pole of the thyroid and the the superior vascular pedicle, superiorly by the attachment of the strap muscle, and medially by the midline (Figure 2.14).

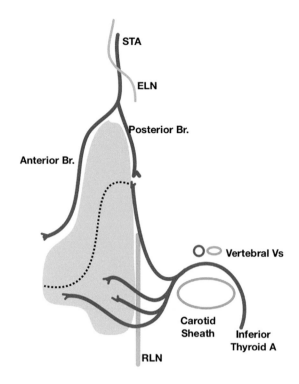

Figure 2.14 Relation of the superior thyroid artery to the external branch of superior laryngeal nerve.

Reeves's space is the avascular space between the superior pole of the thyroid and the cricothyroid muscle. This is also one of the landmarks by which to identify the EBSLN.

RECURRENT LARYNGEAL NERVE
This is a branch from the vagus nerve. It winds around the subclavian artery on the right side and the arch of the aorta on the left side. After winding around, it runs upward and medially in the neck. In the neck, the RLN runs in a tracheoesophageal groove.

There are many landmarks to identify the RLN:

1. Beahr's triangle
2. Lore's triangle
3. Nodule of Zuckerkandl
4. Cricothyroid joint
5. Berry's ligament

BEAHR'S TRIANGLE
Beahr's triangle is bounded laterally by the common carotid artery, superiorly by the inferior thyroid artery, and medially by the recurrent laryngeal nerve (Figure 2.15).

LORE'S TRIANGLE
Lore's triangle is bounded medially by the trachea/esophagus, laterally by the carotid artery, and superiorly by the surface of the inferior pole of the thyroid.

NODULE OF ZUCKERKANDL
Emil Zuckerkandl (1849–1910), an Austrian anatomist in 1902, described a protuberance arising from the posterior border of the thyroid lobes. This protuberance was termed as *processus posterior glandulae thyroidea*. It is a thickening or a nodule in the posterior aspect of the gland. Whenever the nodule of Zuckerkandl is present and identified, it is one of the important and reliable landmarks in identifying the RLN. The nodule of Zuckerkandl directly points toward the RLN (Figure 2.16).

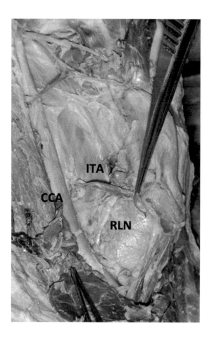

Figure 2.15 Anatomy of Beahr's triangle.

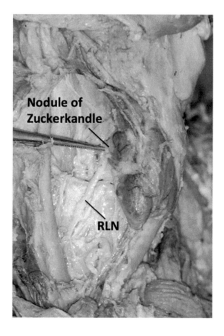

Figure 2.16 Relationship of the RLN to the nodule of Zuckerkandl.

CRICOTHYROID JOINT

The relation of the cricothyroid joint and the RLN is constant and very much reliable. Many surgeons prefer this as the first landmark to identify the RLN. This landmark is considered to be reliable because the nerve enters inside the larynx from this joint.

BERRY'S LIGAMENT

Berry's ligament is not exactly a landmark for identifying the RLN, but it is the region where damage can be done if the relation of the

RLN with Berry's ligament is not known. The RLN can be superficial to Berry's ligament, deep to it, or sometimes split around Berry's ligament.

After identifying the RLN, it is very important that it should not be traced throughout the course of surgery, as this may jeopardize the blood supply and leave the patient with RLN palsy.

NON-RECURRENT LARYNGEAL NERVE (NRLN)

Whenever the RLN is not identified via the landmarks mentioned previously, the possibility of non-recurrent laryngeal nerve should be considered. The possibility of non-recurrent laryngeal nerve is more on the right side because it is associated with an anomaly of the right subclavian artery. The embryologically right NRLN is secondary to a vascular disorder called *arteria lusoria,* in which the fourth arch on the right involutes instead of persisting on the right as the subclavian artery. Three types of variations are described for the NRLN:

Type 1: The NRLN arises directly from the vagus and travels with the superior thyroid pedicle vessels.

Type 2A: The NRLN travels transversely, parallel, and superficially in relation to the trunk of the inferior thyroid artery.

Type 2B: The nerve travels transversely parallel, but deep to or between the branches of the inferior thyroid artery.

LIGAMENT OF BERRY

The ligament of Berry or suspensory ligament, which is nothing but condensation of deep cervical fascia, is attached to the trachea. This attachment is responsible for the movement of the thyroid gland during deglutition.

PYRAMIDAL LOBE

This structure is often ignored, and therefore it is the most common cause of residual tissue after total thyroidectomy. It is more commonly seen on the right side and sometimes it is bilateral. The pyramidal lobe has a dedicated artery—pyramidal artery—and runs postero-lateral to the *levator glandulae thyroidae.*

REFERENCES

1. Mangalgiri AS, Mahore D, Kapre M. Study of a unique 'inverted u' shaped thyroid gland and its clinical importance. *Indian J Otolaryngol Head Neck Surg.* 2014 Jun;66(2):224–5.

2. Mangalgiri A, Mahore D, Kapre M. Pyramidal artery: An artery to pyramidal lobe-A new nomenclature. *Indian J Otolaryngol Head Neck Surg.* 2018 Jun;70(2):313–8.

3. Cernea CR, Ferraz AR, Nishio S, Dutra A Jr, Hojaij FC, dos Santos LR. Surgical anatomy of the external branch of the superior laryngeal nerve. *Head Neck.* 1992 Sep-Oct;14(5):380–3.

Chapter 3

CLINICAL ASSESSMENT OF THE THYROID NODULE

Madan Laxman Kapre, Shripal Jani, and Priya Dubey

CONTENTS

History Taking   15
Physical Examination   17

HISTORY TAKING

History taking is a scientific art. The science and art in deciphering the information that the patient volunteers about their illness are asking the right questions, in the right sequence, and with empathy, to begin forming a clinical picture. The patient often narrates his/her own diagnosis if you have the patience to listen to their complaints. We shall endeavor to provide our question algorithm to achieve this in this chapter. Coupled with appropriate clinical examination, we often come to a reasonably accurate diagnosis that enables us to apply appropriate investigations.

Firstly, as mundane as it may be, age, sex, family history, and geographical location of our patient is very relevant as it will help us understand risk stratification, which shall be dealt with in appropriate sections of well differentiated thyroid carcinomas. Then we can focus our attention on extracting symptoms which will be relevant to the function of the thyroid gland.

Loss of appetite, weight gain, lethargy, loss of hair, and roughness of skin point to hypofunction of the gland; increased appetite yet weight loss, restlessness, and sweaty palms point to hyperfunction. Proptosis, ecchymosis, and recurrent corneal ulceration clearly point to a thyro-toxic state (Figures 3.1 and 3.2). While a hypofunctioning gland with a nodule indicates possible malignancy, a hyperfunctioning gland with a nodule is usually benign.

Additionally, in female patients, the thyroid hormone produces symptoms due to activity on estrogen-dependent physiology. The thyroid gland is generally enlarged at puberty, pregnancy, and menopause. Menstrual cycle irregularities are to be enquired into to exclude hypo- or hyperthyroidism.

Children also need special attention as aberrant thyroid glands and anomalies of the thyroglossal duct ranging from lingual thyroid to thyroglossal cysts occur in this age group (Figure 3.3). Previously drained midline tuberculous abscesses in an Indian context leading to sinus formation is often confused with the congenital variety (Figures 3.4 and 3.5).

In long standing nodules, recent onset of pain, rapid increase in size, voice changes, and dysphagia indicate malignant transformation in the pre-existing thyroid nodule. By their location in the tracheoesophageal groove, posteriorly located nodules may cause dysphagia. However, acute bleeding in benign goiterous nodules can cause pain. Intense pain and severe odynophagia spell acute thyroiditis like autoimmune thyroiditis or chronic or acute suppurative infection of the thyroid gland (Figures 3.6 and 3.7).

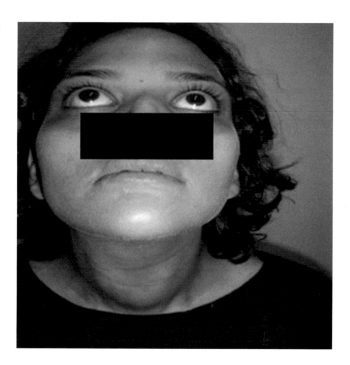

Figure 3.1 Thyrotoxic state.

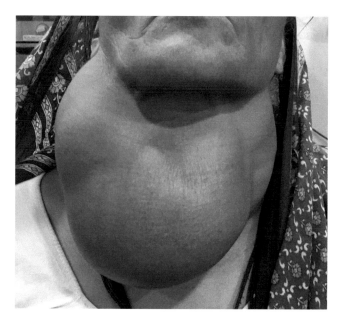

Figure 3.2 Thyrotoxic state.

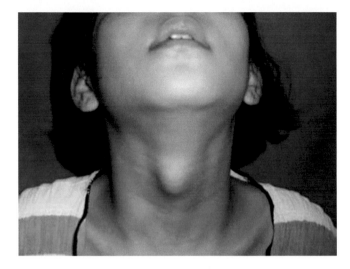

Figure 3.3 Thyroglossal cyst.

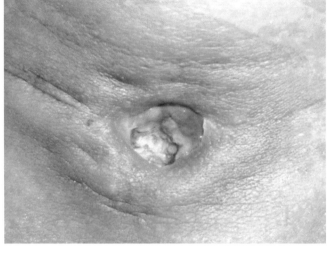

Figure 3.5 Midline tuberculous abscess.

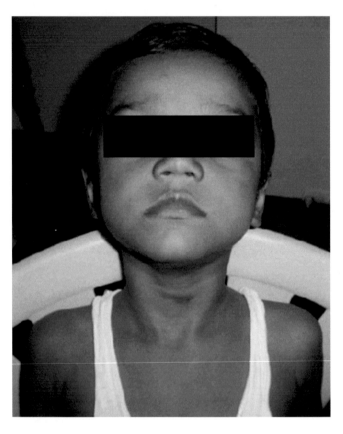

Figure 3.4 Midline tuberculous abscess.

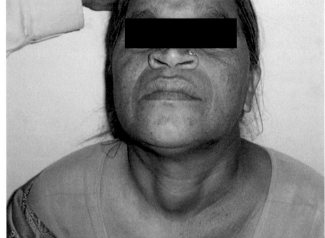

Figure 3.6 Suppurative infection of the thyroid gland.

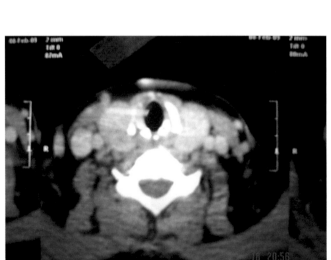

Figure 3.7 Suppurative infection of the thyroid gland.

Voice changes are attributed to two mechanisms. It could be because of the structural changes within the vocal folds as in the edematous cords of hypothyroidism. Or, more ominously, it could be due to altered vocal cord dynamics, i.e., vocal cord palsy or fixation due to infiltration of the RLN and/or the cricothyroid joint by malignant disease. Slow and insidious involvement of the RLN due to malignant infiltration gives adequate time for compensation by the opposite vocal cord, and there may not be voice alteration.

Malignant infiltration of the upper trachea may cause hemoptysis in case of obvious thyroid disease. Retro-sternal extension and mediastinal crowding by goiter causes difficulty in breathing, particularly when lying down in a supine position. It could also be due to bilateral abductor palsy in a rare situation of advanced thyroid cancer. Prominent neck veins and centripetal blood flow indicates superior mediastinal obstruction.

PHYSICAL EXAMINATION

The physical examination also requires a disciplined approach. General examination is directed towards signs of thyroid dysfunction in distant organs where the thyroid hormone acts. Subclinical hypofunction would be considered in an obese patient with a gruffy fatigued voice and edematous looking facies. An anxious look, prominent eyes, exposed cornea, sweaty handshake, and tremors observed in the patient would indicate a thyrotoxic state. The rapid, often collapsing pulse of hyperthyroidism is unmistakable.

A local examination should begin with the inspection of the neck. Enlarged neck veins and their direction of flow should forewarn the clinician about superior mediastinal obstruction by benign retrosternal goiter or metastatic lymph nodes of papillary carcinoma of the thyroid. The external jugular veins on either side indicate lateral most extent of the benign large thyroid which the authors have encountered in many of their rural tribal practices.

As patients range from incidentally imaged small nodules to massive neck masses shouting their presence as a patient enters the room, we should have some uniform way of describing the goiter size. We follow a grading system that is quite easy to communicate among treating colleagues, from surgeon to anesthetist to operating room support staff, so that an appropriate preparatory schedule can be made. Grade I goiter is seen only when the patient hyperextends the neck. Grade II goiter is one that is seen as the patient sits in a neutral neck position. Grade III goiter is seen as obvious nodular projection on the anterior neck, yet their lower borders can be seen on swallowing movements. Grade IV goiters are as in grade III, but where their lower border is not seen on swallowing movements.

Simple as it may sound, palpation of the thyroid should be performed using the following special method and not only by a cursory "neck feel" of an experienced senior surgeon. We stand behind the patient with the neck relaxed and flexed to examine the thyroid nodules. A soft and uniformly enlarged thyroid can be due to physiological enlargements, as mentioned earlier, or a dysfunctional gland (Figure 3.8). Late stage Hashimoto's thyroiditis will have hard and smallish gland. On the other hand, in early stages of the disease, the gland is tender and markedly nodular. Uniform, yet firm, non-tender glands are usually present in lymphomas. Nodularity of the gland, either unilaterally or bilaterally, can best be assessed with patience and with effort to locate the laryngeal framework and trachea first. In the perspective of the trachea, the nodule can be conveniently lateralized, even when some of these large nodules may appear bilateral in the beginning. One large dominant nodule may hide smaller nodules located posteriorly. We then focus our attention towards the mobility of the gland on swallowing. If the thyroid moves on deglutition, however large it may be, it is within the confines of its fascia and not breaking out to get fixed to adjoining structures. This is important as benign lesions, however big they are, will not breach fascia, while malignant nodules might breach and invade into adjoining soft tissue like muscle, RLN, trachea, or the esophagus.

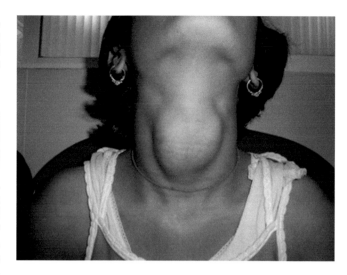

Figure 3.8   Dysfunctional gland or physiological enlargement.

The authors wish to make an important observation on demonstration of tenderness of the thyroid gland. Sitting across the patient, putting the flat of the fingers on the thyroid gland firmly, and asking the patient to swallow, wincing of the face will give away tenderness and the diagnosis. The outcome of such a clinical maneuver in the authors' opinion will with relative certainty be a diagnosis that *Globus hystericus* is truly thyroiditis.

The presence of nodes in the lateral compartment is an obvious indicator for malignancies of the thyroid. Neck nodes in higher levels, i.e., grades II and III, indicate papillary carcinomas whereas nodes in level V point toward the possibility of medullary carcinomas.

The assessment of retrosternal extension is performed by a few bedside clinical maneuvers (Figures 3.9 and 3.10). The more common one is having the patient in a supine position with a hyperextended neck. Upon swallowing, the clinician tries to insinuate their fingers across the lower border of the thyroid swelling. The ability to do so gives the clinician confidence of cervical delivery of the retrosternal goiter. Pemberton's sign is demonstrated in the following manner. The patient stands and slowly takes his/her arms up to full stretch. This will narrow the superior mediastinum.

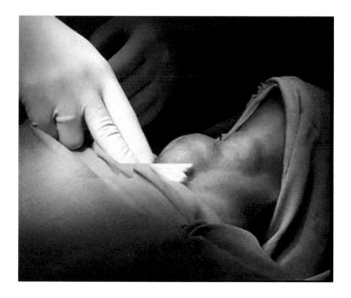

Figure 3.9   Bedside clinical maneuvers for assessment of retrosternal extension.

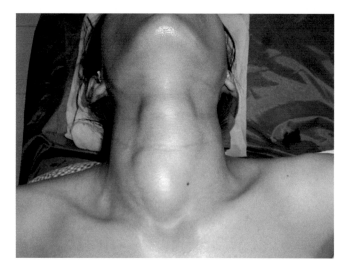

Figure 3.10   Bedside clinical maneuvers for assessment of retrosternal extension.

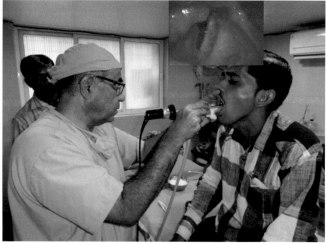

Figure 3.11   Telelaryngoscope to assess the mobility of the vocal cords.

A mass lesion already compromising the venous return will exaggerate the effect leading to facial puffiness and fullness of neck veins and difficulty in breathing. Respiratory symptoms must be enquired into. Hoarseness of voice with difficulty in breathing would indicate unilateral RLN palsy with or without laryngotracheal invasion. However, a normal voice and difficulty in breathing is a rather more sinister symptom as it would indicate bilateral involvement of the RLN with or without laryngotracheal invasion.

Patients who will provide a history of changed sleeping patterns, either taking additional pillows or preferring to sleep in lateral positions, probably have retrosternal extension causing compression.

Morbid obesity and thick, bull necks pose considerable difficulties in the assessment of necks. A thorough patient history paired with suitable clinical examination often comes to the rescue of the surgeon. In resource restricted situations, a very focused investigation and avoiding unnecessary tests help economizing on time and cost.

Last, but not least, is the assessment of the functionality of the recurrent laryngeal nerves. All thyroid surgeons must train themselves either using old-fashioned bullseye lamps and indirect laryngoscopy mirrors or modern-day telelaryngoscopes to assess the mobility of the vocal cords both before and after surgery. A normal voice is no insurance for normally mobile cords as slow and insidious RLN involvement can so often get compensated. (Figure 3.11) The authors will insist on full endoscopic evaluation of the upper airways and the pharyngoesophageal segment where a laryngotracheal or upper esophageal invasion is suspected.

Recommended clinical questionnaire for thyroid swellings:

- Duration of the nodule
- Bilateral or unilateral
- Recent change in size
- Recent onset of pain
- Recent change in voice
- Onset of dysphagia
- Breathing difficulty
- Presence of lateral neck mass
- Cough or hemoptysis
- Positive Pemberton's sign
- Inability to sleep supine

Clinical questionnaire for functionality:

- Weight gain
- Weight loss
- Hair loss
- Appetite
- Sleep
- Sweating
- Palpitation
- Eye symptoms
- Menstrual irregularity
- Tremors

Suggested proforma for clinical documentation:

1. Size of the nodule
2. Location of the nodule

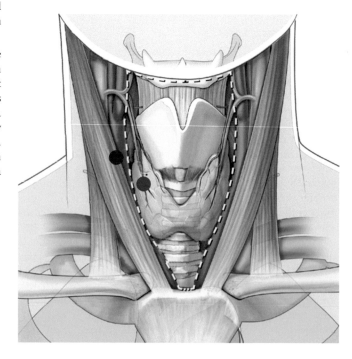

Figure 3.12   Diagrammatic representation of right sided solitary thyroid nodule located at the superior pole with an ipsilateral level III lymph node.

3. Number of nodules
4. Unilateral or bilateral
5. Position and centrality of laryngotracheal framework
6. Consistency: Soft/Firm/Hard
7. Mobility
8. Ability to palpate the lower border of the thyroid gland
9. Condition of the overlying skin
10. Cervical lymphadenopathy
11. Documentation of vocal fold mobility

Diagrammatic representations may help to standardize the depiction and communication of relevant clinical examination findings of a thyroid nodule (Figure 3.12).

Chapter 4

IMAGING OF THE THYROID

Alka Ashmita Singhal

CONTENTS

Introduction	21
Thyroid Ultrasound	21
Thyroid Nodules	26
Follicular Neoplasm	29
Papillary Thyroid Carcinoma	29
Papillary Thyroid Microcarcinoma	30
Medullary Thyroid Carcinoma	30
Anaplastic Carcinoma	31
Metastasis to the Thyroid	40
Conclusion	42
References	42

INTRODUCTION

Thyroid ultrasound and radionuclide imaging are the most common diagnostic modalities used in the management of thyroid disorders. Nuclear scintigraphy is used for the evaluation of metabolic activity of the nodules and the physiologic thyroid function. Ultrasound is the mainstay of thyroid imaging and helps in evaluation of both diffuse thyroid disorders and focal thyroid nodules. Advanced Doppler evaluation along with sono-elastography and contrast-enhanced ultrasound are useful adjuncts. TIRADS scoring, ultrasound guided fine needle aspiration, and Bethesda cytopathology are combined to give a risk stratification for thyroid nodules. Computed tomography (CT), magnetic resonance imaging (MRI), and positron emission tomography (PET) are advised in select cases.

THYROID ULTRASOUND

HISTORY AND EVOLUTION

The thyroid gland, owing to its superficial location in the neck, was one of the first organs to be studied by ultrasound, as early as 1960 [1,2]. Since then ultrasound has gone through a dynamic change with evolving technology and has added elements of Doppler, elastography, and contrast-enhanced ultrasound.

ULTRASOUND PRINCIPLE AND PHYSICS

Modern ultrasound equipment consists of a sensitive transducer containing a piezoelectric crystal [3], keyboard, software, hardware, and display. A piezoelectric crystal emits sound waves in response to electric stimulation and receives the reflected echo, which is processed to produce a corresponding display image. Sound waves need a material medium to transfer. Ultrasound gel is used as a basic coupling medium to enable transfer of the sound waves into the body by overcoming the air barrier. The degree of attenuation of the sound waves into the body depends on the intrinsic tissue properties through which sound travels into the medium and the echoes reflected back to

the transducer. Gray-scale imaging is combined with Doppler [4–6] ultrasound. Color, power, and spectral Doppler give the vascularity information. We aim to use the highest possible transducer frequency to achieve the required depth of imaging. The basic determinant of resolution and image quality is the transducer frequency. Appropriate focus must be adjusted to have a narrower beam width at the area of interest and hence improved resolution. Gain settings, including Doppler settings, should be optimum, not under- or overwritten. Ultrasound artifacts could be inherent due to the modality itself or due to an improper technique. Inherent ultrasound artifacts are related to the ultrasound beam characteristics, the propagation of sound in the various tissues, and the assumptions made in image processing. Some of the artifacts [7] in ultrasound imaging are used as a valuable tool in image interpretation. Notable artifacts for thyroid ultrasound are posterior enhancement or cystic enhancement (Figure 4.1) distal to a fluid-filled cystic structure, posterior acoustic shadowing (Figure 4.2) distal to calcifications, reverberations, and comet tail. Both cystic enhancement and posterior acoustic

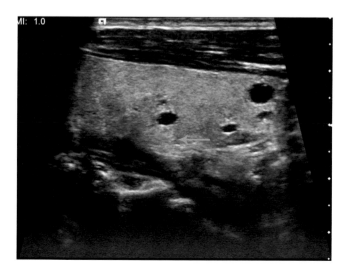

Figure 4.1 Posterior enhancement (yellow arrow) posterior to a colloid cyst, suggesting uniform character and minimal attenuation of sound through it.

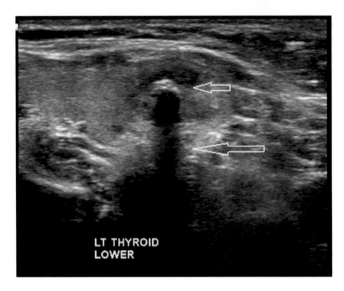

Figure 4.2 Posterior acoustic shadowing (blue arrow) noted distal to calcification (yellow arrow). As most of the sound is reflected back from dense calcifications, very little penetrates through, the area posterior to them is not insonated, and appears dark (shadows).

shadowing are attenuation errors related to the sound beam and tissue properties. When a strongly reflective (example: calculus) or a highly reflective (example: bone) structure comes in the path of an ultrasound beam, the amplitude of the beam distal to the structure is diminished, hence the echoes returning from the area behind the structure are also diminished and appear as dark areas or "shadows." Conversely, when a weakly attenuating structure (example: a clear cyst) is in the path of an ultrasound beam, the sound is attenuated to a lesser extent as compared to adjacent tissues at the same level, hence more amplitude sound waves reach the area and are returned leading to an increased transmission seen as a bright band beyond the low attenuating structure. This artifact helps in understanding the composition of the tissue, and when present, posterior enhancement suggests a cystic structure.

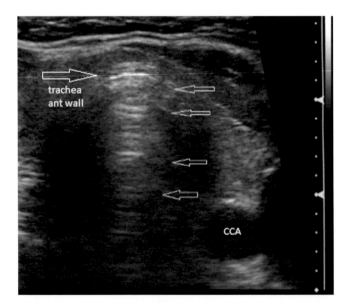

Figure 4.3 Reverberation artifacts (white arrows) from the anterior wall of trachea (yellow arrow). These occur due to sound waves reflecting many times from a sharp acoustic interface into the deeper tissues with diminishing intensity.

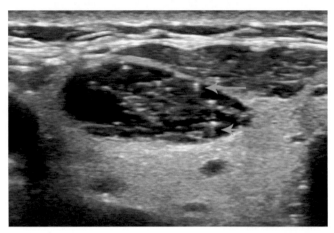

Figure 4.4 Comet tail artifact. A type of reverberation artifact seen due to crystallization of the colloid which gives a tiny sharp interface and leads to a triangular tapering echo (yellow arrows).

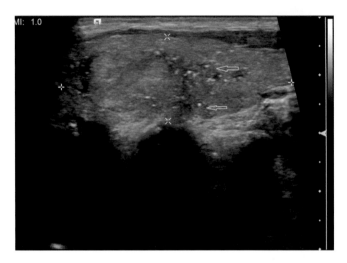

Figure 4.5 Tiny punctate echogenic foci (yellow open arrows) or microcalcifications which are seen in papillary thyroid carcinoma are due to the psammoma bodies. These do not show the comet tail artifact or any posterior shadowing.

Reverberation artifacts (Figure 4.3) occur when ultrasound echoes are repeatedly reflected between two highly reflective surfaces resulting in an image display having multiple equally spaced signals in the far field, as in the case of tracheal surface in the neck. The comet tail artifact (Figure 4.4) is a small triangular reverberation artifact noted characteristically posterior to the colloid particles, and it fades distally. Here the sequential echoes are very close to each other and not perceived separately, and as they diminish in intensity in the far field they give a tapering "triangular" appearance. The tiny punctate echogenic foci seen in the papillary carcinoma thyroid do not show this artifact (Figure 4.5).

THYROID ULTRASOUND ANATOMY

The normal thyroid gland [8] is an H-shaped gland draped over the trachea with the right and left lobes connected by a narrow isthmus and on ultrasound shows a smooth homogenous hyperechoic echotexture with a thin echogenic peripheral thyroid capsule (Figure 4.6a–e). On color Doppler, few vessels can be identified, mainly the superior and the inferior thyroid arteries at the poles.

The sternocleidomastoid and the strap muscles sternothyroid and sternohyoid are seen antero-laterally and appear as hypoechoic structures. The carotid sheath (containing the common carotid

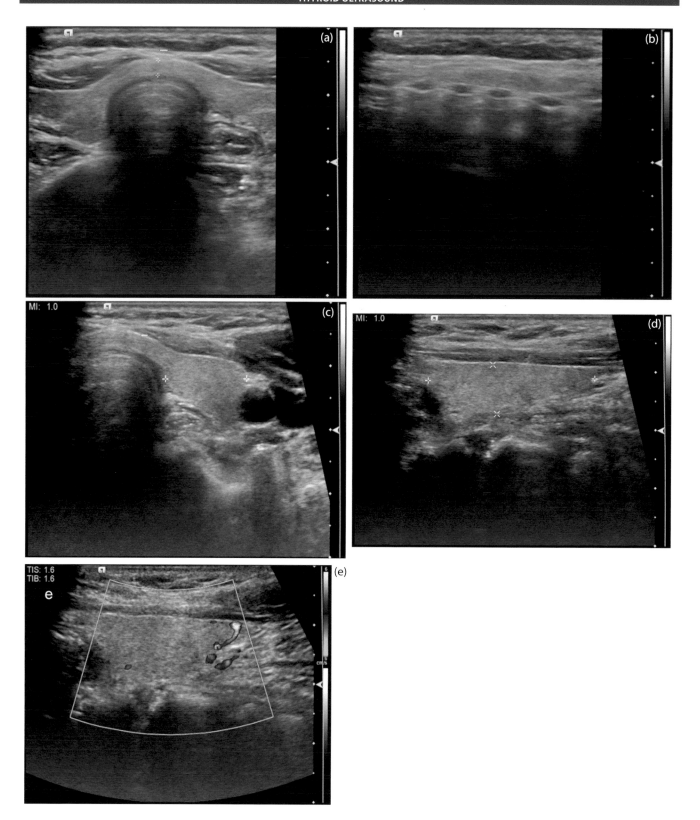

Figure 4.6 (a–e) Normal thyroid (isthmus and lobes) transverse and longitudinal and scan with color Doppler showing the smooth homogenous hyperechoic echotexture and a few vessels on color Doppler.

artery [CCA], the internal jugular vein [IJV], and the vagus nerve) and scalenus anterior muscles are seen postero-laterally. The esophagus is seen posteriorly. A normal adult gland measures 40–50 mm in craniocaudal length, 12–18 mm in transverse width, and 10–12 mm in anterio-posterior depth. The gland is supplied by the superior thyroid artery, a branch of the external carotid artery, and the inferior thyroid artery, a branch of the subclavian artery. The

superior and inferior thyroid artery may be well seen at the poles. Venous drainage is mainly to the IJV. The thyroid has an extensive subcapsular and intrathyroidal lymphatic network. Metastasis from the thyroid primary are common in level 6 and level 2–4. The recurrent laryngeal nerve [9] lies in the posterior relation to the mid-part of the thyroid gland along with the inferior thyroid artery. The ectopic superior parathyroids [10] are usually located behind the

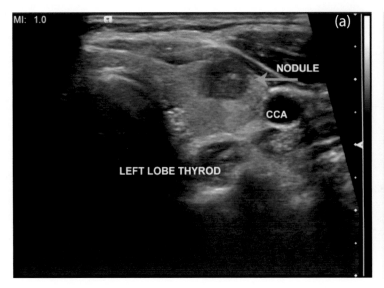
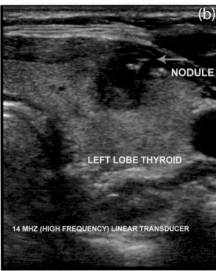

Figure 4.7 (a) Image of thyroid nodule taken with 7–11 MHz transducer showing a heterogeneous hypoechoic nodule. (b) Image of the same thyroid nodule taken with 12–14 MHz transducer showing additional image clarity with well delineated punctate echogenic foci and anterior capsular breach (arrow). Biopsy proved papillary carcinoma thyroid.

mid-thyroid at the point of the crossing of the inferior thyroid artery and the recurrent laryngeal nerve. The ectopic inferior parathyroids are located around the lower pole of the thyroid glands. The nodule of Zuckerkandl may appear as a prominent pseudomass behind the mid-part of thyroid [11].

EMBRYOLOGY AND ECTOPIC THYROID GLANDS
The thyroid gland is a mesodermal derivative originating from the floor of the mouth at the level of the foramen cecum [12,13]. The thyroglossal duct invaginates and descends anterior to the trachea, bifurcating to form the two thyroid lobes. Ectopic thyroid tissue and abnormalities of the thyroglossal duct are found along this path. The pyramidal lobe is formed from the last part of the thyroglossal duct.

ULTRASOUND TECHNIQUE AND PATIENT POSITION
The thyroid gland is located very superficially in the anterior upper neck and easily amenable to ultrasound; however, it is dependent on proper technique [14] and experience of the examiner. Adequate exposure of the neck area and proper patient positioning is important. The patient is placed in a supine position with a pillow behind the shoulders to slightly extend the neck; however, caution must be observed in elderly patients. Alternative positions such as a tilted sitting position may also be adopted. A variety of transducers may be needed to be used for one scan to achieve a comprehensive and a detailed image. A linear 7–11 MHz transducer may be adequate for most examinations; however, the use of a higher frequency 12–14 MHz and even 14–16 MHz small footprint transducer provides further details of very superficial nodules (Figure 4.7a and b).

An additional advantage of small footprint transducers is that they are better to maneuver around the trachea and clavicles to look for lymph nodes and other pathology. For large multinodular goiters and masses, a curved C4-6 transducer with deeper penetration is required. Use of panoramic view (Figure 4.8) is preferred over the split screen merge technique to measure large thyroids and to give pictorial representation of and relation of any abnormality with the neck structures. A systematic approach to scan the entire neck area from under the jaw line up to the clavicles must be done in all cases for complete assessment of the lymph nodes and other neck structures. Scanning is done in both longitudinal and transverse directions. Color and power Doppler are used to assess vascularity. Color flow gives a graphic display of both speed and direction, while power Doppler is the sum of the total flow, hence increased sensitivity to low flow, though more prone to flash artifacts. Sono-elastography can be applied for stiffness information of the nodules.

ULTRASOUND IN DIFFUSE THYROID DISORDERS
AUTOIMMUNE THYROIDITIS
The common forms of thyroiditis are chronic lymphocytic and Graves' disease. Chronic lymphocytic thyroiditis could be atrophic thyroiditis or goitrous Hashimoto's thyroiditis. Postpartum thyroiditis and silent thyroiditis are usually self-limiting.

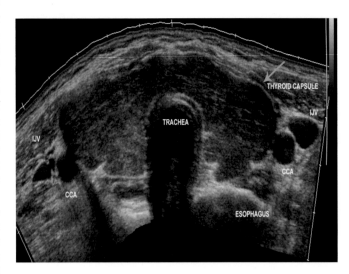

Figure 4.8 A panoramic view of the thyroid can be used to give a pictorial representation of the whole gland in one image and help communicate the anatomical relation of the structures in the neck and of any associated pathology.

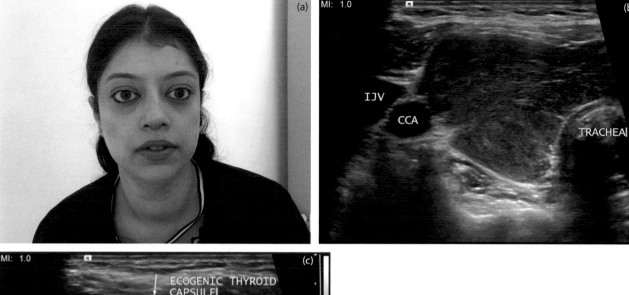

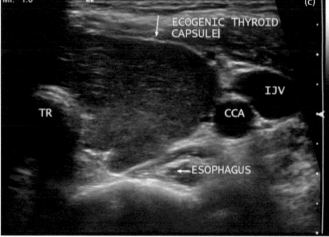

Figure 4.9 (a) A 35-year-old female with thyrotoxicosis. Patient photograph showing exophthalmos and diffuse swelling in the anterior neck suggesting thyroid enlargement. (b and c) Gray-scale ultrasound showing diffuse enlargement of both the lobe of the thyroid with decreased echogenicity or hypoechoic echotexture, involving the whole of the thyroid. The hypoechogenicity is similar to the overlying strap muscles.

ULTRASOUND FINDINGS IN THYROIDITIS

A diffuse or multifocal decrease in echogenicity (Figure 4.9a–c) demonstrated on ultrasound is the hallmark of many types of thyroiditis [15,16]. This decrease in echogenicity may be due to an increase in the intrathyroidal blood flow, increased cellularity of the thyroid follicles with decreased colloid production, or lymphocytic infiltration. The decrease in echogenicity occurs even before the bio-clinical abnormality and correlates with the circulating level of thyroid antibodies [17,18]. On color and power Doppler studies, increased blood flow is noted throughout the gland (Figure 4.10a–c). Return of the normal thyroid echogenicity and blood flow is noted on resolution of the disease. However, heterogeneity may persist if the chronic thyroiditis ensues and fibrosis may set in within the gland, resulting in a coarsened echotexture.

Graves' disease is an autoimmune thyroid disease and is the most common cause of thyrotoxicosis. On ultrasound, the thyroid gland is mildly enlarged with a hypoechoic and slightly heterogeneous echotexture. Ultrasound is required to evaluate size, echotexture, vascularity, and nodules. A characteristic hypervascular "thyroid inferno" pattern is noted on color Doppler in Graves thyrotoxicosis. Ultrasound is also used in evaluating the response to treatment as the degree of hypoechogenicity and vascularity corresponds to the level of circulating antithyroid antibodies. Small reactive cervical lymph nodes may be seen.

HASHIMOTO'S THYROIDITIS

Hashimoto's thyroiditis [17,18], also known as lymphocytic thyroiditis or chronic autoimmune thyroiditis, is a subtype of autoimmune thyroiditis. Patients are usually hypothyroid, although there may be a brief hyperthyroid early phase. Ultrasound features (Figure 4.11a–d) depend on the severity and phase of the disease. Generally, the gland is diffusely enlarged with a heterogeneous echotexture. The presence of hypoechoic micronodules (1–6 mm) with surrounding echogenic septation is also considered to have a relatively high positive predictive value. Color Doppler usually shows normal or decreased flow, but occasionally hypervascular flow may be seen. Associated prominent reactive cervical nodes may be present, especially in level VI. Large nodules may be present in nodular Hashimoto's thyroiditis. In long standing cases, a typical nodular "swiss-cheese" appearance (Figure 4.12a–d) is seen. There is a higher reported risk for papillary thyroid carcinoma, hence nodules need to be carefully evaluated and suspicious nodules should be biopsied [19,20].

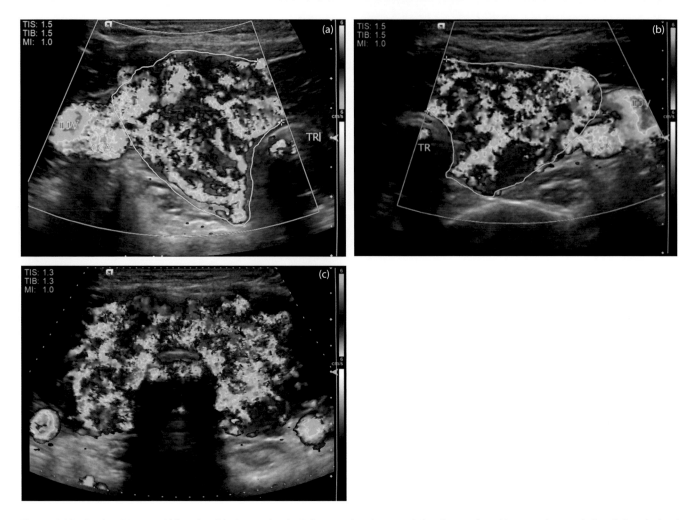

Figure 4.10 (a–c) A 35-year-old female with thyrotoxicosis. Color Doppler ultrasound showing profound increase in vascularity of the whole of the thyroid, giving the appearance of "thyroid inferno." (a) Right lobe. (b) Left lobe. (c) Panoramic view.

In Riedel thyroiditis, inflammation extends beyond the confines of the gland into adjacent tissues and typically presents as a hard goiter with compression symptoms on the trachea.

THYROID NODULES

A thyroid nodule is defined as a region of parenchyma sonographically distinct from the remainder of the thyroid. Incidence of thyroid nodules is on the rise with the advent of high resolution transducers and incidental nodules detected on CT, MRI, or PET-CT done for other indications. Thyroid nodules [21,22] could be solitary or multiple as in multinodular goiter. Most thyroid nodules are benign. To screen out and select suspicious nodules for FNAC (fine needle aspiration cytology) is still a challenge and various methods of ultrasound TIRADS (Thyroid Imaging, Reporting, and Data System) scoring are currently being used. TIRADS [23] scoring is done by choosing the correct lexicon, and risk stratification is done to select the nodules for FNA or follow up depending on the appropriate size criteria. With multiple nodules, each nodule should be scrutinized for suspicious features and selected for FNA on the basis of sonographic features. Scoring is determined from five categories of ultrasound findings. The higher the cumulative score, the higher the TIRADS level and the likelihood of malignancy.

Each nodule is evaluated for its size:

Composition: [cystic/almost completely cystic (0), spongiform (0), mixed cystic and solid (1), solid/almost completely solid (2), cannot determine (2)].
Echogenicity: [anechoic (0), hyperechoic (1), isoechoic (1), hypoechoic (2), very hypoechoic (3), cannot determine (1)].
Shape: [not taller than wide (0), taller than wide (3)].
Margins: [smooth (0), ill-defined (0), lobulated/irregular (2), extra-thyroidal extension (3), cannot determine (0)].
Echogenic foci: [none (0), large comet tail artifacts (0), macrocalcifications (1), peripheral calcifications (2), punctate echogenic foci (3)].

Thorough cervical lymph node assessment is done. Color Doppler to assess vascularity and elastography to assess the stiffness of the nodules is done. Correlation with cytopathology and Bethesda scoring is done.

TIRADS risk category: [TR1 (0 points), TR2 (2 points), TR3 (3 points), TR4 (4–6 points), TR5 (≥7 points)].

The recommendations for FNA/follow up as per size and TIRADS [24] category are as follows.

No	IMAGES	SIZE (mm)		COMPOSITION			ECHOGENICITY			TALLER-THAN-WIDE		MARGINS			ECHOGENIC FOCI			TOTAL POINTS		TI-RADS LEVEL
		X	X																	
		X	X																	
		X	X																	
		X	X																	
		X	X																	
TWO largest nodules and any with IMPORTANT FEATURES		C	Cystic		0	A	Anechoic	0	No	0	S	Smooth	0	N	None	0	0 Pts	TR1	Benign
		Sp	Spongiform		0	↑	Hyperechoic	1	Yes	3	ID	Ill-defined	0	CT	Comet-Tail	0	2 Pts	TR2	Not Suspicious
		M	Mixed cystic and nodule		1	=	Isoechoic	1			L	Lobulated	2	M	Macrocaks	1	3 Pts	TR3	Mildly Suspicious
		S	Solid		2	↓	Hypoechoic	2			I	Irregular	2	PC	Periph calc	2	4–6 Pts	TR4	Mod Suspicious
						↓↓	Very hypoechoic	3			E	Extra-thyroidal ext	3	P	Punctate	3	7+	TR5	Highly Suspicious
		*If cystic or spongiform, do not add further points for other categories																		

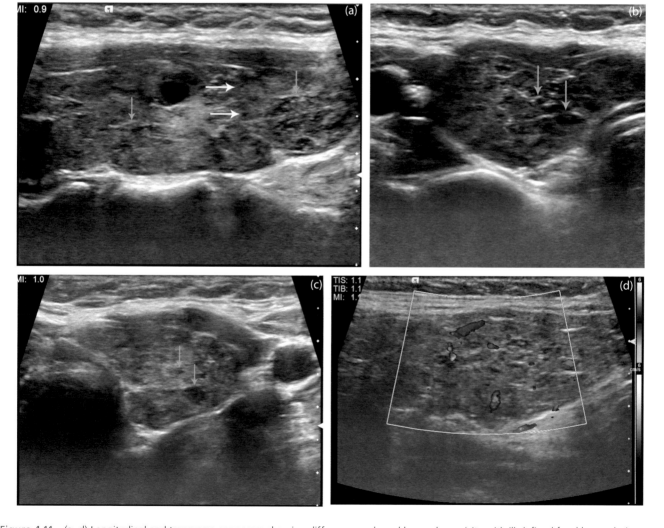

Figure 4.11 (a–d) Longitudinal and transverse sonogram showing diffuse parenchymal hypoechogenicity with ill-defined focal hypoechoic areas (yellow arrows) and echogenic lines due to fibrosis (white arrows). On color Doppler only minimal vascularity is seen. Patient is clinically hypothyroid.

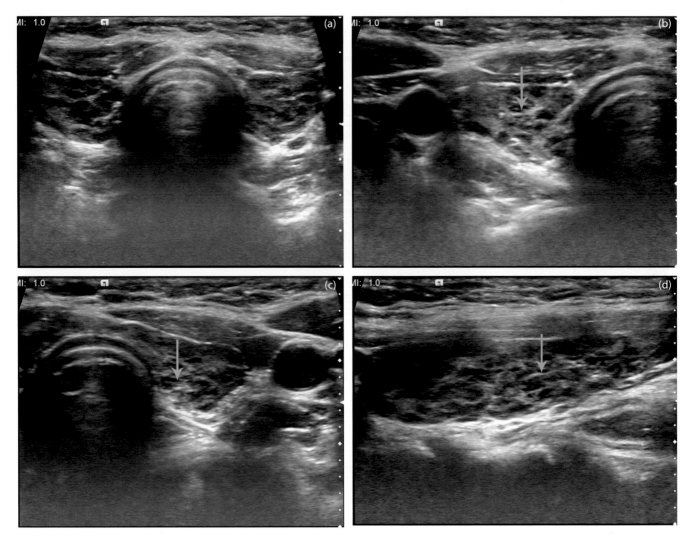

Figure 4.12 (a–d) Transverse and longitudinal sonogram in patient with long standing hypothyroidism due to Hashimoto's disease showing the marked hypoechogenicity with echogenic fibrous septa, giving the gland a characteristic "swiss-cheese" appearance.

TR1 and TR2: no FNA required
TR3: ≥1.5 cm, follow-up, ≥2.5 cm FNA
- *follow-up:* 1, 3, and 5 years
TR4: ≥1.0 cm, follow-up, ≥1.5 cm FNA
- *follow-up:* 1, 2, 3, and 5 years
TR5: ≥0.5 cm, follow-up, ≥1.0 cm FNA
- annual follow-up for up to 5 years

Biopsy is recommended for suspicious lesions (TR3 – TR5) with the above size criteria.

The cancer risk as per ACR TIRADS is 0.3% for TR1, 1.5% for TR2, 4.8% for TR3, 9.1% for TR4, and 35% for TR5.

BENIGN THYROID NODULES

Purely cystic nodules (Figure 4.13a and b) are well defined anechoic cysts within the capsule of the thyroid. They show smooth walls and characteristic posterior acoustic enhancement. They are scored as TIRADS 1. Spongiform nodules (Figure 4.14) composed of >50% aggregates of microcystic component are specific for benign thyroid nodules. Colloid nodules (Figure 4.15) are the most common benign thyroid nodules. They can be as small as 3–4 mm or be as large as to be completely replacing the thyroid gland. They are usually well defined cystic or mixed solid cystic (Figure 4.16a and b), iso- to hypoechoic nodules. A characteristic feature of colloid nodules is tiny echogenic or a bright focus with a posterior triangular shadowing known as a comet tail artifact. The comet tail artifact is likely due to the presence of microcrystals and is a classical feature of colloid nodules. Colloid nodules are also known as adenomatous nodules or colloid nodular goiter. Although they may grow to be large multinodular thyroids (Figure 4.17a and b), they will usually not spread beyond the thyroid gland. A thorough scrutiny of each nodule is done for any suspicious features [25].

MALIGNANT THYROID NODULES

The main objective of the management of thyroid nodules is to identify the suspicious nodules for malignancy and do the FNA [26]. The suspicious ultrasound features include: solid composition; marked hypoechogenicity; irregular or microlobulated margins; taller than wide nodule; presence of microcalcification, punctate echogenic foci, or broken rim calcifications; abnormal heterogeneous vascularity on color Doppler [27]; presence of local invasion; and metastasis. When multiple nodules (≥4) are present, only the four highest scoring nodules, not necessarily the largest, should be scored, reported, and followed up. Interval enlargement [28–30] on follow-up is felt to be significant if there is an increase of 20% and 2 mm in two dimensions, or a 50% increase in volume. Further CT, MRI, or PET-CT may be required for complete evaluation. Papillary thyroid cancer and follicular carcinoma comprise the majority of

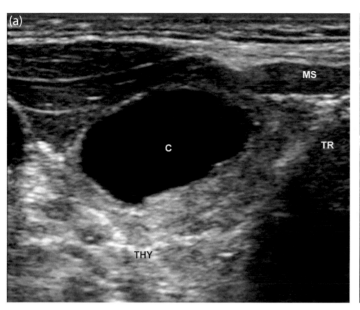

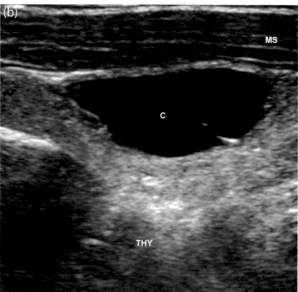

Figure 4.13 (a and b) Transverse and longitudinal gray-scale sonogram showing a well-defined clear anechoic cyst, located within the confines of the thyroid capsule. TIRADS 1. (tr: trachea, ms: strap muscles, thy: thyroid, C: cyst).

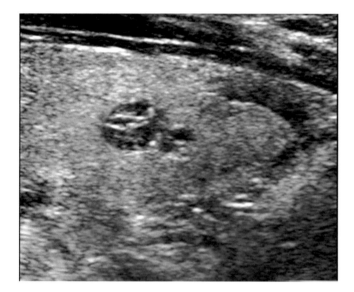

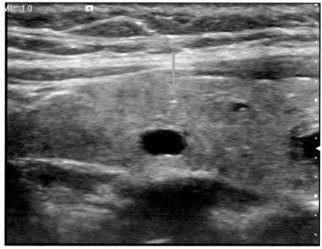

Figure 4.14 Longitudinal gray scale sonogram showing a typical spongiform thyroid nodule consisting of aggregates of microcystic components of at least 50% of nodule volume. These nodules are benign and do not need any further investigations.

Figure 4.15 Gray-scale ultrasound right lobe thyroid sonogram showing a small well-defined clear hypoechoic cyst typical of a colloid nodule (a comet tail artifact may be seen in them).

cases. Other common subtypes are Hurthle cell neoplasm, anaplastic carcinoma, and medullary carcinoma. Lymphoma and metastasis are rarely seen.

FOLLICULAR NEOPLASM

Follicular adenomas are encapsulated true neoplasms of the thyroid gland. On ultrasound they are seen as solid well-defined isoechoic to hyperechoic nodules. Features of loss of halo and more hypoechoic echotexture are suggestive of carcinoma. The differentiation of follicular adenoma from a follicular carcinoma (Figure 4.18) is based on the presence of capsular or vascular invasion

on histologic examination and thus cannot be made by ultrasound or by FNA cytology [31–33].

HURTHLE CELL NEOPLASM

Hurthle cell neoplasm [34] on ultrasound (Figure 4.19a–d) imaging is predominantly solid with mixed internal echogenicity with both hyperechoic and hypoechoic components. They have ill-defined margins with partial halo.

PAPILLARY THYROID CARCINOMA

Papillary thyroid carcinoma accounts for 60%–70% of thyroid cancer [35–38]. It can be seen as a multicentric form and may be micro-nodular (<1 cm size nodule). It spreads along lymphatics to regional lymph nodes, and distant metastasis is

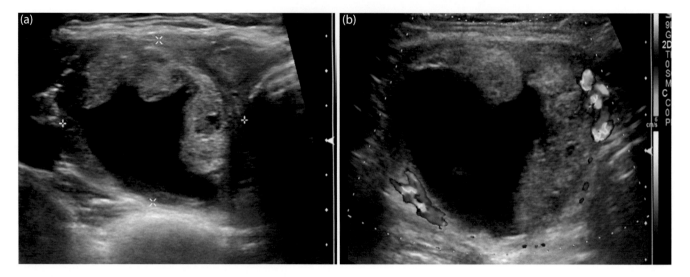

Figure 4.16 (a and b) Transverse sonogram. (a) Gray scale and (b) color Doppler showing a mixed solid cystic, iso- to hypoechoic nodule, located within the confines of the thyroid capsule. On color Doppler minimal peripheral vascularity is seen. TIRADS 2.

commonly to lung and bone. Characteristic ultrasound features (Figures 4.20 through 4.22) are a solid or a mixed solid cystic hypoechoic or very hypoechoic mass lesion with punctate (Figure 4.23) echogenic foci within. The margins may be lobulated or irregular or ill-defined. Extrathyroidal extension and metastatic lymph nodes show features similar to primary lesions such as hypoechoic texture and punctate foci and cystic changes. On color Doppler, central heterogeneous vascularity is seen (Figures 4.24 through 4.26).

PAPILLARY THYROID MICROCARCINOMA

Papillary thyroid microcarcinoma (PTMC) [39–41] by definition includes papillary thyroid carcinoma with the nodule measuring less than 10 mm in greatest dimension (Figure 4.27a and b). Most of these are often incidental diagnoses on imaging (ultrasound or CT) done for other abnormalities. They often present with cervical masses which may be metastatic lymph nodes (Figure 4.28a–e). FNA is needed to establish the diagnosis. As these are frequently multifocal, total

or near total thyroidectomy is often advised. The evaluation of the cervical lymph nodes, both lateral and central compartments, needs to be very thorough and detailed. Availability and use of a small footprint transducer is helpful in evaluating the central compartment as it can be maneuvered around to the trachea along the lower pole of thyroid with ease due to its smaller size. The lymph nodes must be measured in three dimensions and evaluated with color Doppler and sono-elastography.

MEDULLARY THYROID CARCINOMA

Medullary thyroid carcinoma (MTC) [42–45] comprises 3%–5% of thyroid cancers and can be sporadic or familial (autosomal dominant pattern of transmission), associated with multiple endocrine neoplasia (MEN) 2a and MEN 2b. RET proto-oncogene mutation is found in almost all of the hereditary cases. It arises from parafollicular cells, or C cells. Serum calcitonin levels are elevated which is used both in diagnosis and follow-up. Ultrasound features overlap with papillary carcinoma and comprise a solid ill-defined

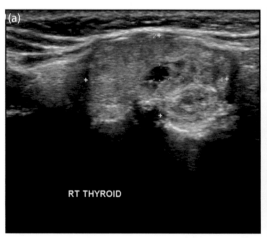

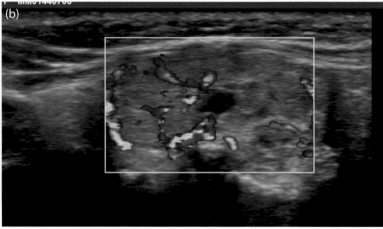

Figure 4.17 (a and b) A 45-year-old female with multinodular goiter. Longitudinal sonogram of the thyroid showing a well-defined almost solid hypoechoic nodule with minimal vascularity on color Doppler. TIRADS 3. Biopsy showed benign follicular adenoma.

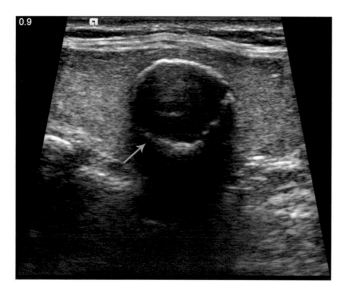

Figure 4.18 Ultrasound right thyroid of a 43-year-old female showing a well-defined solid 3.1 × 3.0 cm solid, iso- to hyperechoic nodule with peripheral calcifications (arrow). TIRADS 5 (S/solid/2, ≈/Isoechoic/1, S/smooth/0, PC/peripheral Calc/2, 5 pts/TR4/moderately suspicious). Biopsy showed follicular carcinoma thyroid.

heterogeneous hypoechoic nodule. The calcifications seen here are often coarser. On color Doppler they show heterogeneous vascularity, and often cervical (paratracheal and lateral cervical) metastasis are seen at presentation (Figures 4.29 and 4.30). Distant metastasis occurs to liver, lungs, bone, and to brain and skin. The risk of distant metastasis increases with the size of the thyroid tumor, extension of the tumor beyond the thyroid capsule, and presence and extent of lymph node metastasis. PET-CT is needed for further evaluation.

ANAPLASTIC CARCINOMA

Anaplastic carcinoma [46–48] is one of the most aggressive malignancies and usually presents as a rapidly enlarging mass with local compressive symptoms, often with distant metastasis via the bloodstream to brain, liver, lungs, and bone. On ultrasound there is often a large very hypoechoic mass (Figure 4.31) involving the whole of the gland and possibly extending beyond with local invasion and metastasis.

Anaplastic carcinoma is rare (<1% of all thyroid masses) but extremely aggressive. Patients are usually elderly with a history of goiter and present with a rapidly growing neck mass. The tumor

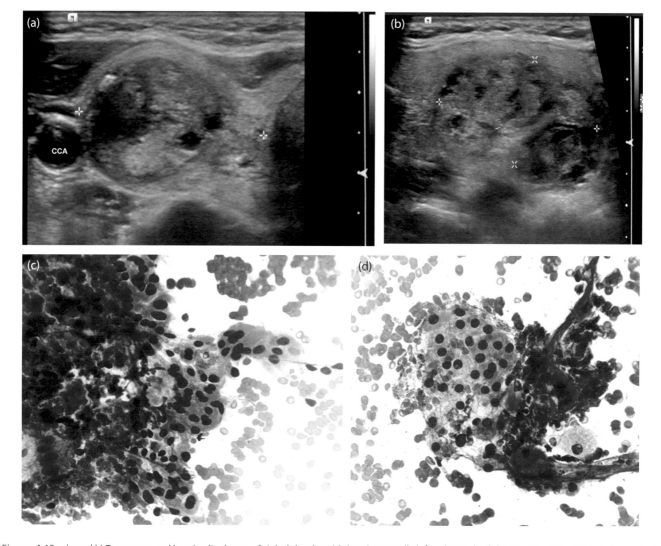

Figure 4.19 (a and b) Transverse and longitudinal scan of right lobe thyroid showing a well-defined mixed solid cystic 31 × 17 × 25 mm hypoechoic nodule with ill-defined margins. TIRADS 4 (mixed cystic and solid/1, ↓/hypoechoic/2, No/0, ID/ill-defined/0, PC/peripheral Calc/2 = 5 pts/TR4/mod suspicious). (c and d) FNAC showed Bethesda III AUS with Hurthle cell predominance.

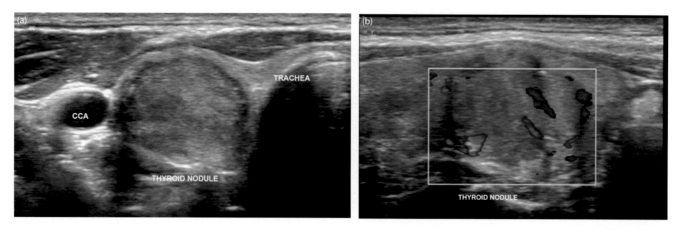

Figure 4.20 (a and b) Transverse and longitudinal scan of right lobe thyroid with color Doppler showing a well-defined solid hypoechoic nodule with lobulated margins. TIRADS 4 (S/solid/2, ↓/hypoechoic/2, L/lobulated/2, N/none/0 = 6 pts/TR4/mod suspicious). On FNA, few smears showed small crowded groups with enlarged hyperchromatic, slightly irregular nuclei (? Papillary tips) with scant colloid and focal cytological and architectural atypia, *suspicious of follicular neoplasm with possibility of follicular adenoma/FVPTC/NIFTP.*

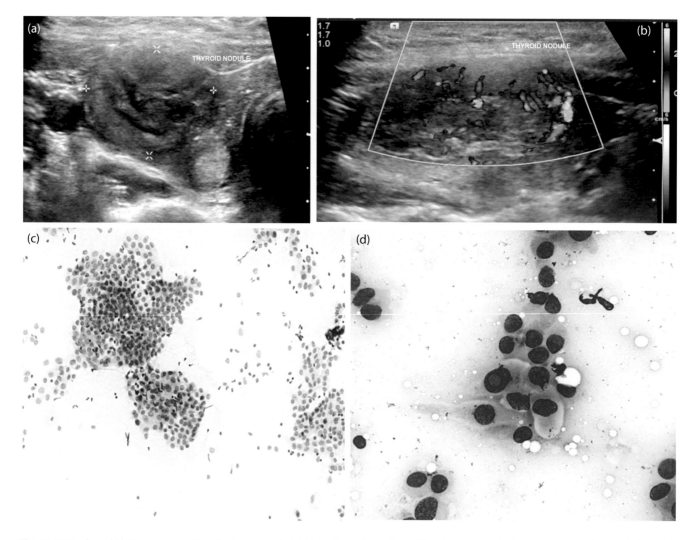

Figure 4.21 (a and b) Transverse and longitudinal scan of right lobe thyroid showing a 28 × 11 mm exophytic heterogeneous hypoechoic nodule with likely ETE (extrathyroidal extension, curved arrow) along the anterior capsular surface. On color Doppler heterogeneous vascularity is seen within the nodule. TIRADS 5 (S/solid/2, ↓/hypoechoic/2, No/0, ETE/3, N/None/0 = 7pts/TR5/suspicious). (c and d) FNAC showed papillary Ca. Pap stained smear shows crowded sheets and papillary clusters of thyroid follicular cells with intranuclear cytoplasmic inclusion.

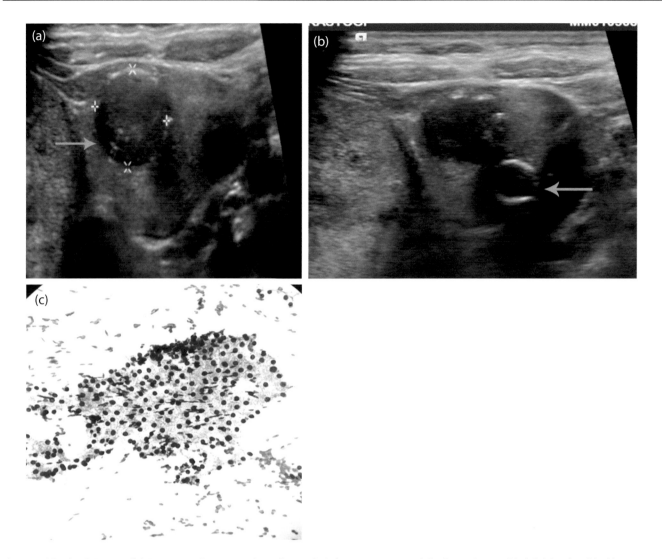

Figure 4.22   (a–c) Two small (12 × 11 mm & 7 × 6 mm) very hypoechoic heterogeneous nodules (curved arrows) in left lobe thyroid with punctate foci and peripheral broken rim calcifications. TIRADS 5 (S/solid/2, ↓↓/very hypoechoic/3, No/0, ID/Ill-defined/0, P/Punctate/3, 8 pts/TR5/suspicious). FNAC showed papillary carcinoma (multicentric PTC).

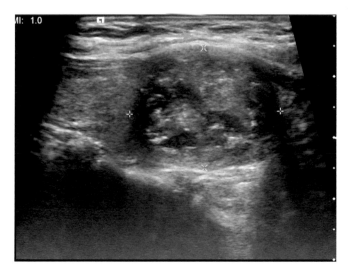

Figure 4.23   Transverse sonogram of the right lobe thyroid showing a heterogeneous hypoechoic nodule (curved arrow) with numerous punctate echogenic foci. TIRADS 5 (S/solid/2, ↓/hypoechoic/2, No/0, ID/ill-defined/0, P/punctate/3, 7+/TR5/Highly suspicious). FNAC Bethesda VI: PTC.

invades locally and distant metastases most commonly involve the lungs, bones, brain, and liver. Mean survival is 6 months, with a 5-year survival rate of 7%. CT is needed for full assessment.

PRIMARY THYROID LYMPHOMA
Primary thyroid lymphoma [49,50] is rare (<2% of thyroid cancers). The peak incidence is during the seventh decade, and the male/female ratio is 1:3. Clinically patients present with a rapidly enlarging painless mass, often with compressive symptoms. History of preceding long-standing auto-immune thyroiditis or Hashimoto's disease may be given. Most patients have elevated anti-thyroglobulin antibodies. Ultrasound features comprise solid hypoechoic, often pseudocystic masses on a background of thyroiditis.

ULTRASOUND ELASTOGRAPHY
Ultrasound elastography [51–53] measures tissue elasticity or stiffness, which is in turn used as an adjunct to characterize the lesions. The technique involves application of a small mechanical force during scanning, and the degree of distortion is used to estimate the stiffness of the tissue of interest (Figures 4.32 and 4.33)

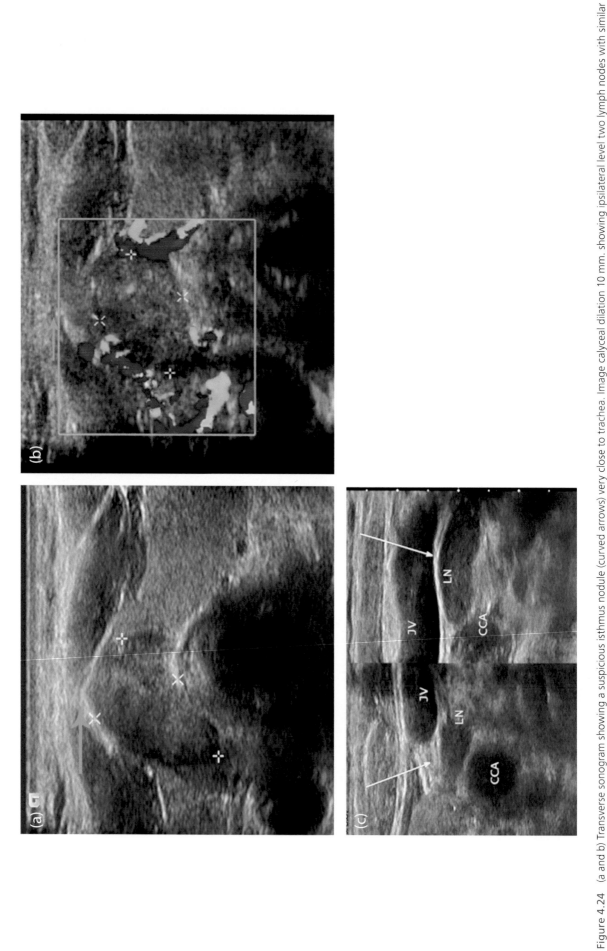

Figure 4.24 (a and b) Transverse sonogram showing a suspicious isthmus nodule (curved arrows) very close to trachea. Image calyceal dilation 10 mm. showing ipsilateral level two lymph nodes with similar punctate echogenic foci within. Ln + TIRADS 5 (S/solid/2, ⊥⊥/very hypoechoic/3, N/none/0, E/extrathyroidal ext/3, N/none/0, LN+, 9+/TR5/Highly suspicious). Biopsy: papillary CA.

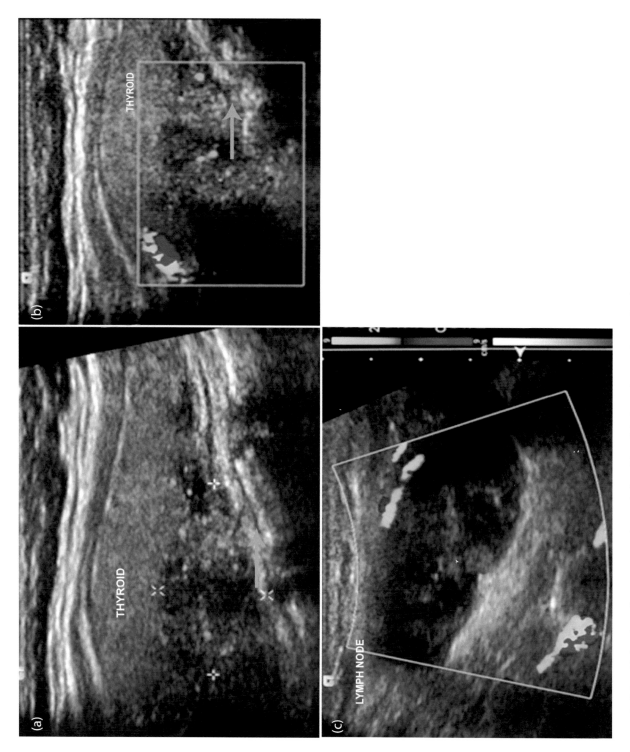

Figure 4.25 (a–c) Ultrasound of thyroid showing a heterogeneous hypoechoic solid nodule (curved arrows) with ill-defined/irregular margins and multiple tiny punctate echogenic foci. TIRADS 5. Biopsy papillary carcinoma. Image calyceal dilation 10 mm. Showing associated ipsilateral metastatic left level 3 lymph node.

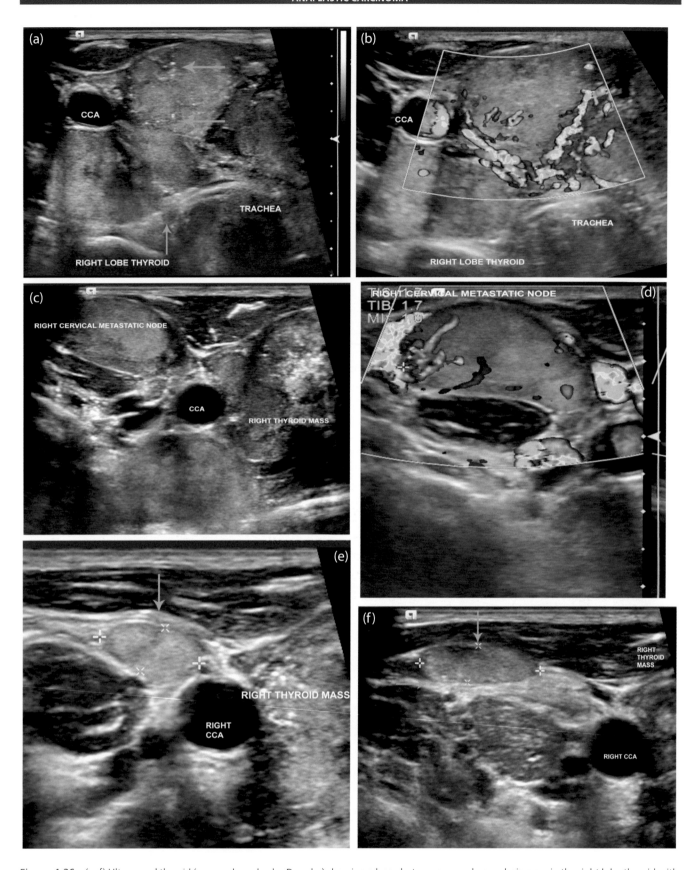

Figure 4.26 (a–f) Ultrasound thyroid (gray scale and color Doppler) showing a large heterogeneous hypoechoic mass in the right lobe thyroid with multiple tiny punctate echogenic foci. TIRADS 5. Biopsy papillary carcinoma. Associated multiple metastatic left level 3 and level 4 lymph nodes.

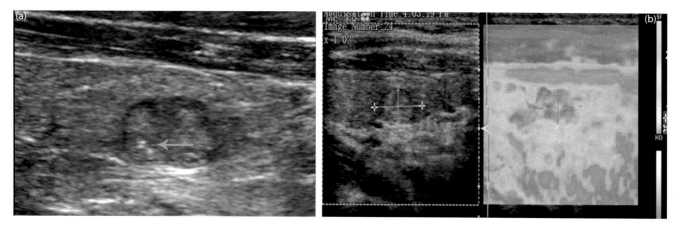

Figure 4.27 (a and b) Micronodular papillary thyroid carcinoma in a 35-year-old female. Biopsy proven. Longitudinal sonogram showing a heterogeneous hypoechoic nodule with few tiny punctate echogenic foci. On elastography the lesion appears hard in stiffness.

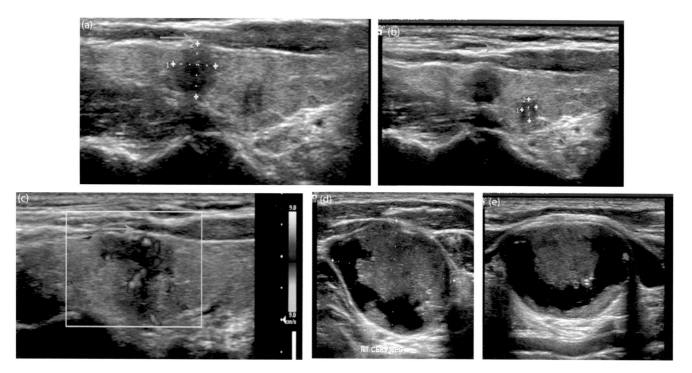

Figure 4.28 (a–e) Micronodular multicentric papillary thyroid carcinoma in a 41-year-old female with (c and d) large cervical metastatic lymph nodes (level 3) at presentation. Biopsy proven. Longitudinal sonogram showing two sub-centimeter heterogeneous ill-defined hypoechoic nodules (curved arrows) with heterogeneous vascularity. Note the tiny punctate echogenic foci in the cervical metastatic nodes.

and is color-coded as per the manufacturer. Soft tissues deform more than hard tissues. There are various studies on this technique's role in predicting malignancy; however, currently it is being used as an adjunct in both thyroid nodule and lymph node assessment.

LYMPHADENOPATHY

The presence of local lymphadenopathy with any suspicious features for malignancy must be noted [54]. A typical reactive lymph node may be ovoid to rounded hypoechoic and show hilar vascularity on color Doppler (Figure 4.34).

Microcalcification and cystic changes [55,56] in regional lymph nodes are highly suspicious (Figure 4.35a and b). Loss of normal fatty hilum, irregular, or rounded appearance with irregular internal hypervascularity (Figure 4.36a and b) are suspicious features. A thorough evaluation of both the central [57,58] and lateral compartment must be done in all cases. Availability of a small footprint transducer is helpful in evaluating the spaces around the trachea and bones. Biopsy is suggested for suspicious lymph nodes. Post-thyroidectomy assessment of the thyroid bed and the nodal compartments must be very thorough and meticulous. Further cross sectional imaging may be advised for detailed mapping.

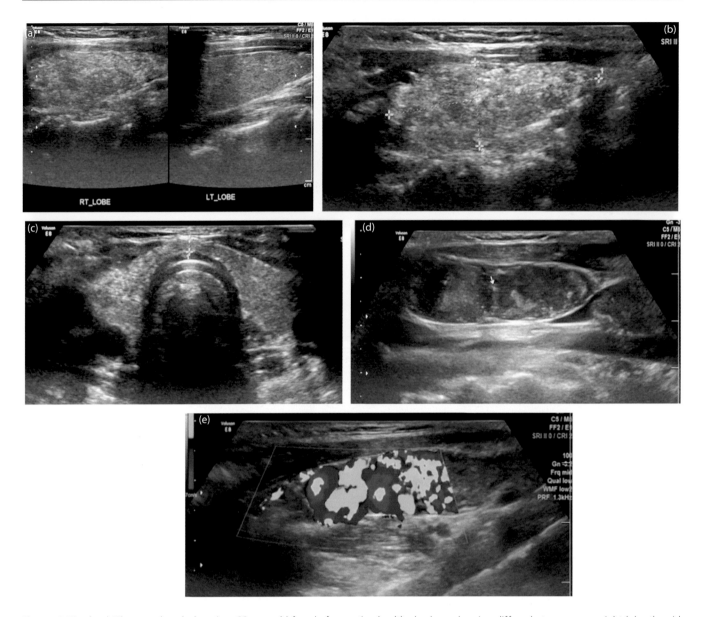

Figure 4.29   (a–e) Ultrasound neck done in a 33-year-old female for routine health check-up showing diffuse heterogeneous right lobe thyroid echotexture as compared to contralateral side. Associated large heterogeneous hypoechoic masses in neck with increased vascularity on color Doppler. Biopsy findings were Bethesda VI, medullary carcinoma, with associated metastatic right level 3 and 4 lymph nodes with calcification at diagnosis.

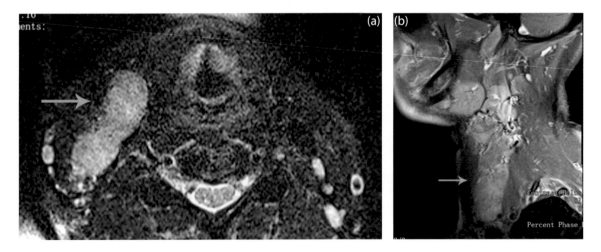

Figure 4.30   (a and b) CEMRI in the same patient as in Figure 4.29. T1 weighted image axial and coronal scan showing multiple well defined lobulated homogenous masses in the neck along the jugulo-diagastric chain (extending from level II to V regions) with mild to intense enhancement on contrast images. Biopsy confirmed metastatic medullary carcinoma thyroid.

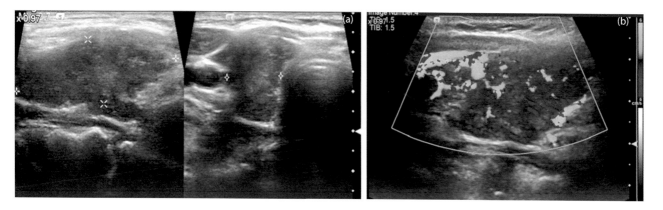

Figure 4.31 (a and b) A 73-year-male. Gray-scale ultrasound showing a large, solid lobulated very hypoechoic mass involving isthmus and left lobe thyroid. Color Doppler showing mild vascularity in this case. Extrathyroidal extension (ETE) is suggested. Biopsy: Anaplastic carcinoma.

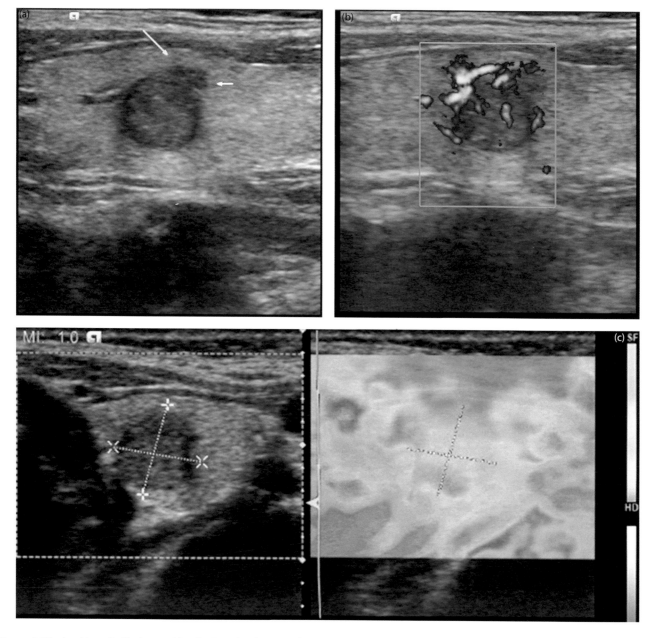

Figure 4.32 (a–c) Longitudinal scan with color Doppler showing a heterogeneous hypoechoic nodule with lobulated margins and internal vascularity on color Doppler. Corresponding real-time qualitative elastogram showing the lesion in the yellow to red zone, suggesting a moderately stiff nodule, suggesting malignancy on elastography. FNA showed Bethesda V, papillary thyroid carcinoma.

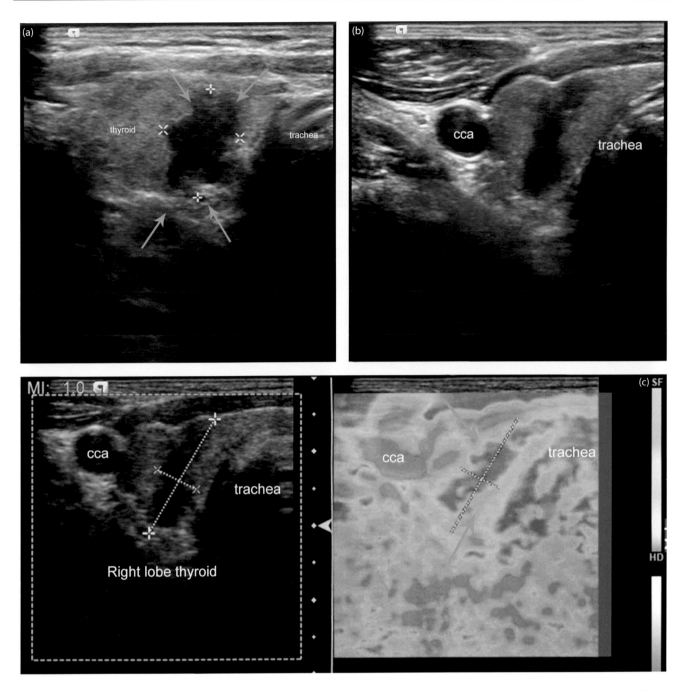

Figure 4.33 (a–c) Longitudinal and transverse sonogram of right lobe showing a suspicious hypoechoic taller than wide right thyroid nodule/ n + TIRADS 5 (S/solid/2, ↓↓/very hypoechoic/3, Yes/3, L/lobulated/2, N/none/0, LN+, 10+/TR5/Highly suspicious). Biopsy: Papillary CA.

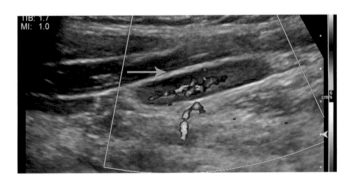

Figure 4.34 Longitudinal ultrasound of left upper neck (Level II) showing a typical ovoid reactive lymph node with hilar vascularity on color Doppler.

METASTASIS TO THE THYROID

Metastasis to the thyroid is rare and is a part of disseminated metastasis from breast, colon, kidney, lung, and melanoma. These cases are often detected as incidentalomas on PET-CT (Figure 4.37) and are sent for ultrasound. Ultrasound features are usually of a non-specific solid heterogeneous hypoechoic mass with disorganized vascularity. Associated other regional and distant metastases are seen. FNA is usually indicated for definitive assessment.

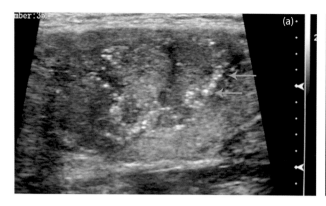
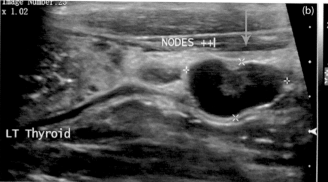

Figure 4.35 (a and b) Longitudinal sonogram of left neck showing a heterogeneous hypoechoic ill-defined thyroid nodule at lower pole with multiple punctate echogenic foci (straight arrows) and associated cystic metastatic cervical lymph node (curved arrow) in the central compartment (level VI). FNA confirmed papillary thyroid carcinoma.

CONTRAST-ENHANCED ULTRASOUND IMAGING

Contrast-enhanced ultrasound (CEUS) is a very promising diagnostic technique that could improve the diagnostic accuracy of identifying benign thyroid lesions to spare a large number of patients an unnecessary invasive procedure. Contrast-enhanced ultrasound enhancement patterns are different in benign and malignant lesions [59,60]. Ring enhancement was predictive of benign lesions, whereas heterogeneous enhancement was helpful for detecting malignant lesions. Currently, contrast-enhanced ultrasound and ultrasound

elastography have been gradually applied to the diagnosis of cervical lymph node metastasis. However, it is not clear whether contrast-enhanced ultrasound and elastography combined with conventional ultrasound improve the accuracy of lymph node metastasis diagnosis.

COMPUTED TOMOGRAPHY (CT), MAGNETIC RESONANCE IMAGING (MRI), AND PET-CT

Further cross sectional imaging like CT [61,62] and MRI [63–66] must be advised in patients with clinical symptoms of hoarseness

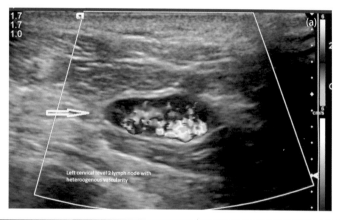

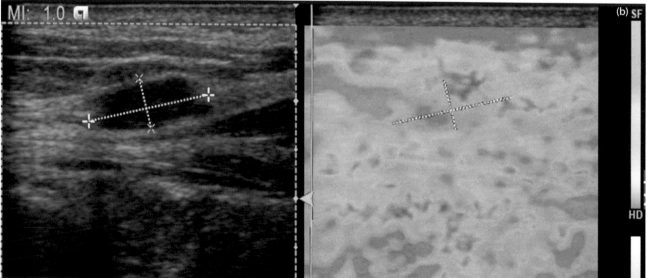

Figure 4.36 (a and b) Longitudinal sonogram of left upper neck in a post-operative PTC patient showing a hypoechoic level 3 lymph node with heterogeneous vascularity. FNA confirmed papillary thyroid carcinoma. Sono-elastography of the lymph node showing intermediate stiffness.

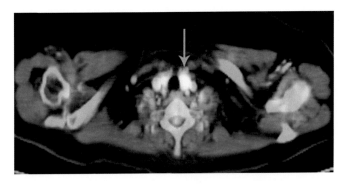

Figure 4.37 FDG-PET-CECT. Axial scan showing subtle hypodensity with increased FDG uptake (SUVmax-9.9) in the left lobe of the thyroid. (These thyroid incidental nodules account for a significant number of detected thyroid nodules).

of voice with or without vocal cord paresis or paralysis, progressive dysphagia or odynophagia, mass fixation to surrounding structures on palpation, respiratory symptoms, hemoptysis, stridor, or positional dyspnea. Other indications would be large size of tumor or mediastinal extension, incompletely imaged on ultrasound;

ultrasound suspicion for significant ETE (extrathyroidal extension), bulky, posteriorly located, or inferiorly located lymph nodes incompletely imaged by ultrasound; and cases of rapid progression or enlargement. In locally invasive thyroid malignancy (such as anaplastic carcinoma), the imaging modalities help to evaluate the extrathyroidal spread of a tumor to the larynx, trachea, and adjacent major vessels and provide evidence of regional or distant metastases. On contrast-enhanced CT (CECT), heterogeneous masses with or without calcifications or enhancement are seen in thyroid cancer (Figure 4.38a–c). A systematic approach to evaluate neck lymph nodes and mapping must be done as nodal metastasis and its extent affects the management planning and prognosis significantly [67–69].

^{18}F-FDG PET-CT [70] is suggested to evaluate for distant metastasis. Diffusion-weighted MRI (DWI) and perfusion imaging with dynamic contrast-enhanced MRI (DCE-MRI) are other techniques to evaluate for metastatic lesions.

POST-THYROIDECTOMY/HEMI-THYROIDECTOMY

The postoperative thyroid bed should appear as a narrow area of increased echogenicity between the common carotid artery laterally and the trachea medially. Any abnormality in the area should be carefully evaluated to differentiate between sequelae of surgery, residual thyroid, or recurrence.

CONCLUSION

Ultrasound evaluation of the thyroid is the fundamental basis of diagnosis and management of thyroid pathologies. A lot of care, detail, and experience is required to do a meticulous neck ultrasound using proper technique for both gray scale and Doppler. A thorough reference to the patient clinical information and correlation must be made. Examination includes and extends beyond the thyroid to complete neck evaluation in all cases. Choose the correct lexicon and give a TIRADS score for the thyroid nodules. Use elastography as an adjunct. Advise of further imaging if suggested. Give a well-documented report. Get a Bethesda score correlation and follow up.

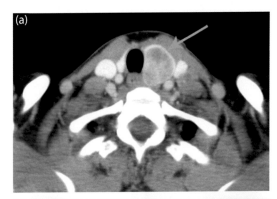

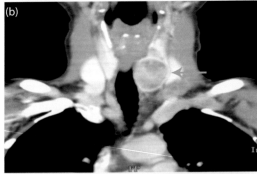

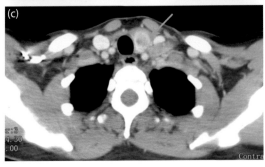

Figure 4.38 (a–c) CECT neck axial and coronal scans showing a heterogeneously enhancing nodule (curved arrows) in the left lobe of the thyroid measuring 2 × 2.5 × 3.3 cm. A heterogeneously enhancing left level 4 lymph node is seen measuring 2.8 × 1.1 cm.

REFERENCES

1. Fujimoto F, Oka A, Omoto R, Hirsoe M. Ultrasonic scanning of the thyroid gland as a new diagnostic approach. *Ultrasonics.* 1967;5:177–80.

2. Orloff L. *Head and Neck Ultrasonography.* San Diego: Plural Publishing Inc; 2008:6–7.

3. Genesis Ultrasound. Breakthrough in ultrasound physics comes from Pierre Curie www.genesisultrasound.com/ultrasound-physics.html. Accessed on January 15, 2019.

4. White DN. Johann Christian Doppler and his effect: A brief history. *Ultrasound Med Biol.* 1982;8(6):583–91.

5. Kainberger F, Leodolter S. Christian Doppler and the influence of his work on modern medicine. *Wien Klin Wochenschr.* 2004;116(4):107–9.

6. Cerbone G et al. Power Doppler improves the diagnostic accuracy of color Doppler ultrasonography in cold thyroid nodules: Follow-up results. *Horm Res.* 1999;52:19–24.

7. Physics and principles of ultrasound. In: Kremkau FW (ed.) *Diagnostic ultrasound*, 6th ed. Philadelphia: WB Saunders; 2002:10, 18–37, 62–64, 71–76, 86–92, 167–194, 273–318.

8. Chaudhary V, Bano S. Thyroid ultrasound. *Indian J Endocr Metab*. 2013;17(2):219–27.

9. Xu W, Iv Z, Wang H. Relationship between RLN and inferior thyroid artery. *Otolaryngol Head Neck Surg*. 2010;143(2 Suppl):199–200.

10. Kapre N. Preservation of the parathyroids in thyroid surgery. *Ear Nose Throat J*. 2009;2-1.

11. Irkorucu O. Zuckerkandl tubercle in thyroid surgery: Is it a reality or a myth? *Annal Med Surg (2012)*. 2016;7:92–6.

12. Fancy T, Gallagher D 3rd, Hornig JD. Surgical anatomy of the thyroid and parathyroid glands. *Otolaryngol Clin North Am*. 2010;43(2):221–7, vii.

13. Nilsson M, Williams D. On the origin of cells and derivation of thyroid cancer: C cell story revisited. *Eur Thyroid J*. 2016;5(2):79–93.

14. Choi SH, Kim EK, Kim SJ, Kwak JY. Thyroid ultrasonography: Pitfalls and techniques. *Korean J Radiol*. 2014;15(2):267–76.

15. Vitti P. Grey scale thyroid ultrasonography in the evaluation of patients with Graves' disease. *Eur J Endocrinol*. 2000;142:22–4.

16. Arslan H, Unal O, Algün E, Harman M, Sakarya ME. Power Doppler sonography in the diagnosis of Graves' disease. *Eur J Ultrasound*. 2000;11:117–22.

17. Pedersen OM et al. The value of ultrasonography in predicting autoimmune thyroid disease. *Thyroid*. 2000;10:251–9.

18. Rago T, Chiovato L, Grasso L, Pinchera A, Vitti P. Thyroid ultrasonography as a tool for detecting thyroid autoimmune diseases and predicting thyroid dysfunction in apparently healthy subjects. *J Endocrinol Invest*. 2001;24:763–9.

19. Cipolla C et al. Hashimoto thyroiditis coexistent with papillary thyroid carcinoma. *Am Surg*. 2005;71:874–8.

20. Ott RA et al. The incidence of thyroid carcinoma in Hashimoto's thyroiditis. *Am Surg*. 1987;53:442–5.

21. Marqusee E et al. Usefulness of ultrasonography in the management of nodular thyroid disease. *Ann Intern Med*. 2000;133:696–700.

22. Moon WJ et al. Thyroid Study Group, Korean Society of Neuro- and Head and Neck Radiology. Benign and malignant thyroid.

23. Grant EG et al. Thyroid ultrasound reporting lexicon: White paper of the ACR Thyroid Imaging, Reporting, and Data System (TIRADS) committee. *J Am College Radiol*. 2015;12(12):1272–9.

24. Tessler FN, Middleton WD, Grant EG. Thyroid Imaging, Reporting, and Data System (TIRADS): A User's Guide. *Radiology*. 2018;287(1):29–36.

25. Bonavita JA et al. Pattern recognition of benign nodules at ultrasound of the thyroid: Which nodules can be left alone? *AJR Am J Roentgenol*. 2009;193:207–13.

26. American Thyroid Association (ATA) Guidelines Taskforce on Thyroid Nodules and Differentiated Thyroid Cancer, Cooper DS et al. Revised American Thyroid Association management guidelines for patients with thyroid nodules and differentiated thyroid cancer. *Thyroid*. 2009;19:1167–214.

27. Papini E et al. Risk of malignancy in nonpalpable thyroid nodules: Predictive value of ultrasound and color-Doppler features. *J Clin Endocrinol Metab*. 2002;87:1941–6.

28. Quadbeck B et al. Long-term follow-up of thyroid nodule growth. *Exp Clin Endocrinol Diabetes*. 2002;110:348–54.

29. Negro R. What happens in a 5-year follow-up of benign thyroid nodules. *J Thyroid Res*. 2014;2014:459791.

30. Frates MC et al. Prevalence and distribution of carcinoma in patients with solitary and multiple thyroid nodules on sonography. *J Clin Endocrinol Metab*. 2006;91:3411–7.

31. DeMay RM. Follicular lesions of the thyroid. W(h)ither follicular carcinoma? *Am J Clin Pathol*. 2000;114:681–3.

32. Greaves TS et al. Follicular lesions of thyroid: A 5-year fine-needle aspiration experience. *Cancer*. 2000;90:335–41.

33. Huangg C, Hsueh C, Liu FH, Chao TC, Lin JD. Diagnostic and therapeutic strategies for minimally and widely invasive follicular thyroid carcinomas. *Surg Oncol*. 2011;20:1–6.

34. Caplan RH, Abellera RM, Kisken WA. Hürthle cell tumors of the thyroid gland. A clinicopathologic review and long-term follow-up. *JAMA*. 1984;251:3114–7.

35. Shin JH. Ultrasonographic imaging of papillary thyroid carcinoma variants. *Ultrasonography*. 2017;36(2):103–10. (Review Article).

36. Stulak JM et al. Value of preoperative ultrasonography in the surgical management of initial and reoperative papillary thyroid cancer. *Arch Surg*. 2006;141(5):489–96.

37. Lew JI, Solorzano CC. Use of ultrasound in the management of thyroid cancer. *Oncologist*. 2010;15(3):253–8.

38. Hahn SY, Shin JH, Oh YL, Kim TH, Lim Y, Choi JS. Role of ultrasound in predicting tumor invasiveness in follicular variant of papillary thyroid carcinoma. *Thyroid*. 2017;27(9):1177–84.

39. Ardito G et al. Aggressive papillary thyroid microcarcinoma: Prognostic factors and therapeutic strategy. *Clin Nucl Med*. 2013;38:25–8.

40. Hughes DT, Hymart MR, Miller BS, Gauger PG, Doherty GM. The most commonly occurring papillary thyroid cancer in the United States is now a microcarcinoma in a patient older than 45 years. *Thyroid*. 2011;21:231–6.

41. Hay ID et al. Papillary thyroid microcarcinoma: A study of 900 cases observed in a 60-year period. *Surgery*. 2008;144(6):980–8.

42. Cohen R et al. Preoperative calcitonin levels are predictive of tumour size and postoperative calcitonin normalization in medullary thyroid carcinoma. *J Clin Endocrinol Metab*. 2000;85:919–22.

43. Kebebew E, Ituarte PH, Siperstein AE, Duh QY, Clark OH. Medullary thyroid carcinoma: Clinical characteristics, treatment, prognostic factors, and a comparison of staging systems. *Cancer*. 2000;88:1139–48.

44. Pelizzo MR et al. Natural history, diagnosis, treatment and outcome of medullary thyroid cancer: 37-year experience on 157 patients. *Eur J Surg Oncol*. 2007;33:493–7.

45. Lee S, Shin JH, Han BK, Ko EY. Medullary thyroid carcinoma: Comparison with papillary thyroid carcinoma and application of current sonographic criteria. *AJR Am J Roentgenol*. 2010;194:1090–4.

46. Ain KB. Anaplastic thyroid carcinoma: Behavior, biology and therapeutic approaches. *Thyroid*. 1998;8:715–26.

47. Bogsrud TV et al. 18F-FDG PET in the management of patients with anaplastic thyroid carcinoma. *Thyroid*. 2008;18:713–9.

48. Smallridge RC. Approach to the patient with anaplastic thyroid carcinoma. *J Clin Endocrinol Metab*. 2012;97:2566–72.

49. Stein SA, Wartofsky L. Primary thyroid lymphoma: A clinical review. *J Clin Endocrinol Metab*. 2013;98:3131–8.

50. Thieblemont C et al. Primary thyroid lymphoma is a heterogenous disease. *J Clin Endocrinol Metab*. 2002;87:105–11.

51. Kwak JY, Kim EK. Ultrasound elastography for thyroid nodules: Recent advances. *Ultrasonography*. 2014;33(2):75–82.

52. Ghajarzadeh M, Sodagari F, Shakiba M. Diagnostic accuracy of sonoelastography in detecting malignant thyroid nodules: A systematic review and meta-analysis. *Am J Roentgenol*. 2014;202(4):W379–89.

53. Cantisani V et al. Strain US elastography for the characterization of thyroid nodules: Advantages and limitation. *Int J Endocrinol*. 2015;2015:8. Article ID 908575.

54. Kuna SK et al. Ultrasonographic differentiation of benign from malignant neck lymphadenopathy in thyroid cancer. *J Ultrasound Med*. 2006;25:1531–7.

55. Leboulleux S et al. Ultrasound criteria of malignancy for cervical lymph nodes in patients followed up for differentiated thyroid cancer. *J Clin Endocrinol Metab*. 2007;92:3590–4.

56. Kessler A, Rappaport Y, Blank A, Marmor S, Weiss J, Graif M. Cystic appearance of cervical lymph nodes is characteristic of metastatic papillary thyroid carcinoma. *J Clin Ultrasound*. 2003;31:21–5.

57. Selberherr A, Riss P, Scheuba C, Niederle B. Prophylactic "first-step" central neck dissection (level 6) does not increase morbidity after (total) thyroidectomy. *Ann Surg Oncol*. 2016;23(12):4016–22.

58. Shirley LA, Jones NB, Phay JE. The role of central neck lymph node dissection in the management of papillary thyroid cancer. *Front Oncol*. 2017;7:122.

59. Zhan J, Ding H. Application of contrast-enhanced ultrasound for evaluation of thyroid nodules. *Ultrasonography*. 2018;37(4):288–97.

60. Bartolotta TV et al. Qualitative and quantitative evaluation of solitary thyroid nodules with contrast-enhanced ultrasound: Initial results. *Eur Radiol*. 2006;16:2234.

61. Ahn JE et al. Diagnostic accuracy of CT and ultrasonography for evaluating metastatic cervical lymph nodes in patients with thyroid cancer. *World J Surg*. 2008;32:1552–8.

62. Bin Saeedan M, Aljohani IM, Khushaim AO, Bukhari SQ, Elnaas ST. Thyroid computed tomography imaging: Pictorial review of variable pathologies. *Insights Imaging*. 2016;7(4):601–17.

63. Frasoldati A, Presenti M, Gallo M, Caroggio A, Salvo D, Valcavi R. Diagnosis of neck recurrences in patients with differentiated thyroid carcinoma. *Cancer*. 2003;97:90–6.

64. Hoang JK, Branstetter BF 4th, Gafton AR, Lee WK, Glastonbury CM. Imaging of thyroid carcinoma with CT and MRI: Approaches to common scenarios. *Cancer Imaging*. 2013;13(1):128–39.

65. Miyakoshi A, Dalley RW, Anzai Y. Magnetic resonance imaging of thyroid cancer. *Top Magn Reson Imaging*. 2007;18(4):293–302.

66. Noda Y, Kanematsu M, Goshima S, Kondo H, Watanabe H, Kawada H, Bae KT. MRI of the thyroid for differential diagnosis of benign thyroid nodules and papillary carcinomas. *Am J Roentgenol*. 2015;204(3):W332–5.

67. Hoang JK, Vanka J, Ludwig BJ, Glastonbury CM. Evaluation of cervical lymph nodes in head and neck cancer with CT and MRI: Tips, traps, and a systematic approach. *Am J Roentgenol*. 2013;200(1):W17–25.

68. Higgins CB, McNamara MT, Fisher MR, Clark OH. MR imaging of the thyroid. *Am J Roentgenol*. 1986; 147(6):1255–61.

69. Chong V. Cervical lymphadenopathy: What radiologists need to know. *Cancer Imaging*. 2004;4(2):116–20.

70. Marcus C, Whitworth PW, Surasi DS, Pai SI, Subramaniam RM. PET/CT in the management of thyroid cancers. *Am J Roentgenol*. 2014;202(6):1316–29.

Chapter 5

PATHOLOGY OF THE THYROID

R. Ravi

CONTENTS

Non-Neoplastic Lesions of the Thyroid 46
Neoplastic Lesions 47
Reference 50
Suggested Reading 50

Fine needle aspiration cytology (FNAC) has been commonly practiced all over the world for more than five decades. A solitary thyroid nodule is frequently encountered in clinical practice and is four times more common in females than in males. Malignancy in the thyroid is also more common in females. The majority of the clinically palpable solitary thyroid nodules are dominant nodules in a multinodular goiter. As cancer is more common in solitary nodules, all solitary thyroid nodules (STNs) are viewed with suspicion. USG (ultrasonography) and thyroid scinti-scanning are non-invasive screening techniques used. Malignancy incidence of solitary cold nodules varies from 10.4%–44.7%. In the context of thyrotoxic Graves' disease, 50% of clinically apparent cold nodules have been shown to be malignant with very aggressive behavior.

FNA cytology has the advantage of being more rapid, less traumatic, and cost effective (economical). Sampling is also more representative (due to ease of several needle passes). Complications are practically non-existent, and diagnostic accuracy is as good or better than core biopsy. Diagnostic pitfalls nevertheless exist.

This chapter briefly discusses the utility of fine needle aspiration cytology in thyroid lesions and also summarizes the management protocol in thyroid lesions in relation with cytology findings. To minimize the disparity in diagnosis by clinicians, radiologists, and cytopathologists/pathologists, the Bethesda system for reporting of thyroid cytopathology (BSRTC) is presently the most popular and worldwide accepted reporting system. There are six diagnostic categories of FNAC of the thyroid with special emphasis on risk of malignancy (ROM).

Coming to consensus on the definition of adequate cytology in the thyroid has been a difficult task. Cytologically benign appearing lesions can be deemed adequate if each of a minimum of two smears contain six clusters of benign cells; others go to the extent of recommending at least six smears, with each smear containing no less than 10 to 15 clusters of benign follicular cells. There are cases on record where just a few clusters of cells have been sufficient to arrive at a diagnosis. The best judge of specimen adequacy is a cytologically diagnostic sample in which it has been possible to give a clinically relevant cytological diagnosis. This is possible in the hands of an experienced cytopathologist.

Adequate cytology can be further subdivided into four groups: benign, undetermined, suspicious (IV and V), and malignant (VI). Benign categories include normal thyroid, goiter, and inflammatory lesions like lymphocytic thyroiditis and deQuervans' thyroiditis. The malignant smears are papillary, medullary, poorly differentiated, undifferentiated carcinoma lymphoma, and metastasis. The suspicious categories include follicular neoplasm and oncocytic lesions (Tables 5.1 and 5.2).

Common lesions encountered in day to day practice are as follows:

goiter, cysts, thyroiditis, follicular neoplasia (including HN), papillary carcinoma, medullary carcinoma, poorly differentiated follicular carcinoma (including insular carcinoma), squamous carcinoma in thyroid, Non Hodgkin Lymphoma (NHL), and parathyroid cysts.

Table 5.1 The Bethesda System for reporting of Thyroid Cytopathology (recommended diagnostic categories and risk of malignancy according to SZ Ali and ES Cibas modified)

Diagnostic categories of FNA thyroid	Risk of malignancy
I. Non-diagnostic or unsatisfactory	
II. Benign Consistent with benign follicular nodule (goiter, colloid nodule, etc.) Consistent with lymphocytic thyroiditis Consistent with granulomatous thyroiditis (sub-acute)	0%–3%
III. Atypia of undetermined significance or follicular Lesion of undetermined significance (AUS/FLUS)	5%–15%
IV. Follicular neoplasm or suspicious for a follicular neoplasm (specifying for Hurthle cell type of neoplasm recommended) Figure 5.1a and b	15%–30%
V. Suspicious for malignancy (suspicious for papillary carcinoma, medullary carcinoma, metastasis, lymphoma)	60%–75%
VI. Malignant (papillary carcinoma, poorly differentiated carcinoma, medullary carcinoma, anaplastic carcinoma, squamous carcinoma, metastatic, and lymphoma)	97%–99%

Table 5.2 Bethesda System—Relationship to clinical algorithms [1]

Category	Malignancy R (%)	Management
ND	1 to 4	Repeat FNA w/US
Benign	<1	Follow-up
AUS	5 to 10	Repeat FNA
SUS FN	5 to 30	Lobectomy
SUS FN HN	15 to 45	Lobectomy
SUS MALIG	60 to 75	Lobectomy or total
Malignancy	97 to 99	Total thyroidectomy

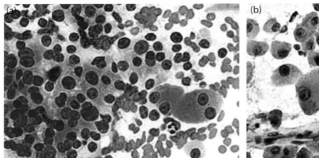
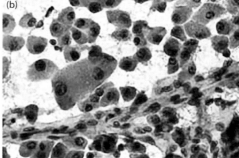

Figure 5.1 (a,b) Papanicolaou stain. Hurthle cell neoplasm.

Uncommon lesions are:

sarcomas, SEETLE (spindle cell tumor with thymic like differentiation), CASTLE (carcinoma with thymic like differentiation), mucoepidermoid carcinoma, teratoma, etc. It is beyond the scope of this chapter to include all the lesions. The commonly encountered lesions are dealt with within this chapter.

NON-NEOPLASTIC LESIONS OF THE THYROID

COLLOID GOITER

Aspirate yields thick or thin brownish fluid. There is abundant colloid with or without blood. Follicular cells are seen in monolayered groups, cells appear uniform, and do not show any nuclear abnormal features. The pitfall is the entire aspirate may not show any follicular cells; only cyst macrophages may be seen. In cases where the radiology is colloid goiter, a cytological diagnosis of colloid goiter with cystic degeneration may be given. Nodular goiter might show both monolayered sheets of follicular cells and cells in

acinar or microfollicular patterns. Fire flair cells may be seen in toxic goiter. Presence of Hurthle cells in smears of nodular goiter makes a distinction from Hurthle cell neoplasm difficult. If Hurthle cells are few and the background is colloid with monomorphic follicular cellist, it is likely to be Hurthle cell change in a goiter. Otherwise, Hurthle cell changes compatible with Hurthle cell neoplasm/ nodular goiter may be given as differential diagnosis. If fire flair cells appear in more than 50% of follicular cells, toxic goiter or Graves' disease are a possibility.

THYROIDITIS

Clinical presentation is of paramount importance. In thyroiditis, the background is bloody with many lymphoid cells, epitheloid cells, granuloma, and multinucleated giant cells with scattered follicular epithelial cell groups. Occasional follicular cells may show nuclear grooves and inclusions. However, nuclear overlap is seldom seen. In all such instances, clinical and radiological impression plays a very important role. Anti-microsomal antibodies are also very useful. Sub-acute thyroiditis is clinical, and cytology may show many multinucleate giant cells with neutrophils and lymphocytes in a dirty background (Figure 5.2).

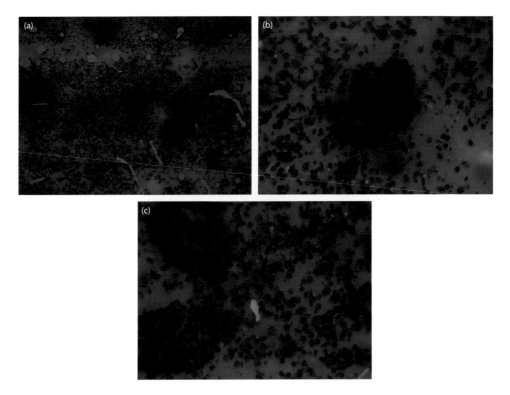

Figure 5.2 Lymphocytic thyroiditis. (a) Thyroid follicles with sheets of lymphocytes; (b) thyroid follicles, lymphocytes, and occasional giant cell; (c) thyroid follicles with sheets of Lymphoid cells.

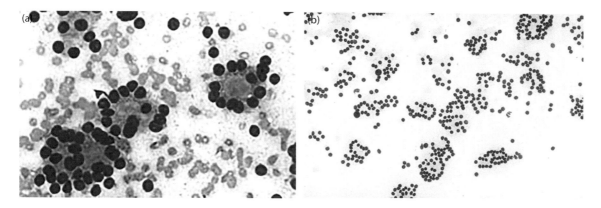

Figure 5.3   (a,b) H and E stain. Follicular neoplasia.

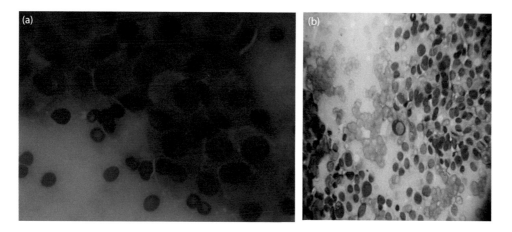

Figure 5.4   (a,b) Nuclear inclusions in a case of NIFTP.

NEOPLASTIC LESIONS

FOLLICULAR NEOPLASIA

Differentiating follicular adenoma from carcinoma is not cytologically possible because of strict criteria of diagnosis of follicular carcinoma by capsular and vascular invasion. FNA helps to identify lesions that can be picked up for surgical excision. There is bloody background, moderate to high cellularity, uniform cells in acinar (follicular), and honey comb pattern. The main problem is distinction of hyperplasia from neoplastic proliferation. Nuclear size is often helpful though not diagnostic in distinguishing follicular hyperplasia from neoplasia (Figure 5.3).

Neoplastic follicles usually would show nuclear enlargement more than 1.5 times the size of cells in non-neoplastic lesions. With the use of the Bethesda reporting system, all such lesions can be reported as Bethesda IV I e Follicular Neoplasia, and the final call regarding the surgical management is made by clinical and USG findings criteria. In 2016, a new entity was introduced: Non-invasive follicular thyroid neoplasm with papillary nuclear features (NIFTP) (Figure 5.4). The article appeared in *JAMA* 2016 as "Nomenclature Revision for Encapsulated Follicular Variant of Papillary Thyroid Carcinoma." Thyroid tumors currently diagnosed as Non-Invasive EFVPTC (Encapsulated Follicular Variant of Papillary Thyroid Carcinoma) have a very low risk of adverse outcome and should be termed NIFTP (Figure 5.5). This reclassification will affect a large population of patients worldwide and result in a significant reduction in psychological and clinical consequences associated with the diagnosis of cancer.

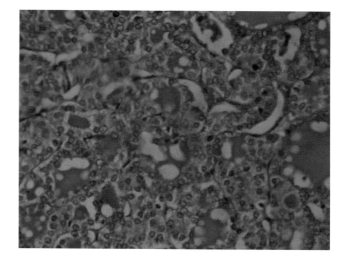

Figure 5.5   EFVPTC or NIFTP histology.

PAPILLARY CARCINOMA

Females are more commonly affected by papillary carcinoma than males, 4:1, and 60% to 80% of thyroid cancers are papillary carcinoma (Figure 5.6). FNAC usually shows papillary arrangement (picket-fencing) (Figure 5.7), intranuclear grooves and inclusions, optically clear nucleus, thick chewing gum like colloid, and few multinucleate giant cells (Figure 5.8). Psammoma bodies may be present. FNAC of 11%–35% cases of papillary carcinoma may show Psammoma bodies. It is important to note that Psammoma bodies are also seen in nodular goiter; however, other cytological criteria are helpful in making a diagnosis.

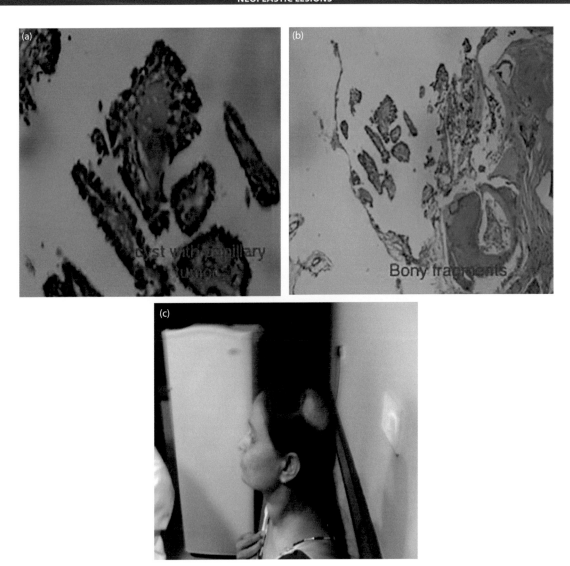

Figure 5.6   (a,b) Bone metastases in papillary carcinoma thyroid; (c) clinical picture of papillary carcinoma thyroid with metastases in skull.

Figure 5.7   Picket-fencing in papillary thyroid lesion.

Figure 5.8   Papillary carcinoma cytopathology.

MEDULLARY CARCINOMA

This represents 10% of all thyroid cancers. Cytological criteria are round cells and plasmacytoid cells, spindle cells, polygonal cells, cells with reddish granular cytoplasm, salt and pepper chromatin, and amorphous pink colloid, which in fact is amyloid (Figure 5.9). In the background, squamous metaplasia may be seen. Serum calcitonin is high and is of great utility in making a diagnosis in absence of immunocytochemistry for calcitonin, chromogranin, and synaptophysin.

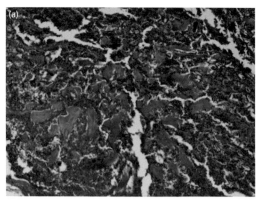
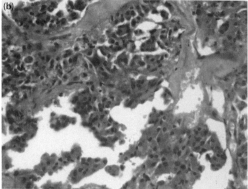

Figure 5.9   (a,b) Medullary carcinoma thyroid.

INSULAR CARCINOMA AND POORLY DIFFERENTIATED CARCINOMAS

Smears are cellular with scant or no colloid. Cells are arranged in monolayered, trabecular, follicular, and dissociated pattern. Necrosis is often present in the background. Tumor cells are small with pale scant cytoplasm and high N C ratio. Nuclear overlap is frequent and intracytoplasmic vacuoles may be seen. Foci of Hurthle cells change and clear cell change may be seen (Figure 5.10).

Other lesions like anaplastic carcinomas (Figure 5.11) and lymphomas (Figure 5.12) are not a diagnostic difficulty in clinical and cytological practice. Possibility of metastasis and systemic diseases are to be excluded clinically and sometimes by immunohistochemistry.

Other rarer lesions are difficult to pick up on cytology alone and are also fortunately of rarer occurrence. For details of these rarer conditions, appropriate relevant text may be referred to (Figures 5.13 and 5.14).

It is also beyond the scope of this chapter to cover every lesion; however, there is emphasis on role of the surgical pathologist in handling the thyroid specimen, proper grossing, and surgical pathology reporting.

It is essential to know all the clinical details before grossing. Age, indication of surgery, pre-operative radiology findings, cytology report, any history of prior surgical procedure, family history of thyroid disease if any (MEN syndrome, etc.), and type of specimen received in pathology laboratory are mostly lobectomy (hemithyroidectomy), near total thyroidectomy, total thyroidectomy, and completion thyroidectomy.

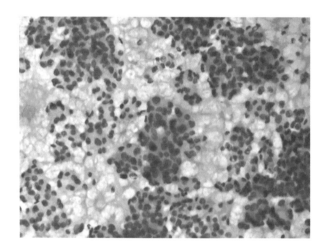

Figure 5.10   Poorly differentiated carcinoma thyroid.

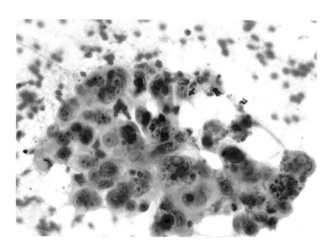

Figure 5.11   Anaplastic carcinoma thyroid.

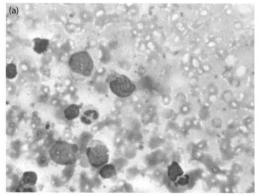
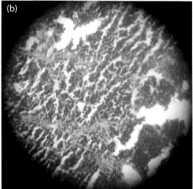

Figure 5.12   (a) Non-Hodgkin's lymphoma (NHL) in thyroid; (b) Cell block of NHL-thyroid.

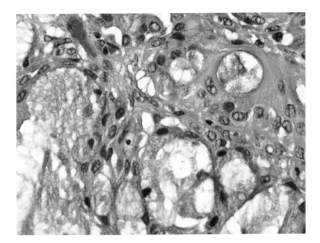

Figure 5.13 Muco-epidermoid carcinoma of thyroid. Muco-epidermoid carcinoma of thyroid and salivary glands develop from ultimobranchial pouch in embryo. Hence all lesions of salivary gland occur in thyroid as well.

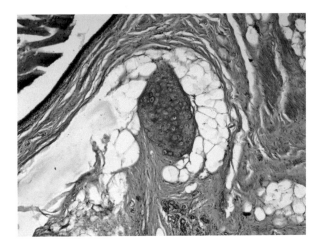

Figure 5.14 Teratoma of thyroid.

STEPS IN GROSSING

Describe the type of specimen, weigh the specimen, measure the dimensions of each lobe, and look for any other masses attached to the gland. Orient the specimen; in case of completion thyroidectomy, identify the residual portion of the thyroid lobe or thyroid bed, describe the external surface, capsule intact or breached, and try to look for parathyroid glands. Ink the thyroid completely from external surface and either slice the lobes transversely from upper to lower lobe (bread loafing) or bisect longitudinally. Observe the cut section, consistency, cystic, hard mass lesion, number of nodules, color of nodule, and any calcification. Look for circumscription of nodule (encapsulated or invasive). Note distance from tumor to inked surface, note presence of any extrathyroid extension. Take following sections: (a) Tumor with capsule; (b) Tumor with adjacent thyroid, isthmus, adjacent normal thyroid of other lobe, and parathyroid gland if any. After the final grossing, the histopathology report may be reported in the following format.

SPECIMEN TYPE

Type of carcinoma (papillary, follicular medullary, poorly differentiated carcinoma).
In case of papillary carcinoma, mention differentiation.

Location of tumor, unifocal or multifocal.
Vascular or lymphatic invasion identified/not identified.
Extrathyroid extension.
Mention the inked surgical margins.
Adjacent thyroid status.
Parathyroid glands.
And the final impression may be done by using WHO TNM classification.
T – Primary Tumor.
TX – Primary Tumor cannot be assessed.
T1 – Tumor 2 cm or less limited to thyroid.
T2 – Tumor more than 2 cm but not more than 4 cm limited to thyroid.
T3 – Tumor more than 4 cm, limited to thyroid or minimal extrathyroid extension.
T4a – Tumor of any size extending beyond thyroid capsule invading subcutaneous soft tissue, larynx, trachea, recurrent laryngeal nerve.
T4b – Tumor invaded paravertebral fascia or encases carotid artery.
All anaplastic thyroid carcinomas are considered T4 (4a intrathyroid and 4b with extrathyroid extension).
Regional lymph nodes (N).
NX – Lymph nodes cannot be assessed.
N0 – No nodal metastasis.
N1 – Regional nodal metastasis.
N1a – Metastasis to Level VI (pretracheal, paratracheal, and prelaryngeal, Delphian lymph node)
N1b – Metastasis to unilateral, bilateral, or contralateral cervical or superior mediastinal lymph nodes.
Distant metastasis (M).
Mx – Cannot be assessed.
M0 – No distant metastasis.
M1 – Distant metastasis.

Of course pathologists and surgeons hand-shake, not only in the diagnostic exercise, or, have a final say in histopathology, but, their mutual exchanges intra-operatively can benefit enormously to make a personalized treatment strategy.

REFERENCE

1. Edmund S, Cibas MD, Syed Z, Ali MD. The Bethesda System for Reporting Thyroid Cytopathology. *Am J Clin Pathol.* 2009;132:658–65.

SUGGESTED READING

Dey P. *Diagnostic Cytology.* Jaypee Brothers.

Greene FL, Komorowski AL, Kazi R, Dwivedi R (eds). *Clinical Approach to Well Differentiated Thyroid Cancers.* Byword Books Private Limited.

Grossing of Surgical Oncology specimens Tata Memorial Hospital department of Pathology.

Jayaram G. *Atlas and Test Book of Thyroid Cytology.* Arya Publications.

Orell SR, Sterrett GF. *Fine Needle Aspiration Cytology.* Churchill Livingstone Elsevier.

World Health Organization. *Classification of Tumours.* Tumours of Endocrine organs.

Chapter 6

MEDICAL MANAGEMENT OF THYROID DISORDERS

Himanshu Patil and Shailesh Pitale

CONTENTS

Graves' Disease   51
Thyroiditis   52
Hypothyroidism   53
Suggested Reading   54

GRAVES' DISEASE

Graves' disease is an autoimmune disorder characterized by the presence of clinical hyperthyroidism and autoimmune antibodies against thyrotropin or thyroid-stimulating hormone (TSH) receptors. The presentation of the disease varies with age. Circulating TSH receptor antibodies are present in at least 90% of patients. An interesting aspect is its association with ophthalmopathy.

Graves' disease is seen commonly in women between ages 20–50 years. The incidence is 1–10 per 100,000, however, it varies with iodine content in geographical areas. Cigarette smoking and stressful life events have also been linked to Graves' disease.

The thyroid glands of patients with Graves' disease are infiltrated with antigen specific T cells. There are abnormalities in T cell function that allow TSH receptor antibodies to develop, which not only stimulate TSH receptor action in thyrocytes but may also cross react with orbital antigens.

The main feature of hyperthyroidism is related to the action of thyroid hormone excess and increased adrenergic activity.

Typical manifestations include weakness, fatigue, anxiety, tremulousness, heat intolerance, and weight loss. Recent studies have shown that elderly patients may develop congestive cardiac failure and reversible cardiomyopathy.

Weight loss despite voracious eating, hyperdefecation, deranged liver functions, vitiligo, and graying of hair may indicate presence of anti-melanocyte antibodies. Elevated thyroid hormones are associated with decreased bone mineral density (more marked in postmenopausal women), and generalized proximal muscle weakness and hand tremors are common.

Central nervous system (CNS) manifestations include irritability, restlessness, nervousness, and impatience. Depression, suicide, and criminal behavior is unusual. Rarely they present with neurological findings like chorea.

Thyroid hormone measurements include total T4, total T3, and TSH. Recent advances now allow direct measurement of free T4 which is a superior technique. Total T4 measurements are affected by hormone blinding proteins, drugs (oral contraceptive pills [OCPs], androgens, and opiates) and medical conditions like hepatitis, cirrhosis, and nephrotic syndrome. Free T4 levels are unchanged in these circumstances. Approximately 5% of patients will have normal serum free T4 levels and elevated serum T3 levels.

Patients with hyperthyroidism will usually present with concentrated higher amounts of radioactive iodine, rather than with normal amounts, reflecting the ability of the gland's concentrated iodine. In addition to radioactive iodine uptake, a scan of the thyroid can provide additional information about the size of the thyroid gland.

TSH receptor antibody measurement can be performed. The advantages of the TSI assay is that it measures TSH receptor-stimulating antibodies which are relevant to hyperthyroidism. Their presence will differentiate Graves' disease from other causes of hyperthyroidism.

Treatment of any medical condition is directed at its cause; unfortunately, the immune dysregulation in Graves' disease remains obscure. Therefore, treatment is directed at the thyroid gland rather than the underlying autoimmunity.

Antithyroid drugs remain the first choice of initial therapy in children, adolescents, and adults. They do not directly affect iodine uptake or hormone release by the thyroid. Within the thyroid both Propylthiouracil (PTU) and Methimazole inhibit thyroid hormone synthesis by interfering with intrathyroidal iodine utilization and iodotyrosine coupling, both of which are catalyzed by thyroid peroxidase (TPO). Extrathyroidally, PTU inhibits conversion of T4 to T3 in peripheral tissues. Serum halflife of PTU and Methimazole is 1 and 4–6 hrs, respectively.

Anti-thyroid drug therapy can be used in two ways: primary therapy can be given for 1–2 years in hopes that the patient will achieve remission, or it can be used for a few months prior to ablative therapy.

Methimazole is the first choice, once-a-day drug, which improves compliance and the toxicity is more predictable. PTU could be considered in patients with mild drug reaction to Methimazole, or in the first trimester of pregnancy.

For patients who are hyperthyroid on low drug doses but hypothyroid on larger doses, some physicians prefer a "block and replace technique" regimen.

Prospective studies on long treatment with antithyroid drugs have not shown to be more effective, therefore 12–18 months duration of therapy is reasonable.

Anti-thyroid drug side effects can be split into minor and major. Minor side effects include rash, arthralgia, hair loss, abnormal taste, and smell sialadenitis. Major side effects include severe polyarthritis, agranulocytosis, aplastic anemia, vasculitis, severe hepatitis, cholestasis, hypoprothrombinemia, and insulin-autoimmune syndrome.

Major side effects are rare. Agranulocytosis is typically seen in the first three months of therapy, but there are notable exceptions.

Liver toxicity is a rare but serious side effect. Hepatic involvement with PTU typically presents as clinical hepatitis with malaise, anorexia, jaundice, and tender hepatomegaly.

Routine assessment of blood cell count is not currently recommended; some clinicians monitor complete blood count and liver functions prior to antithyroid drug titrations.

BETA ADRENERGIC BLOCKERS

Blockade of adrenergic pathways provide patients with considerable relief from adrenergic symptoms such as tremors, palpitations, anxiety, and heat intolerance.

Although Propranolol was the initial choice of drugs used in the dose of 80–160 mg/day in undivided doses, similar effects are produced by 50–200 mg of Atenolol or Metoprolol or 40–80 mg of Nadolol. Propranolol or Esmolol can be used intravenously for patients who are acutely ill.

POTASSIUM IODIDE THERAPY

Potassium iodide (KI) can be used to treat mild hyperthyroidism. Two Japanese studies found that it can be useful in patients who are allergic to antithyroid drugs.

RADIOIODINE THERAPY

I-131 therapy for Graves' disease has been used for more than 70 years. The goal of therapy is to render the patient permanently hypothyroid. This process takes about three months.

There are two approaches to decide the therapeutic dose of radioactive iodine for patients with Graves' disease. The first method is to calculate the size of the thyroid gland and deliver 80–200 μC of I-131 per gram of thyroid tissue. The second method is simple and consists of administering the typical fixed dose of 10–15 μC of I-131. This practice does not account for the size and activity of the thyroid gland.

Typically, radioactive iodine therapy is administered to induce hypothyroidism. 10%–20% of patients will require a second dose and 1% may need a third dose to induce permanent hypothyroidism.

I-131 is believed to exacerbate existing ophthalmopathy. It is important to take a relevant history and perform a thorough clinical examination. If ophthalmopathy is moderately severe or progressive, it is important to include the ophthalmologist and obtain a CT scan or MRI to evaluate the presence or extent of the disease.

Franklin et al. suggested that I-131 was associated with a higher incidence of thyroid cancer. They retrospectively studied 7,417 patients treated in Birmingham, England with radioactive iodine for Graves' disease. On analyzing 72,073 patients at their year of follow-up, 634 cancer diagnoses were found. The relative risk of cancer mortality was also decreased, as well as the incidence of cancers of the pancreas, bronchus, trachea, bladder, and lymphatic-hematipoetic system. However, there was significant increase in the risk of mortality of cancers of the small bowel and thyroid, although the absolute risk of the cancers was small.

Total or near total thyroidectomy is also an option for selected patients with Graves' disease. This therapy is generally reserved for patients not controlled on antithyroid, who are allergic to antithyroid drugs and do not want radioactive therapy, or who have a particular reason for surgery like large goiter with co-existing hyperparathyroidism and solitary nodules with suspicious aspirate.

THYROIDITIS

Thyroiditis is an inflammation of the thyroid gland, of which there are various causes as discussed in the following sections.

- Chronic lymphocytic thyroiditis
- Silent thyroiditis
- Postpartum thyroiditis
- Sub-acute thyroiditis
- Riedel's thyroiditis
- Drug induced thyroiditis
- Radiation thyroiditis

CHRONIC LYMPHOCYTIC THYROIDITIS

This is one of the most common of all autoimmune disorders. In this condition there is enhanced presentation of thyroid antigens and reduction in immune tolerance with an increase in Th-1 lymphocyte activity and destruction of thyroid follicles. This destruction results from several effects of cytokine induced apoptosis and ICAM-1 mediated CD8 + cell mediated cytotoxicity. Almost all patients have antithyroid antibodies in their serum, most commonly anti-thyroid peroxidase (anti-TPO) antibodies, but also anti-thyroglobulin (anti-TG) antibodies. Patients often have thyroid enlargement with normal thyrotropin (TSH). Progression is very slow and occurs over years.

It is estimated that genetic susceptibility contributes 70%–80% towards the disorder. Environmental factors contribute to 20%–30% of chronic thyroiditis.

Low levels of selenium have been associated with Hashimoto's thyroiditis, however, there is no consistent data showing the benefit of selenium supplementation. Presence of thyroid antibodies usually does not in itself warrant treatment. A higher antibody titer may predict the rapidity of progression to hypothyroidism.

Thyroxine replacement is initiated and TSH is maintained in the low one-third of normal to maintain euthyroidism.

INFECTIOUS/POST-INFECTIOUS THYROIDITIS

Infectious thyroiditis is an inflammatory process caused by the invasion of the thyroid gland by mycobacteria, fungi, protozoa, or flat worms. Infectious thyroiditis is rare due to the presence of abundant vascularity, iodine, and hydrogen peroxide and in its encapsulation.

Streptococcus; staphylococcus; escherichia; salmonella; bacteroides; pasturella; treponema; mycobacterium; and several fungi including coccidioides, aspergillus, candida, and nocardia spp have been associated with thyroiditis.

Often the infection is caused by direct extension of an internal fistulous tract between the pyriform sinus and the thyroid. This extension tends to develop more commonly in the left thyroid lobe compared to the right. Infectious thyroiditis with thyrotoxicosis has been reported to occur after repeated FNA of the thyroid gland.

Patients present with pain, swelling, hot, and tender thyroid. They may also have signs of cervical lymphadenopathy and signs of systemic infection. Laboratory data may reveal an elevated white blood cell (WBC) count and increased ESR. Patients may have symptoms of thyrotoxicosis.

In one study's data, 12 out of 56 cases were hyperthyroid; however, most of them were euthyroid biochemically and the radioactive iodine uptake will usually be normal. CT of the neck and thyroid ultrasound may reveal an abscess or pus collection.

Treatment depends on identification of causative agent, and systemic antibiotics tailored to the specific infectious agent. An abscess, if present, will require surgical exploration and drainage.

DE QUERVAIN'S (SUB-ACUTE) THYROIDITIS

De Quervain's (sub-acute) thyroiditis is a painful swelling of the thyroid gland thought to be triggered by a viral infection, such as mumps or the flu. Sub-acute thyroiditis is closely associated with HLA-B35 in 70% of patients, suggesting genetic susceptibility to antecedent viral infections.

It is most commonly seen in women aged 20 to 50. It usually causes fever and pain in the neck, jaw, or ear. The thyroid gland can also release too much thyroid hormone into the blood (thyrotoxicosis), leading to symptoms of an overactive thyroid gland (hyperthyroidism) such as anxiety, insomnia, and heart palpitations. These symptoms settle after a few days. Symptoms of an underactive thyroid gland often follow, lasting weeks or months, before the gland recovers completely.

Non-steroidal anti-inflammatory drugs (NSAIDS) or salicylate are used initially to treat sub-acute thyroiditis. Corticosteroids can be used in severe cases of pain and non-responders. Prednisone is administered in a typical dose of 40 mg/day with a tapering dose of 10 mg/week and withdrawal over four weeks. Beta blockers may control the thyrotoxic symptoms but are rarely needed in presence of NSAIDS and corticosteroids.

POSTPARTUM THYROIDITIS (PPT)
Postpartum thyroiditis only affects a small number of women who have recently given birth.

It is characterized by the presence of transient painless thyrotoxicosis with low radioactive iodine uptake and a hypothyroid phase which is followed by thyroid recovery. However, not every woman with postpartum thyroiditis will go through both these phases.

Women who are prone to develop PPT are likely to have pre-existing asymptomatic thyroiditis. During pregnancy, the maternal immune system may be suppressed with subsequent rebound thyroid antibodies after delivery. Studies have shown that higher levels of thyroid antibodies are associated with higher thyroid dysfunction. Postpartum thyroiditis is associated with HLA types HLA-DR3, HLA-DR4, and HLA-DR5.

One study mentioned significant increase in thyroid volume in 8 to 20 weeks of gestation patients who later developed postpartum thyroiditis. Another study mentioned that the thyroid size before, during, and after pregnancy was not a useful indicator for development of postpartum thyroiditis. Hence, even though postpartum thyroiditis may be associated with a goiter, the presence of goiter is not a predictive indicator of postpartum thyroiditis.

Treatment of thyrotoxic postpartum thyroiditis is often not needed since symptoms are usually mild. Beta blocking agents can be used in symptomatic patients.

Negro et al. studied 85 euthyroid antibody positive patients in the first trimester and supplemented some with Selenium, 200 g starting at 12 weeks of gestation, and some with a placebo. Postpartum thyroiditis developed significantly less in women who received Selenium than in those who received the placebo. However, this study needs further confirmation and determination of adverse events before Selenium therapy is recommended.

DRUG-INDUCED THYROIDITIS
Some examples of drugs are Interferons (used to treat cancer), Amiodarone (for heart-rhythm problems), and Lithium (taken for bipolar disorder).

In patients treated with Interferon-alpha, 5% to 15% develop clinical thyroid disease. Therapy with Interleukin-2 is associated with painless thyroiditis in approximately 2% of patients. The most common side effect of Lithium is development of goiter and hypothyroidism, but it can also induce hyperthyroidism due to thyroiditis.

Tyrosine kinase inhibitors are used in a broad spectrum of malignancies and have been associated with hypo- and hyperfunctioning of the thyroid gland. Thyroid dysfunction is common in patients on Sunitinib, which targets tyrosine kinase and vascular endothelial growth factors.

Amiodarone is a widely used class III antiarrhythmic used for therapy of ventricular and supra-ventricular arrhythmias. Incidence of AIT (Amiodarone induced thyrotoxicosis) varies between 0.003% to 11.5%. In one study of 1,448 patients, 30 developed AIT.

AIT type 1 is caused by increased synthesis in autonomously functioning thyroid tissue due to exposure of high amounts of iodine. AIT type 2 results from cytotoxic destruction of thyrocytes.

Amiodarone should be discontinued, however, this may not be always be possible for patients with life threatening arrhythmia. Patients with AIT type 1 should be treated with Methimazole. For patients with AIT type 2, Prednisone can be used for 1–2 months before tapering.

RADIATION-INDUCED THYROIDITIS
The thyroid gland can sometimes be damaged by radiotherapy treatment or radioactive iodine treatment given for an overactive thyroid gland. This can either lead to symptoms of an overactive or underactive thyroid gland. Low thyroid hormone levels are usually permanent, and require lifelong thyroid hormone replacement treatment.

HYPOTHYROIDISM

Hypothyroidism is a clinical syndrome described in 1894 by Gull under the name of myxedema in view of swollen skin and excess deposition of mucin (myx-). Murray reported the treatment of myxedema by hypodermic injection of sheep thyroid extract; eating ground thyroid extract proved equally beneficial.

Prevalence:

Hypothyroidism: 18/1,000 F, 1/1,000 M
Unsuspected: 3/1,000 F, 0/1,000 M
Known: 15/1,000 F, 1/1,000 M
Subclinical: 75/1,000 F, 28/1,000 M

Incidence:

Hypothyroidism: 4.1/1,000 F/year, 0.6/1,000 M/year

CENTRAL HYPOTHYROIDISM
Reduced Thyroxine in central hypothyroidism is due to a lack of thyroid stimulation by TSH due to lesions of the pituitary gland. Word central hypothyroidism is preferred as lesions may involve both sites. A TSH response to exogenous TRH would suggest a pituitary cause; a delayed response would indicate a hypothalamic cause

CENTRAL (HYPOTHALAMIC/PITUITARY)
- Loss of functional thyroid tissue
    - Tumors
    - Trauma
    - Vascular
    - Infectious
    - Infiltrative
    - Chronic lymphocytic hypophysitis congenital
- Functional defect in TSH release
- Mutation in gene coding for TRH receptor
- Drugs: Dopamine, Glucocorticoids, Levothyroxine withdrawal

PRIMARY HYPOTHYROIDISM
- Loss of functional thyroid tissue
    - Chronic autoimmune thyroiditis
    - Reversible autoimmune hypothyroidism
    - Surgery and irradiation

- Infiltrative and infectious diseases
- Sub-acute thyroiditis
- Thyroid dysgenesis
- Functional defects in thyroid hormone synthesis
  - Congenital defects in thyroid hormone synthesis
  - Iodine deficiency and iodine excess
  - Drugs: antithyroid agents, Lithium, goiterogenic chemicals—natural and synthetic

CLINICAL FEATURES

Energy and Metabolism

Slowing of a wide variety of metabolic processes results in decreased energy expenditure, oxygen consumption, and use of substrate. Reduced thermogenesis is related to characteristic cold intolerance, body weight increases by 10% due to increased body fat, and retention of water and salt.

Increase in cholesterol occurs as a result of increased LDL.

Skin

Skin changes are prevalent among hypothyroid individuals and include dry, pale, thick, rough with scales and the skin feels cold. Pallor is related to reduced skin blood flow and anemia. Hair becomes brittle and coarse.

Nervous System

Thyroid hormones are essential for normal brain development. Congenital hypothyroidism if left untreated leads to mental retardation and neurologic abnormalities. Hypothyroid patients are slow in movements, less alert, and less able to concentrate. Speech can be slow, and hearing impaired patients may sleep longer and report daytime drowsiness. Severe anxiety and agitation occur in a condition called myxedematous madness. Depression that may develop is likely related to reduced synthesis and rarely turnover of 5 HT.

Hashimoto's encephalopathy is an otherwise unexplained clinical manifestation of central nervous system dysfunction and linked to the presence of thyroid antibodies.

Muscles

Myalgia, stiffness, weakness, fatigue, and cramps are prevalent in the hypothyroid patient. Half relaxation time of Achilles tendon reflex is prolonged in many hypothyroid patients, but substantial overlap may be present in euthyroid patients.

Joints

Arthralgia and joint stiffness are common complaints. Synovial effusions are rare.

Bones

Hypothyroidism is associated with reduced bone turnover, increased mineralization, and increased fracture susceptibility. Urinary excretion of hydroxyproline serum, alkali phosphatase, and osteocalcin levels can be decreased. Serum calcium is usually normal.

Cardiovascular System

Cardiovascular dynamics in hypothyroidism include an increased peripheral vascular resistance and reduced cardiac output; aortic stiffness may be increased. Cardiovascular symptoms include dyspnea and decreased exercise tolerance.

Respiratory

Shortness of breath weakens respiratory muscles and impairs pulmonary function.

Urogenital

Renal plasma flow and glomerular filtration rates are reduced. Serum creatinine is increased to 10%–20%. Hyponatremia may occur.

Reproductive

Juvenile hypothyroidism leads to sexual maturation. In adult hypothyroid males, semen analysis is normal, but ED is common but recovers fully. Some women may present with amenorrhea-galactorrhea syndrome, which results from hyperprolactinemia due to thyroid hormone deficiency. Overt hypothyroidism may be associated with increased spontaneous abortion, premature delivery, and/or low birth weight and fatal distress in labor.

Gastrointestinal

Constipation, malabsorption, achlorhydria, B12 deficiency, abnormal liver functions (usually reversible), and hypotonia of gallbladder can present in some patients.

Hematopoetic System

Anemia, microcytic and hypochromic, disappears with thyroxine treatment. Leukocytes, thrombocytes, and granulocyte lymphocytes are normal. Leukopenia may be associated with B12 deficiency.

Endocrine

Low insulin, like growth factor serum concentration, may lead to growth retardation. Hypothyroidism in the presence of a pituitary mass does not always indicate central hypothyroidism. Rarely, this alteration may cause a distinct pituitary macro adenoma in severely hypothyroid patients with high TSH levels, but that shrinks after thyroid hormone replacement.

Adrenal

Metabolic clearance and production of cortisol are decreased in hypothyroidism. Serum cortisol and 24 hour urinary cortisol remain within normal limits.

DIAGNOSIS

One rationale of clinical examination is to increase the likelihood of hypothyroidism which will increase the diagnostic accuracy. Elevated free T4 and low ash indicates primary hypothyroidism.

TREATMENT

All current guidelines recommend Levothyroxine for hypothyroidism, to be taken 30–60 mins prior to breakfast. The halflife of Thyroxine is approximately seven days, hence, skipping dose or single dose omission is of little consequence.

The full replacement dose of Levothyroxine is 1.6 mcg/kg/day, to aim for TSH in the low to normal range.

There is new interest in the combination of Levothyroxine and Liothyronine. Eleven meta-analysis of randomized clinical trials found no difference in the effectiveness of LT4 and LT3 combination therapy versus T4 mono therapy in terms of pain, fatigue, anxiety, depression, and quality of life.

SUGGESTED READING

GRAVES' DISEASE

Bahn RS. Graves Ophtalmopathy. *N Engl J Med.* 2010;362:726–38.

Barbesino G, Tomer Y. Clinical review; Clinical utility of TSH receptor antibodies. *J Clin Endocrinol Metab.* 2013;98: 2247–55.

Bartalena L, Fatourechi V. Extrathyroidal manifestations of Graves' disease: A 2014 update. *J Endocrine Invest*. 2014;37: 691–700.

Lin TY, Shekar AO, Li N, Yeh MW. Incidence of abnormal liver biochemical test in hyperthyroidism. *Clin Endocrinol(Oxf)*. 2017;86:755–9.

Morshed SA, Davies TF. Graves' disease mechanisms; role of stimulating, blocking, and cleavage region TSH receptor antibodies. *Harm Metals Res*. 2015;47:727–34.

Siu CW, Yeung CY, Lau CP, Kung AW, Tse HF. Incidence of clinical characteristics and outcome of congestive heart failure as initial presentation in patients with primary hyperthyroidism. *Heart*. 2007;93:483–7.

Smith TJ, Hegediis LG. Graves' disease. *N Engl J Med*. 2016;375:1552–65.

Wiersinga WM. Advances in treatment of active, moderate to severe Graves' opthalmopathy. *Lancet Diabetes Endocrinol*. 2017;5:134–42.

THYROIDITIS

Amino N et al. High prevalence of transient postpartum thyroiditis and hypothyroidism. *N Eng J Med*. 1982;306:849–52.

Anjan RA, Weetman AP. The pathogenesis of Hashimoto's thyroiditis. *Horm. Metal Res*. 2015;47:702–10.

Fatourechi V, Aniszewski JP, Fatourechi GZ. Clinical features and outcome of subacute thyroiditis in an incidence cohort; Olmsted county. Minnesota, study. *J Clin Endocrinol Metab*. 2003;88:2100–5.

Hennessy JV. Clinical review; Riddle's thyroiditis; clinical review. *J Clin Endocrinol Metab*. 2011;96:3031–41.

Hutfless S. Significance of pre diagnostic thyroid antibodies in women with autoimmune thyroid disease. *J Clin Endocrinol Metab*. 2011;96(9):E1466–71.

Lee HJ, Li CW. Immunogenetics of autoimmune thyroid disease. *Comprehensive Review*. 2015;64:82–90.

Nokolai TF. Lymphocytic thyroiditis with spontaneously resolving hyperthyroidism and subacute thyroiditis, long term follow up. *Arch Intern Med*. 1981 Oct;141(11):1455–8.

Nordyke RA, Gibert Fl, Jr, Lew C. Painful subacute thyroiditis in Hawaii. *West J Med*. 1991;155:61–3.

Woollen LB, Mc Conahey WM, Beahrs OH. Granulomatous thyroiditis (de Quervain's thyroiditis). *J Clin Endocrinol Metab*. 1957;17:1202–21.

HYPOTHYROIDISM

Carle A, Pedersen B, Knudsen N. Gender differences in symptoms of hypothyroidism; a population -based Dan Thyr study. *Clin Endocrinol (Oxf.)*. 2015;83:717–25.

Chaker L, Bianco AC, Jonklass J. Hypothyroidism. *Lancet*. 2017;390:1550–62.

Guglielmi R, Frasoldati A. Association of clinical endocrinologists' statement - Replacement therapy for primary hypothyroidism - brief guide for clinical practice. *Endocr Pract*. 2016;22:1319–26.

Peeters RP. Subclinical hypothyroidism. *N Eng J Med*. 2017;376:2556–65.

Surks MI, Hollowell JG. Age-specific distribution of serum thyrotrophin and antithyroid antibodies in US population; implications of prevalence of subclinical hypotyroidism. *J Clin Endocrinol Metab*. 2007;92:4575–82.

Wichmann J, Winther KH, Bonnema SJ, Hegedus L. Selenium supplementation significantly reduces thyroid autoantibody levels in patients with chronic autoimmune thyroiditis: A systematic review and metaanalysis. *Thyroid*. 2016;26:1681–92.

Wiersinga WM, Duntas L, Fadeyev V, Nygaard B. Guidelines: The use of LT4 + LT3 in treatment of hypothyroidism. *Eur Thyroid J*. 2012;1:55–71.

Chapter 7

ANESTHESIA FOR THYROID SURGERY

Vidula Kapre, Shubhada Deshmukh, Pratibha Deshmukh, Meghna Sarode, and Rajashree Chaudhary

CONTENTS

Introduction	57
Main Content	57
Pre-Operative Preparation	60
Induction of Anesthesia	61
Post-Operative Complications	62
Regional Anesthesia	63
Cervical Epidural Anesthesia	63
Authors' Experience/Pearls of Wisdom	66
Conclusion	66
References	66

INTRODUCTION

While thyroid surgery is the most common endocrine surgery performed across the world [1], it can be very challenging for the surgeons as well as the anesthesiologists. Anesthesia management for thyroid surgery is particularly demanding because it can pose problems to the anesthesiologist during the pre-operative, intra-operative, and post-operative periods.

Pre-operatively, the issues are metabolic if the patient is not euthyroid and airway management in case of large goiters.

Intra-operatively, the main concerns are the cardiovascular changes due to hypo- or hyperthyroidism. They are further compounded by the use of anesthetic drugs and endotracheal intubation. In addition, the requirement of the anesthesiologist during the intra-operative period is to provide stable hemodynamics to reduce the risk of hemorrhage due to the large vessels in the vicinity.

Post-operatively, anesthesiologists are likely to face critical events due to airway compromise either because of a large hematoma or bilateral recurrent laryngeal nerve damage.

For the scope of this chapter, we shall restrict ourselves to anesthesia management as it pertains to thyroid surgery only. We will refrain from detailing the general anesthesia management issues which one would have to deal with for any surgery.

As mentioned previously, anesthesia management for thyroid surgery begins with intense involvement of the anesthesiologist from the pre-operative period, extending to the intra-operative and post-operative periods.

MAIN CONTENT

PRE-OPERATIVE ASSESSMENT

Pre-operative assessment for thyroid surgery focuses on two main aspects:

1. *Metabolic*: The specific purpose here is to assess whether the patient is euthyroid, hypothyroid, or hyperthyroid.

As such, the importance of any co-morbidity in the pre-operative period lies in:

- Its incidence, as in how often we are likely to encounter it in our patients posted for surgery, and
- Its impact on patient outcome and accordingly anesthesia management during the peri-operative period.

The incidence of sub-clinical and overt hypothyroidism is 4.6%–9.5%, while that of sub-clinical and overt hyperthyroidism is 1.3%–2.2% [2], so it is quite likely that patients whom we have to anesthetize for thyroid surgery may be hypo- or hyperthyroid, and we have to be alert to assess this in the pre-operative period, because thyroid dysfunction has a variable clinical presentation depending on the age of the patient, the degree of dysfunction, concomitant disease, and duration of disease [2]. During the pre-operative assessment, chances of picking up an altered thyroid state will depend on thorough knowledge of presentation of altered thyroid function and high degree of suspicion.

Since thyroid hormones stimulate virtually all metabolic processes in the body—synthetic as well as catabolic—altered thyroid function can present itself through varied clinical manifestations outlined in Table 7.1 [2].

As such, in hypothyroidism, there is overall slowing of metabolic activity and hyperthyroidism is a hypermetabolic state.

We can see from Table 7.1 that out of all clinical manifestations, the most significant ones are the cardiovascular changes. They are likely to worsen, even become life threatening in the peri-operative period. Hence during pre-op assessment it is worthwhile to focus on any evidence of cardiovascular changes associated with hypo- or hyperthyroidism.

In hypothyroidism there is bradycardia, decreased cardiac output, and reduced blood volume, which may get further aggravated by cardiac depressant effects of anesthetic drugs and blood loss during surgery. Abnormal baroreceptor function poses problems because if there is a fall in cardiac output, the normal tachycardic response is blunted so the blood pressure cannot be restored and there may be catastrophic hypotension.

Table 7.1   Clinical manifestations of hypothyroidism and hyperthyroidism

Hypothyroidism	System affected	Hyperthyroidism
Weight gain Fatigue Cold intolerance and hypothermia Hyponatremia Elevation of creatine phosphokinase	General	Weight Loss Heat intolerance Anxiety/nervousness Insomnia Muscle weakness
Dry and coarse skin, pretibial myxedema (non-pitting edema) Dry and coarse hair Hair loss	Skin	Excess perspiration Palmer erythema
Goiter Hoarse voice Enlarged tongue Periorbital edema	Head and Neck	Ophthalmopathy (Graves' disease only: proptosis and chemosis)
Constipation	Gastrointestinal	Frequent stools/diarrhea
Myalgia Muscle cramps Carpel tunnel syndrome	Musculoskeletal	Tremor
Depression Decreased concentration Dementia	Nervous System	Anxiety/nervousness Hyperkinesis
Irregular menstrual periods/amenorrhea Menorrhagia Galactorrhea with elevated prolactin levels Infertility Increase risk of miscarriage	Reproductive	Irregular menstrual periods/amenorrhea Light menstrual flow Infertility Gynecomastia (males)
Bradycardia Decreased cardiac output Reduced blood volume Abnormal baroreceptor function Hypercholesterolemia Pericardial effusion Congestive heart failure Increased peripheral vascular resistance	Cardiovascular	Tachycardia Increased myocardial contractility Arrythmias Cardiomegaly Increased cardiac output Palpitations Dyspnea on exertion Bounding pulses Atrial fibrillation

Exactly opposite is the case of hyperthyroidism where there is tachycardia, increased myocardial contractility, and tendency toward arrythmias which may be precipitated due to sympathetic response to intubation, extubation, and arythmogenic volatile anesthetic agents.

With this background comes the importance of detailed clinical history and clinical examination which may give pointers to the metabolic state of the patient.

Routine biochemistry is done for all patients. Calcium estimation is not mandatory but will provide baseline levels. Thyroid-stimulating hormone (TSH) estimation is mandatory in every patient undergoing thyroid surgery. The American Thyroid Association's (ATA) guidelines recommend level A for TSH estimation even if the patient may not exhibit any clinical signs and symptoms of hypo- or hyperthyroidism.

We are all aware of sub-clinical hypo- or hyperthyroidism wherein the thyroid hormone levels are normal but TSH levels may be raised or lowered respectively (Table 7.2).

Although evidence suggests that this group of sub-clinical hypo- or hyperthyroidism does not warrant any treatment pre-operatively, it

Table 7.2   Levels of Thyroid hormones in subclinical thyroid disorders

Sub-clinical hypothyroidism		Sub-clinical hyperthyroidism
Raised	TSH Levels	Lowered
Normal	T3 Levels	Normal
Normal	T4 Levels	Normal

is important to identify them during pre-operative assessment, and our anesthesia management should be as if we were dealing with overt hypo- or hyperthyroidism.

Detailed cardiac evaluation is done if there are any signs of ischemic heart disease or arrythmias.

It is not necessary to highlight for surgeons the importance of pre-operative assessment of vocal cord function.

2. Airway assessment is the second most important aspect in pre-operative assessment for thyroid surgery. In case of unilateral goiters, there may be tracheal deviation (Figures 7.1 and 7.2).

Retrosternal goiters can cause compression of the trachea in that region. Long-standing large goiters can cause tracheal narrowing and tracheomalacia (Figure 7.3).

Large goiters pose a difficult airway situation, right from induction of anesthesia, to bag mask ventilation, to intubation (Figure 7.4).

Upon induction of anesthesia, the sheer size of the gland may cause tracheal compression. Bag mask ventilation may be difficult due to pressure of the gland on the airway. Most importantly, the presence of large goiter in the anterior part of the neck precludes two crucial maneuvers of airway management (Figure 7.5):

● External manipulation in the neck by assistant to bring the larynx into view during laryngoscopy and intubation
● Surgical anterior neck access to the airway

To avoid the situation of an airway emergency, it is very important to do thorough airway assessment in the pre-operative period.

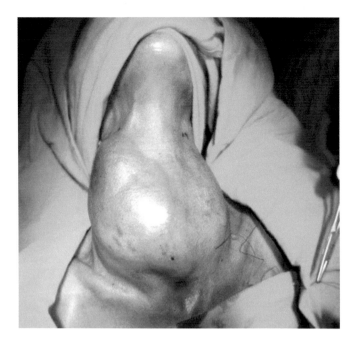

Figure 7.1   A case of large right-sided goiter.

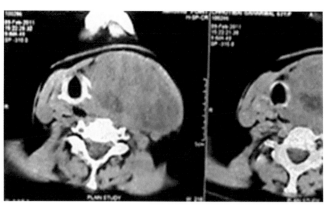

Figure 7.2   Left-sided deviation of the trachea.

HISTORY

- Duration of thyroid enlargement is important because long-standing goiters have a greater likelihood of causing tracheomalacia.
- History of dyspnea, especially with the patient in supine position or lateral position with a unilateral goiter, gives an indication of compression of the trachea.

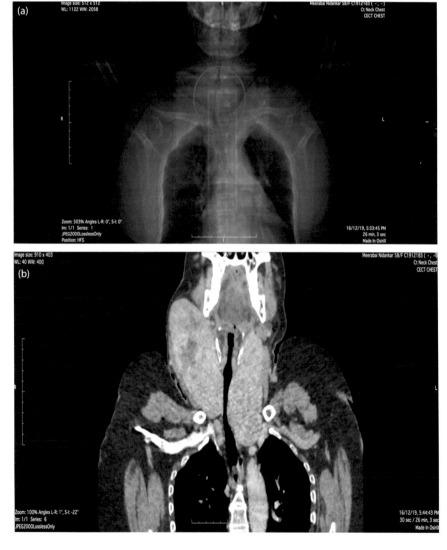

Figure 7.3   (a and b) Tracheal compression by retrosternal goiter.

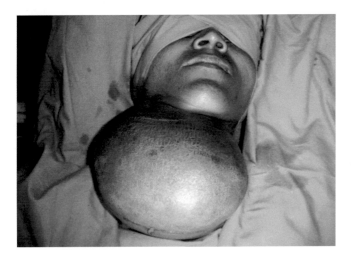

Figure 7.4   Large goiters present an airway risk.

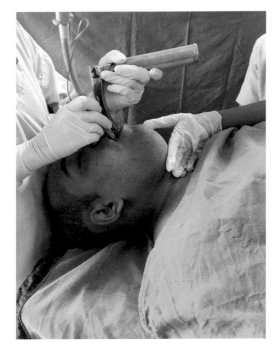

Figure 7.5   External manipulation of neck during laryngoscopy.

- Reduced effort tolerance or dyspnea in a seemingly innocuous thyroid enlargement should ring a bell for possibility of retrosternal extension causing tracheal compression.
- Hoarseness of voice indicates involvement of recurrent laryngeal nerve on one side, and we have to be alert about any possibility of inadvertent damage to recurrent laryngeal nerve on the other side during surgery. This will cause bilateral vocal cord palsy and stridor in the immediate post-operative period.

EXAMINATION

- Initial airway examination should include bedside indices to assess.
- Cervical and atlanto occipital joint function which can be judged by the range of flexion and extension of the neck.
- Temporomandibular joint function which can be assessed by mouth opening and sliding of the mandible.
- Mandibular space determines ease of laryngoscopy and can be evaluated on the basis of thyromental distance, which is the distance between the thyroid notch and symphasis menti when the neck is extended. It should be at least 6 cm.

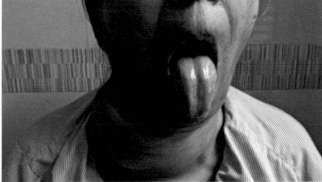

Figure 7.6   Malampatti grading of patient.

- Adequacy of oropharynx for laryngoscopy and intubation which can be graded by universally familiar Malampatti grading. The patient should be made to sit upright, open the mouth as wide as possible, and stick out the tongue without phonation (Figure 7.6).
  - Grade I: Faucial pillars, uvula, soft and hard palate visible.
  - Grade II: Uvula, soft and hard palate visible.
  - Grade III: Base of uvula, soft and hard palate visible.
  - Grade IV: Only hard palate visible.

Grade III and IV are indicators for difficult intubation. If these parameters suggest a difficult airway, we have to remember that the presence of an enlarged thyroid will compound the difficulty.

Airway assessment vis-à-vis the enlarged thyroid should focus on:

- Size of the gland
- Retrosternal extension
- Whether trachea is palpable
- Tracheal deviation

In a multivariate analysis by Bouaggad, factors for difficult intubation in thyroid surgery were assessed. The conclusion was that the presence of large goiter alone is not associated with higher incidence of difficult intubation. However, a cancerous thyroid may pose difficulty during intubation because of tracheal invasion and laryngeal fibrosis [3].

RADIOLOGICAL ASSESSMENT

A plain lateral neck x-ray gives an idea of effective mandibular length and posterior depth of the mandible. An increase in posterior depth of the mandible more than 2.5 cm poses problems during laryngoscopy and intubation [4]. Computed tomography (CT) of the neck will show tracheal deviation or compression caused by the enlarged thyroid gland (Figure 7.7).

The observations of airway assessment will determine the preparation and approach towards airway management.

PRE-OPERATIVE PREPARATION

The main goal of pre-operative preparation is to render the patient euthyroid if they are not already so.

Management of hypo- or hyperthyroidism is best done by an endocrinologist. Hypothyroidism is treated with an oral supplement of the synthetic form of LT4 [2]. Thyroid hormone levels will reach normal range in a few weeks, but TSH level normalization takes up to three weeks. Treatment for primary hyperthyroidism is achieved by antithyroid medication like Methimazole and Propylthiouranil. B blockers are used to ameliorate cardiovascular and neuromuscular

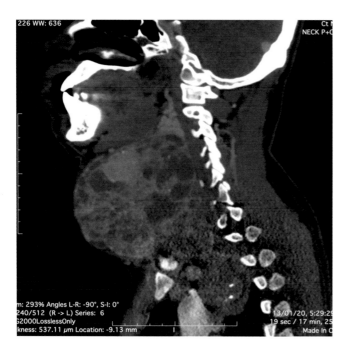

Figure 7.7   Tracheal deviation and compression.

symptoms of thyrotoxicosis. Any of the thyroid-related medications should be administered on the day of surgery.

PREPARATION OF AIRWAY MANAGEMENT

Pre-operative airway assessment will give an idea of the degree of difficulty. In patients found to have difficult airways further compounded by the goiter or patients with large or retrosternal goiters causing tracheal compression, it is safest to prepare for awake intubation. Preparing a patient for awake intubation requires thorough counseling in order to gain the confidence and cooperation of the patient.

Before embarking upon intubation for thyroid surgery, all difficult airway aids should be readily available, in working condition, and well laid out (Figure 7.8):

- Laryngoscope with long blade, McCoy blade
- Video laryngoscope
- Intubating LMA
- Stilette, bougies
- Rigid laryngoscope
- Intubating fiberoptic bronchoscope

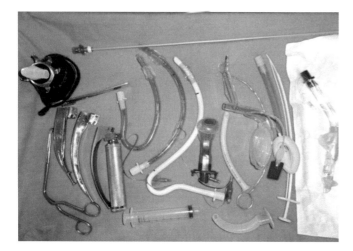

Figure 7.8   Difficult airway aids.

These are some of the aids which will help during intubation or aid in oxygenating the patient in a difficult airway situation.

INDUCTION OF ANESTHESIA

AWAKE INTUBATION

Patients for awake intubation can be administered a mild anxiolytic, like Alpraxolam 0.25 mg, the night prior to surgery. On the day of surgery, Glycopyrolate 0.2 mg is administered as antisialogogue. Airway anesthesia is achieved by nebulization with 4% lignocaine. Bilateral superior laryngeal nerve blocks and transtracheal injection of local anesthetic solution is desirable but may not be possible due to the goiter. In the operating theater, with all monitors attached, the patient is pre-oxygenated and sedated with IV Fentanyl 50 mg and midazolam 1 mg. Intubation can be achieved with the help of a fiberoptic bronchoscope (Figure 7.9). If it is not available and the anesthesiologist is skilled, blind nasal intubation is an alternative.

GENERAL ANESTHESIA

For the scope of this chapter it will suffice to mention drugs of choice that are used in the context of thyroid surgery and the reasoning behind it. For pre-medication, Glycopyrolate is used as it does not produce tachycardia. Midazolam is a good sedative with anterograde amnesia. Fentanyl is a potent analgesic which prevents surges of heart rate and blood pressure. Propofol is useful as an induction agent because it blunts the sympathetic response to laryngoscopy and intubation. Most importantly it causes some relaxation of the pharyngeal muscles so that while the patient is breathing spontaneously, we can perform laryngoscopy and assess whether we will be able to intubate the patient. This will avoid a disastrous situation where after administering a muscle relaxant, we are not able to intubate or ventilate the patient.

A muscle relaxant is injected to facilitate intubation only if the anesthesiologist has confidence of intubating the patient and certainty of ventilating the patient with bag and mask. The muscle relaxant of choice in case of difficult intubation is Succinylcholine because it is short acting.

Flexometallic reinforced endotracheal tubes are preferred because they will not kink during any surgical manipulation or changing of head or neck position.

MAINTENANCE OF ANESTHESIA

The goals during maintenance of the anesthesia are to provide stable hemodynamics and avoiding surges of heart rate or blood pressure. Maintaining the deep plane of anesthesia, and avoiding hypoxia and hypercarbia will reduce the chances of arrhythmias.

In hyperthyroid patients there are chances of arrythmias, which are further compounded by sympathetic responses to laryngoscopy and intubation and use of volatile anesthetic agents. To avoid this,

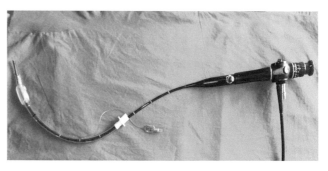

Figure 7.9   Fiberoptic bronchoscope.

the plane of anesthesia should be deep, with good analgesia, and use of volatile anesthetic agents with less arrhythmogenicity like Sevoflourane and Desflurane. Dexmedetomidine is a useful drug which can be used intra-operatively. It has the benefit of maintaining heart rate, blood pressure, and provides analgesia. It also reduces post-operative nausea and vomiting [5–7].

In hypothyroid patients, the low cardiac output and reduced blood volume with the additional cardiac depressant effect of anesthetic agents may cause precipitous hypotension. To avoid this we should use a judicious dosage of anesthetic agents, adequate fluid replacement, and use of cardiovascular stable muscle relaxant like Vecuronium.

Use of balanced anesthesia with the agents mentioned in this section, and anti-Trendelenburg tilt will provide a good operating field and reduce surgical blood loss.

MONITORING

Routine monitoring should include monitoring of the heart rate, non-invasive blood pressure (NIBP), O2 saturation, end-tidal CO_2 (EtCO$_2$) concentration, electrocardiogram (ECG), and temperature. These parameters should be watched vigilantly during the entire peri-operative period.

Any derangement in these parameters can give early indications of hemodynamic instability, respirating inadequacy, onset of arrythmias, and hypo- or hyperthermia in case of hypo- or hyperthyroidism.

RECOVERY FROM ANESTHESIA

Once the surgeon has ensured hemostasis and surgery is complete, the esthetic agents are switched off, the effect of the neuromuscular blocking agent is reversed, and the patient is ventilated with 100% oxygen.

The following guidelines should be followed during extubation:

- There is complete reversal of neuromuscular paralysis and the patient's respiratory efforts are adequate according to oxygen saturation (SpO$_2$) and EtCO$_2$.
- The patient should be extubated in a slightly deep plane of anesthesia to avoid surges in heart rate and blood pressure which can cause hemorrhage in the post-operative period. The deep plane of anesthesia also protects against the possibility of arrythmias due to sympathetic stimulation during laryngoscopy and extubation.
- It is desirable that the anesthesiologist be able to note and document normal functioning of both vocal cords at the time of extubation.
- If there is any suspicion of tracheomalacia or bilateral RLN damage, extubation should be over an airway exchanger so that the patient can be oxygenated and if there are any signs of respiratory distress can be intubated immediately over the airway exchanger.

Post-operative pain can be controlled with the help of systemic NSAIDs or use of local anesthetic injected in the area of superficial cervical plexus and suture line [8].

Post-operative nausea and vomiting can be controlled with the help of Ondansetron, Palanosetron, or Metocloparamide. As mentioned, Dexmedetomidine used intra-operatively contributes toward antiemetic effect.

POST-OPERATIVE COMPLICATIONS

For the anesthesiologist, the dreaded post-operative complication after thyroid surgery is airway obstruction due to:

- Large hematoma causing direct compression of airway
- Laryngeal edema due to venous obstruction caused by hematoma [9]
- Bilateral recurrent laryngeal nerve damage [10,11]
- Tracheomalacia

To guard against complications of a large hematoma, the patient should be closely monitored during the post-operative period. In case of acute stridor, drastic measures of removing sutures at bedside to release hematoma can be life-saving. For definitive airway management, the patient may need to be intubated.

If the surgeon is aware or in doubt of bilateral recurrent nerve damage or tracheomalacia, the anesthesiologist should extubate the patient over a tube exchanger (Figure 7.10).

The patient should be monitored closely, and if there are any signs of airway obstruction the patient can be intubated over the tube exchanger. If there is unanticipated acute stridor due to bilateral recurrent laryngeal nerve damage or tracheal collapse due to tracheomalacia, tracheostomy may be the only answer. Definitive procedures can be carried out later in a planned manner.

SPECIAL SITUATIONS

1. *Intra-operative nerve monitoring*: In case surgeons want to use intra-operative nerve monitoring, the anesthesiologist will have to use special endotracheal tubes with integrated electrodes. Tube placement should be such that the electrodes are at the level of the vocal cords.

   During surgery the surgeon can confirm presence of the recurrent laryngeal nerve by stimulating any structure resembling it. If there is significant deflection on the monitoring screen, it indicates that it is the recurrent laryngeal nerve and the surgeon should take care to protect it.

   Anesthesia management should be such that at the time of stimulation of the recurrent laryngeal nerve the patient is not under the influence of muscle relaxants. For this the anesthesia may be maintained with the patient under spontaneous ventilation. If the size of the thyroid gland is very large, the patient is obese, or there are other co-morbidities, it is advisable to maintain the patient under a short acting muscle relaxant like Cisatracurium and allow the action to wear off nearer to the time of stimulation of the RLN.

2. Although it is the rule that all patients are rendered euthyroid before thyroid surgery, for the sake of completeness it is worthwhile to outline the management in case of myxedema coma and thyroid storm.

   Myxedema coma: Signs of myxedema coma are severe bradycardia, hypotension, hypothermia, and hyponatremia eventually leading to coma.

   Management involves:

   - Tracheal intubation and controlled ventilation.
   - Levothyroxine 200–300 ugm IV over 5–10 min followed by 100 ugm IV in 24 hrs.
   - Hydrocortisone 100 mg IV followed by 25 mg IV 6 hrly.
   - Fluid and electrolyte therapy as indicated.
   - Measures to raise patient's body temperature.

3. *Thyrotoxic storm*: Thyroid storm will manifest as severe tachycardia, hyperthermia, atrial fibrillation, and cardiac failure.

   Management includes administration of:

   - Cold IV fluids.
   - Sodium Iodide either through nasogastric tube or IV 6 hrly.

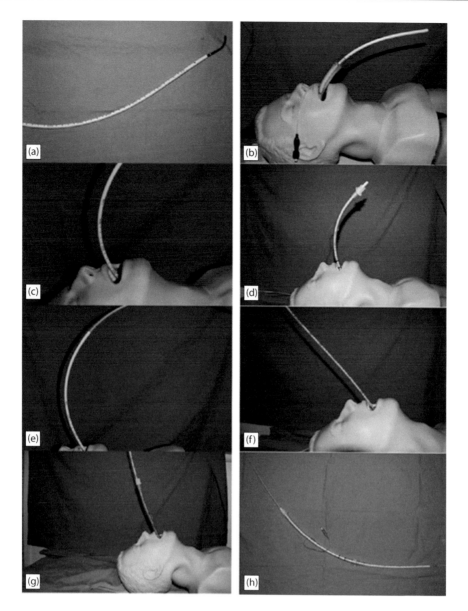

Figure 7.10   Extubation over tube exchanger.

- Propylthiouracil 200–400 mg through nasogastric tube.
- Hydrocortisone 100 mg IV 6 hrly.
- Propranolol 10–40 mg 6 hrly through nasogastric tube or Esmolol infusion
- Cooling body temperature.
- Meperidine 25–50 mg IV 6 hrly to prevent shivering.
- Digoxin for heart failure, especially in case of atrial fibrillation with rapid ventricular rate.

REGIONAL ANESTHESIA

Thyroid surgery can be performed under regional anesthesia if

- General anesthesia is contraindicated
- Significant risk is anticipated with respect to difficult intubation or likelihood of arrhythmias
- Or in special situations

Although thyroid surgeries have been reported under superficial and deep cervical plexus blocks, they can be considered for unilateral goiters that are too small in size. The risks involved with deep cervical plexus block does not make it an attractive proposition.

CERVICAL EPIDURAL ANESTHESIA

The past couple of decades have shown a resurgence in the use of cervical epidural anesthesia for thyroid surgery.

There are some studies in literature, albeit not a very large sample size, with the unanimous conclusion that the "cervical epidural route can be safely used for surgery on thyroid gland and should be considered in patients where difficult endotracheal intubation is anticipated and in whom altered thyroid functional status makes them vulnerable to cardiovascular complications under general anesthesia" [12].

Due to the relative uniqueness of this technique and the authors' vast experience with it, it is in order to give a detailed account of cervical epidural anesthesia for thyroid surgery.

It is a regional anesthesia technique wherein local anesthetic solution is injected into the cervical epidural space. Usually C7-T1 or C6-C7.

This achieves a block of the cervical and brachial plexus which is adequate for thyroid surgery [13].

INDICATIONS

- Difficult endotracheal intubation in case of large goiters
- Altered thyroid functional status
- Surgery on ASA III, IV patients
- Special situations where general anesthesia may be contraindicated or undesirable

COUNSELING

Patients found suitable for cervical epidural anesthesia are thoroughly counseled. Pre-operative counseling specially for cervical epidural anesthesia is essential to gain the patient's confidence and cooperation. Although the anesthesia technique blocks pain fibers from the surgical site, the neck extended position of the patient and tracheal manipulation during surgery can be discomforting. The patient should be made aware of this, while at the same time be reassured that they will be administered sedation to take care of the discomfort.

During counseling, emphasis is on the following points:

- The patient is informed of the block that will be administered.
- They are told about the neck extension position in which they will be lying during surgery.
- They are also told they may have some cough when surgeons handle the trachea.
- They are assured that they will be sedated and, if need arises, can be put under general anesthesia.

PRE-MEDICATION

Patients are given anxiolytic in the form of T. Alprazolam 0.25 mg and T. Ranitidine the night prior and on the day of surgery.

METHOD

Patients are pre-loaded with intravenous (IV) crystalloid solution. IV Glycopyrrolate is administered. A monitor is attached. The patient is in a sitting position with the height adjusted so that the patient's neck is at waist level of the anesthesiologist. The patient is made to hold a pillow with both arms. This gives them stability, and while both arms hold the pillow across the chest, the back becomes relaxed (Figures 7.11–7.17).

With all aseptic precautions, the anesthesiologist prepares the epidural trolley. The solution used is 9 mL of 0.25% preservative free Bupivacaine + 1 mL fentanyl. This solution is used to prime the epidural catheter. The patient's back of the neck is cleaned and draped. The space chosen is C7-T1, C7 spinous process (vertebra prominence) being easy to palpate. 2% Lignocaine with Adrenaline is injected in the skin and subcutaneous tissue. An 18/16 G epidural needle is introduced at the C7-T1 space, with the direction being perpendicular to the spine with bevel facing cranially. The needle is advanced until it is gripped in the ligamentum flavum. The epidural space is located by loss of resistance to the injection of air technique. Once the epidural space is entered, the stilette is removed and the epidural catheter is introduced through the needle. The catheter should go in very smoothly without any force required. About 15 cm of catheter is introduced to be sure that it is freely going into the epidural space. Keeping the catheter steady, the epidural needle is withdrawn. Markings on the needle give an idea of the depth of the epidural space from the skin. It is usually 3–4 cm. An additional 4 cm catheter is left in the space and the rest of the catheter is withdrawn. Sterile clear dressing is given at the entry point of the catheter making a loop of the catheter to avoid kinking and accidental pull on the catheter. The catheter is taped along the shoulder and down the forearm on the same side as the IV cannula. After checking for aspiration of blood or cerebrospinal fluid (CSF), 2 mL of test dose is administered. After observation for 15 min, the

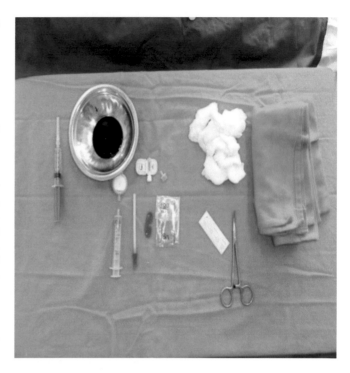

Figure 7.11 Epidural anesthesia tray.

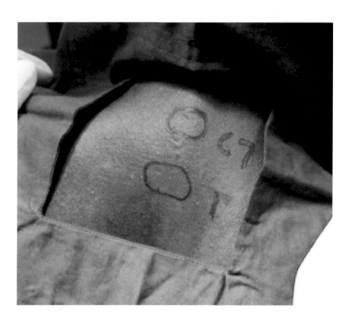

Figure 7.12 Surface landmarks for epidural block.

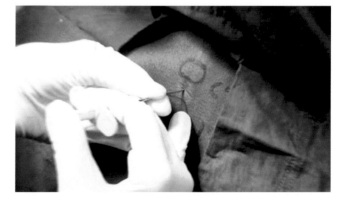

Figure 7.13 Insertion of the epidural needle.

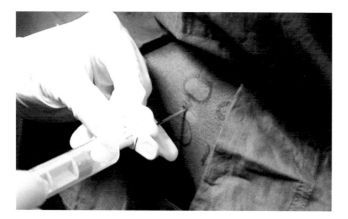

Figure 7.14   Identifying the epidural space.

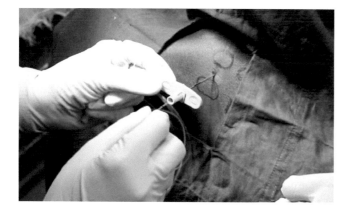

Figure 7.15   Introduction of the epidural catheter.

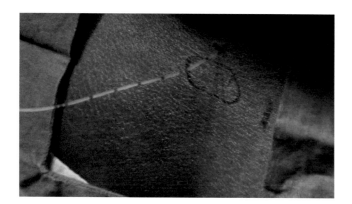

Figure 7.16   Adjusting the length of the catheter in epidural space.

rest of the local anesthetic solution is injected. After another 15 min the patient is given a neck extension position with a shoulder pillow. Oxygen is administered by nasal prongs. The patient is sedated with IM 2 mg Butorphanol and 2 mg Midazolam. After checking the adequacy of the anesthesia, the surgery begins.

INTRA-OPERATIVE MANAGEMENT

The patient's heart rate, NIBP, Sp02, and ECG are monitored. IV fluids are administered as per the surgical demand and BP of the patient. Every hour 4 mL of top-up of the same are given (Figures 7.18–7.21).

POST-OPERATIVE PAIN MANAGEMENT

At the end of the surgical procedure, 4 mL of 0.125% preservative free Bupivacaine is injected through the catheter for post-operative

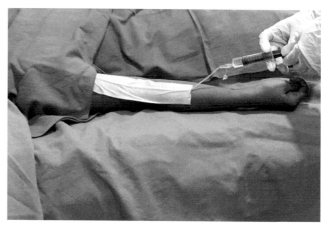

Figure 7.17   Injection port of the catheter.

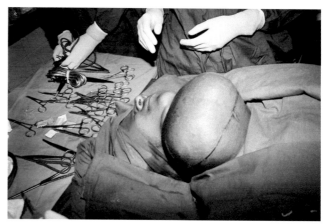

Figure 7.18   Patient ready for surgery.

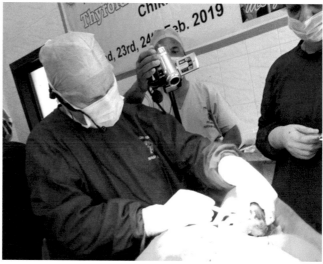

Figure 7.19   Surgery in progress.

pain relief. At our practice we remove the catheter after this first dose of post-operative analgesia as the patients are managed in the wards of rural hospitals where strict asepsis may not be followed. Also, the nursing staff at the rural hospitals are not trained to manage epidural catheters. As it is a regional anesthesia technique, the patient does not require much monitoring post-operatively in the ward.

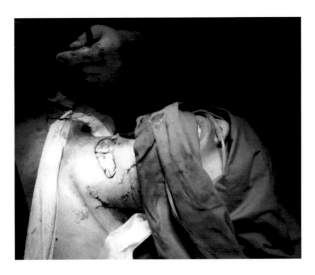

Figure 7.20   Surgery completed under epidural anesthesia.

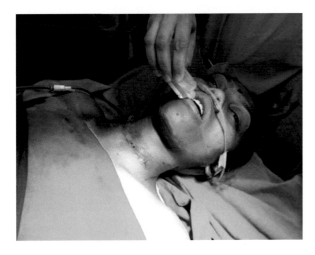

Figure 7.21   Patient can drink water at the end of surgery.

AUTHORS' EXPERIENCE/PEARLS OF WISDOM

General anesthesia is the standard and chosen technique for thyroid surgery.

Cornerstones for success in anesthesia management are:

- Optimization of the patient's metabolic status pre-operatively.
- Airway assessment and preparation management of the difficult airway.
- Cardiovascular stability during the intra-operative period so as to minimize blood loss and provide a good operating field for the surgeon.
- Preparedness for management of airway obstruction in the post-operative period in eventuality of bilateral recurrent laryngeal nerve palsy, large hematoma, or tracheomalacia.

CONCLUSION

Anesthesia management for thyroid surgery requires:

- Knowledge of metabolic issues in patients with thyroid disorder and their effect on the cardiovascular system of the patient.

- Skill in airway management, especially in case of large goiters.
- Understanding and cooperation between surgical and anesthesia teams.

The anesthesiologist should be able to adapt their technique to facilitate surgeons' requirements, e.g., intra-operative nerve monitoring.

It helps if anesthesiologists are familiar with and experienced in awake fiberoptic intubation in case of anticipated difficult intubation.

The authors' experience suggests that it also helps to be conversant in an alternative anesthesia technique such as cervical epidural block. When administered with due precaution and skill, it is absolutely safe. Although not a technique of choice in routine cases, it is a useful tool for the anesthesiologists managing complex thyroid surgeries.

REFERENCES

1. Bajwa SJ, Sehgal V. Anesthesia and thyroid surgery: The never ending challenges. *Indian J Endocrinol Metab.* 2013 Mar;17(2):228.

2. Gregory W. Randolf. *Textbook on Surgery of Thyroid and Parathyroid Glands.* Chapter 3, pp. 25–33.

3. Bacuzzi A, Cuffari S, Anesthesia for thyroid surgery: Perioperative management. *Int J Surg.* 2008;6(Suppl. 1):S82–S85.

4. Khan R. Airway Management. Chapter 4. Paras medical publisher, pp. 18–21.

5. Bajwa SJ et al. Dexmedetomidine and clonidine in epidural anaesthesia: A comparative evaluation. *Indian J Anaesth.* 2011 Mar;55(2):116.

6. Bajwa SJ, Arora V, Kaur J, Singh A, Parmar SS. Comparative evaluation of dexmedetomidine and fentanyl for epidural analgesia in lower limb orthopedic surgeries. *Saudi J Anaesth.* 2011 Oct;5(4):365.

7. Bajwa SJ, Gupta S, Kaur J, Singh A, Parmar SS. Reduction in the incidence of shivering with perioperative dexmedetomidine: A randomized prospective study. *J Anaesthesiol, Clin Pharmacol.* 2012 Jan;28(1):86.

8. Dieudonne N, Gomola A, Bonnichon P, Ozier YM. Prevention of postoperative pain after thyroid surgery: A double-blind randomized study of bilateral superficial cervical plexus blocks. *Anesth Analg.* 2001 Jun 1;92(6):1538–42.

9. Rovó L, Jóri J, Brzózka M, Czigner J. Airway complication after thyroid surgery: Minimally invasive management of bilateral recurrent nerve injury. *Laryngoscope.* 2000 Jan;110(1):140–4.

10. Ozbas S, kocak S, Aydintug S, Cakmak A, Demirkiran MA, Wishart GC. Comparison of the complications of subtotal, near total and total thyroidectomy in the surgical management of multinodular goitre. *Endocr J.* 2005;52(2):199–205.

11. Timmermann W, Dralle H, Hamelmann W, Thomusch O, Sekulla C, Meyer T, Timm S, Thiede A. Does intraoperative nerve monitoring reduce the rate of recurrent nerve palsies during thyroid surgery? *Zentralbl Chir.* 2002 May;127(5):395–9.

12. Khanna R, Singh DK. Cervical epidural anaesthesia for thyroid surgery. *Kathmandu Univ Med J.* 2009;7(3):242–5.

13. Dhummansure D, Kamtikar S, Haq MM, Patil SG. Efficacy and safety of cervical epidural anaesthesia for thyroid surgery. *Int J Sci Stud.* 2015 Oct 1;3(7):245–50.

Chapter 8

SAFE THYROIDECTOMY

Madan Laxman Kapre, Sankar Viswanath, Rajendra Deshmukh, and Neeti Kapre Gupta

CONTENTS

Who Is at Risk?   67
The Size   67
Anesthesia   68
Appliances and Technology   68
Learning Curve   69
Identifying the Injuries   73
References   73

Nowhere was it as rewarding as visiting the archives of thyroid surgery in the making of a safe thyroid surgeon. From being labeled as butchery (Samuel Gross) and being banned in Europe as an extremely unsafe surgical procedure, it has come a long way to be a safe and most gratifying surgery. In 1846, Robert Liston called thyroid surgery "a proceeding by no means to be thought of" after performing five thyroidectomies [1]. Two years later, Samuel Gross wrote: "Can the thyroid in the state of enlargement be removed? Emphatically, experience answers no. Should the surgeon be so foolhardy to undertake it…every stroke of the knife will be followed by a torrent of blood and lucky it would be for him if his victim lived long enough for him to finish his horrid butchery. No honest and sensible surgeon would ever engage in it." [2].

Surgery progressed further with newer methods of infection prophylaxis, such as the use of carbolic acid in antisepsis by Joseph Lister of Glasgow in 1867 [3]. The introduction of steam sterilization of instruments by Ernst von Bergmann in 1886 [4] and intra-operative antisepsis with a cap and gown by Gustav Neubar in 1883 [5] reduced the incidence of infection significantly in the post-operative period. In 1874, Spencer Wells and Jules Pear reached a landmark in surgery by introducing the first effective hemostatic forceps.

Theodor Billroth performed 36 thyroidectomies experiencing 16 deaths, in Zurich and Vienna [6]. With the use of newer methods of antisepsis and hemostasis between 1877 and 1881, Billroth performed 48 thyroidectomies and was able to decrease the mortality to 8.3% [7]. Theodor Kocher, a pupil of Billroth, during his first 10 years in Berne, had performed 101 thyroidectomies, experiencing a mortality of 2.4%. By 1895, the mortality rate improved to about 1% [8].

Thyroidectomy is now considered as a surgical triumph and most skilled craftsmanship among all surgical procedures.

The incidence of permanent complications after thyroidectomy is low [9–12]. Two classical complications specific to thyroidectomy arise due to the close anatomic proximity of the thyroid gland with the recurrent laryngeal nerves (RLN) and with the parathyroid glands: temporary dysphonia occurs in 5%–11% of cases and may be permanent in 1%–3.5% of cases, and temporary hypoparathyroidism occurs in 20%–30% of cases and may be permanent in 1%–4% of cases [9]. These data are drawn from the largest published series and reflect the rate of complications seen at centers of expertise [9–12]. Post-operative compressive hematoma with acute dyspnea is a rare but severe complication that may result in death or severe long-term sequelae. Death after thyroidectomy is very uncommon (0.065%)

and most often results from a combination of advanced age, giant goiters, and upper airway complications [13].

While as many as a third of the patients succumbed to this surgery in past, it would be a matter of grave concern should such eventuality occur now. Not understanding the importance of Spencer Wells' hemostatic forceps and the discovery of antibiotics and thyroid hormones, the surgical training scenario backed up with newer technological advances have made thyroid surgery one of the safest yet skilled surgical maneuvers. An attempt is made to share our learning curves and make this chapter a good read for the learner and learned alike. In the preceding pages we have categorized the importance of being safer surgeons as paying adequate attention to the old dictum "forewarned is forearmed." Skilled surgeons treat their patients by repair/removal/cutting/alteration/replacement of the diseased part/organ. So before starting to make an incision on a patient, the surgeon requires not only confidence, a sound knowledge of the organization of macro- or microforms and structures and their shapes, sizes, and locations, and the correct diagnosis of the disease, but also the anatomical relationship to the disease [14].

WHO IS AT RISK?

Let us first identify the patients who are more likely to have either intra-operative or post-operative problems. This will help us not only to take appropriate preventive measures but also prepare and counsel our patients adequately.

There are two aspects of this: One is the issue of functionality or physiology and the other is anatomy. The altered physiology, i.e., hyperthyroidism or hypothyroidism, is best resolved with the help of our endocrinology colleagues and should be operated only on well-prepared euthyroid patients [15]. Actual details of this are beyond the realm of this chapter.

THE SIZE

It is ironic that large benign thyroid masses are relatively easy to operate as they alter past the structures rather than invade them [16] (Figure 8.1). The real issue lies in the delivery of these large

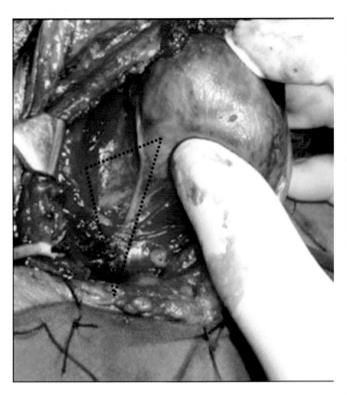

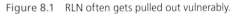

Figure 8.1   RLN often gets pulled out vulnerably.

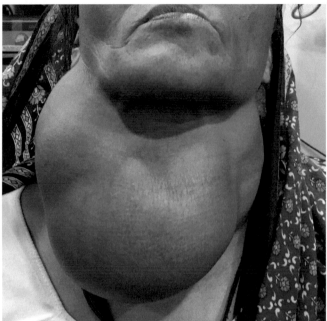

Figure 8.2   Large multinodular goiters in short neck individuals.

goitrous masses. The next structural issue is the invasion and fixity of the thyroid masses to neighboring anatomical structures. Loss of mobility of the thyroid and dysfunction of the structure involved, i.e., cord palsy or dysphagia, will appropriately suggest spreading.

Any history of aspiration or reflex cough on drinking liquids may suggest invasion of the external branch of the superior laryngeal nerve (EBSLN), and one needs to warn the patient of the possibility of worsening of this symptom. Pre-operative ultrasonography (USG) or computed tomography (CT) of the chest may indicate an aberrant subclavian artery and thus a non-recurrent RLN [17]. Prominent neck veins with retrograde venous flow is an indication of venous obstruction in the superior mediastinum [18]. Retrosternal goiter if benign has its blood supply from the neck but retrosternal malignant thyroid may have additional vessels from the adjoining superior mediastinum.

Hemoptysis or respiratory difficulty in a malignant thyroid would forewarn the surgeon about tracheal invasion [19], and one needs to get prepared for such eventuality.

A short neck, an obese patient, or a cervical spine abnormality will need larger incisions and adequate surgical exposure (Figures 8.2 and 8.3).

The pathology of goiter malignant thyroid lesion would force the surgeon to anticipate and plan the surgical procedure. Papillary cancers would mean addressing the neck nodes while follicular lesions may have an embolus in the jugular vein [20]. As there is no proven fall back plan for medullary cancers arising from parafollicular cells, the best surgical procedure can be summed up as "wherever the disease takes you" and hence aggressive excision has to be planned.

ANESTHESIA

Although there is a separate chapter on this aspect of safe thyroid surgery, the authors cannot emphasize enough the importance of establishing a sound rapport between the anesthesia team and the

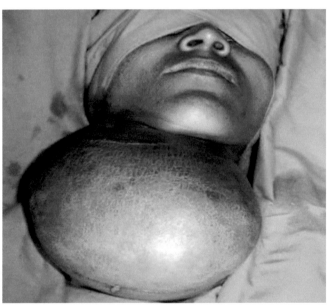

Figure 8.3   Large multinodular goiters in short neck individuals.

surgical team. Hypotensive anesthesia [21] is an advantage, while accurate placement of the endotracheal tube will avoid a lot of anxiety about loss of signal later. While operating a hyperthyroid adenoma or Graves' disease, it is best to divide the muscle and avoid unnecessary handling of the gland. Needless to say the various out flow channels for blood should be ligated at the earliest (Figure 8.4).

APPLIANCES AND TECHNOLOGY

As there are separate chapters on the aspect of safety, the authors prefer to use more easily available and practiced technological support. The first on the list, of course, is accurate mapping of the disease with available imaging techniques. This gives very important

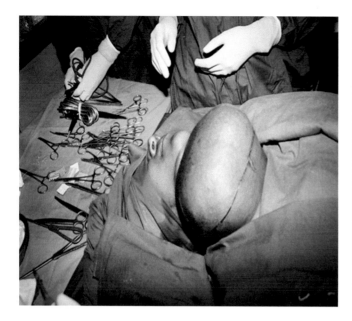

Figure 8.4   A unique technique of cervical epidural anesthesia.

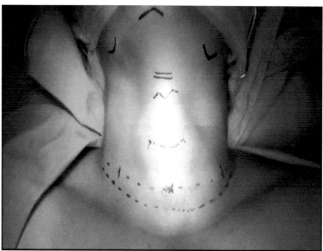

Figure 8.5   Position for thyroid surgery.

information regarding the presence of lymph nodes, embolism of the jugular vein with malignant thrombus, or the presence of non-recurrent RLN.

Hypotensive anesthesia and judicious use of electrosurgical devices will minimize blood loss.

Magnification by way of optical loupe [22] or microscope offers a clear advantage. However, there is considerable learning involved in getting used to these devices. Endoscopes and their application in thyroid surgery are adequately dealt with elsewhere in this book.

LEARNING CURVE

Before one endeavors thyroid surgery in the operating room, modern day surgical apprentices are fortunate to have access to several other learning opportunities. Video demonstration, cadaveric dissection, and hands-on surgical workshops are a few to mention which can prepare an apprentice for thyroid surgery. We cannot emphasize enough the sound anatomical knowledge of the area of concern. The authors believe that a surgeon is primarily an applied anatomist [14].

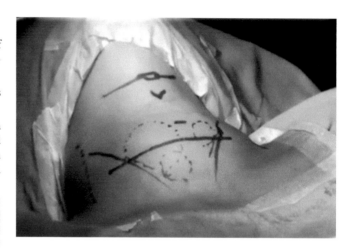

Figure 8.6   Incision planning.

STEPS OF SAFE THYROID SURGERY

1. *Position*: The patient is placed supine with pillow or roll under the shoulder to give maximum possible head extension. This allows the thyroid to be brought up in the neck and to be made fairly superficial (Figure 8.5).

2. *Incision*: Ideally, it is marked up in the sitting position in a suitable skin crease before anesthesia. It is generally placed two-fingers breadth above the suprasternal notch or midway between the cricoid prominence and suprasternal notch. The width of the incision is tailored according to the size of the thyroid, rarely beyond the sternocleidomastoid muscle and equal on either side (Figure 8.6).

3. *Midline dissection*: The sizable number of the goiter is unilateral, and hence the surgical procedure of choice may be hemithyroidectomy. It is crucial to identify and divide the deep fascia from the suprasternal notch to the thyroid notch superiorly (Figures 8.7 and 8.8).

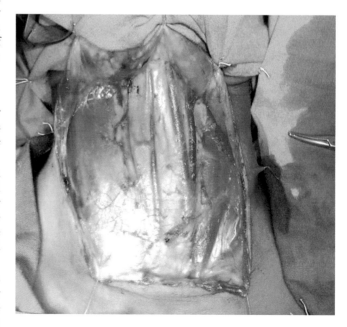

Figure 8.7   Midline dissection LGT (*Levator glandulae thyroidea*).

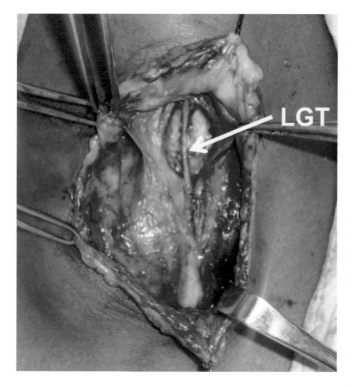

Figure 8.8   Midline dissection LGT (*Levator glandulae thyroidea*).

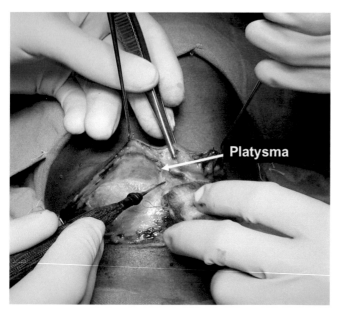

Figure 8.9   Platysma is deficient in midline.

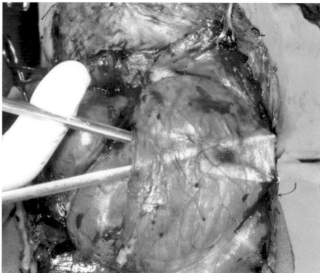

Figure 8.10   Management of strap muscles.

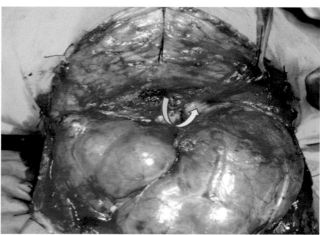

Figure 8.11   Management of strap muscles.

4. *Elevation of flap*: The skin flaps are raised on either side subplatysmally in a relatively avascular loose areolar tissue plane. Upwards the flap elevation reaches the hyoid bone and downwards it exposes the suprasternal notch (Figure 8.9).

5. *Management of strap muscles*: There is no pride lost if one has to divide the strap muscles to get a safe, unhanded delivery of the thyroid in the wound. The lateral extent is the carotid sheath, ligating the middle thyroid vein away, if present. If one should decide to divide the strap muscles, it is done above the insertion of ansa cervicalis into the straps muscles. In such case both muscles are raised upwards and downwards in unison up to their bony/cartilage attachments (Figures 8.10 and 8.11).

6. *Management of upper pole*: The key here is again adequate exposure and ligating the superior thyroid vessels by skeletonizing each. This avoids injury to the external branch of the superior laryngeal nerve whatever may be the course of the nerve. It exposes and helps release the upper pole displaying the whole breadth of the cricopharyngeal muscles and the EBSLN (Figure 8.12).

7. *Dissecting the superior parathyroid*: The next step is to identify and separate the thyroid gland in the sub-capsular plane. The upper parathyroids are encountered, and care is taken not to dissect the fascia lateral to the parathyroids. Hereafter a branch of posterior division of the superior thyroid artery is seen to supply the parathyroid before entering the post aspect of the upper pole (Figure 8.13).

8. *Dissecting the lower pole*: Some authors advise releasing the lower pole before moving to the upper pole for a very good reason. At this point, the surgeon is fresh, and the best chance to encounter any variation of the inferior parathyroid gland is usually now. The inferior parathyroid could be anywhere from within the thyroid gland to anywhere in the superior mediastinum. Great care is taken to preserve both anterior as well as venous drainage of the parathyroids at the lower pole (Figures 8.14 and 8.15).

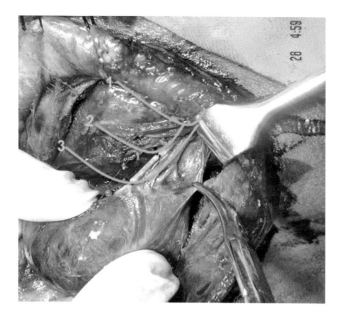

Figure 8.12   Management of the upper pole.

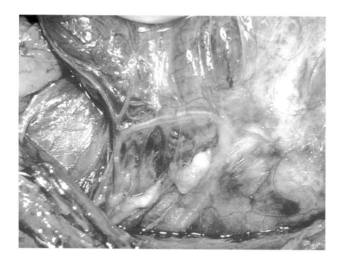

Figure 8.13   Dissecting the superior parathyroid.

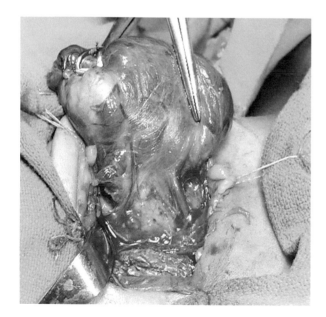

Figure 8.14   Dissecting the lower pole.

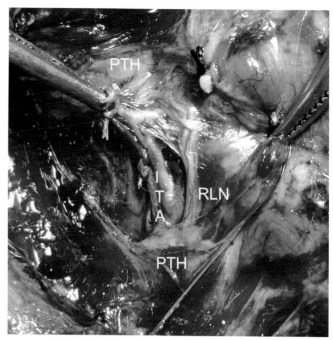

Figure 8.15   Dissecting the lower pole.

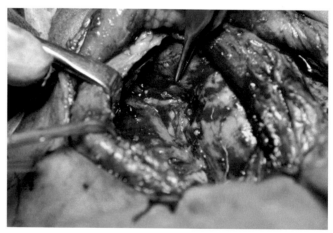

Figure 8.16   Right non-recurrent RLN.

9. *Managing the RLN (Recurrent Laryngeal Nerve)*: Having secured both sets of parathyroid, surgical focus now shifts to the RLN. Author recommends demonstration rather than dissection between the two major branches of the inferior thyroid artery. There are several anatomical landmarks for identification of the RLN. However, the authors rely on and recommend identifying the RLN under the nodule of Zuckerkandl. This is safe, secure, and avoids unnecessary exposures of the RLN (Figures 8.16 through 8.20).

10. *Berry's ligament*: Once the RLN is traced up to its insertion in the larynx at the cricothyroid joint, the width of Berry's ligament, the posterior condensation of thyroid fascia is divided completing the procedure on the given side (Figures 8.21 and 8.22).

11. *Dividing the isthmus*: This is the final release of the ipsilateral thyroid lobe. The authors recommend removal of the isthmus and release of the contralateral lobe from trachea in all cases. This avoids an unsightly midline hump should the isthmus hypertrophy as a result of the loss of lobe.

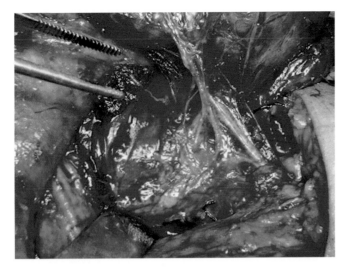

Figure 8.17   Left non-recurrent RLN.

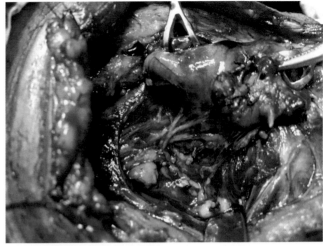

Figure 8.20   Relation of RLN to the inferior thyroid artery.

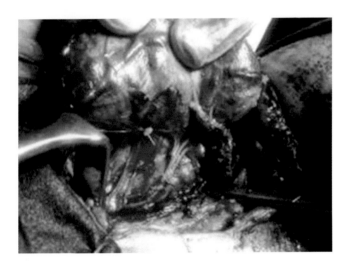

Figure 8.18   RLN with its divisions.

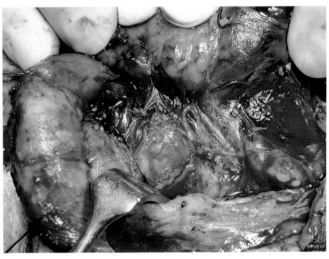

Figure 8.21   Berry's ligament.

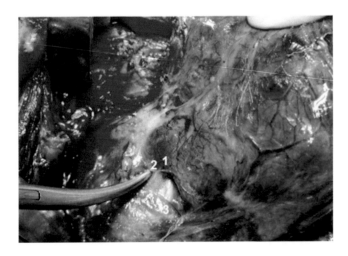

Figure 8.19   (1) Nodule of Zuckerkandl. (2) Cricothyroid joint. (3) RLN.

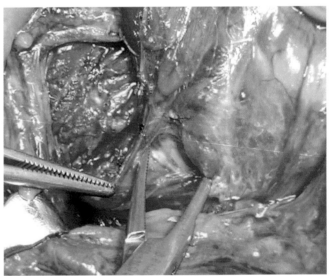

Figure 8.22   Berry's ligament.

IDENTIFYING THE INJURIES

We all make mistakes. They may be caused by a surgeon's judgment, by misadventurous surgical maneuvers, or by a forced error through situations beyond the surgeon's control. But mistakes shall remain mistakes if we do not learn from them. Bad scars, hematomas, and infections are due to violation of basic surgical principles and elaborating on these is beyond the scope of this chapter. We shall restrict ourselves to the RLN/parathyroid.

RLN INJURIES

The RLN may have to be excised for disease clearance. This can be either totally anticipated, i.e., a paralyzed vocal cord is pre-operatively noted, or unanticipated. The authors suggest to work on the opposite side first so that the surgeon is at their best. In an unanticipated situation, the nerve injury may be obvious transection or neuropraxia [23]. Primary approximation and microscopic nerve repair is the procedure of choice if possible. Otherwise, cable nerve grafting is strongly advised.

PARATHYROID INJURIES

These are the real test of thyroid surgeons. Herein lies the real importance of intra-operative recognition of the injury.

The injury can be vascular or accidental extirpation. There could be a simple element on the capsule, which can be quickly and adequately resolved by inching the fibrous capsule of the gland. If the parathyroids [24] are accidentally removed then re-implantation is strongly advised. The technique and rationale is covered elsewhere in the book.

REFERENCES

1. Liston R. *Lectures on the Operations of Surgery and on Diseases and Accidents by Thomas D. Mutter.* Lee & Blanchard, Philadelphia, 1846.

2. Gross SD. *A System of Surgery, Vol. II.* Lea HC, Philadelphia, 1886:394–5.

3. Lister JB, Cameron HC. *The Collected Papers of Joseph Baron Lister…: pt. III. The antiseptic system. pt. IV. Surgery. pt. v. Addresses. Index.* The Clarendon Press, 1909.

4. Garrison FH. *An Introduction to the History of Medicine.* 4th edn. WB Saunders Co, Philadelphia, 1929 Nuland SB.

5. Knopf AA. *Doctors. The Biography of Medicine.* New York, 1988.

6. Becker WF. Presidential address: Pioneers in thyroid surgery. *Ann Surg.* 1977 May;185(5):493.

7. Sarkar S, Banerjee S, Sarkar R, Sikder B. A review on the history of 'thyroid surgery. *Indian J Surg.* 2016 Feb 1;78(1):32–6.

8. Tröhler U. Towards endocrinology: Theodor Kocher's 1883 account of the unexpected effects of total ablation of the thyroid. *J R Soc Med.* 2011;104(3):129–132.

9. Thomusch O, Machens A, Sekulla C, Ukkat J, Lippert H, Gastinger I, Dralle H. Multivariate analysis of risk factors for postoperative complications in benign goiter surgery: Prospective multicenter study in Germany. *World J Surg.* 2000 Nov 1;24(11):1335–41.

10. Bellantone R, Lombardi CP, Bossola M, Boscherini M, De Crea C, Alesina P, Traini E, Princi P, Raffaelli M. Total thyroidectomy for management of benign thyroid disease: Review of 526 cases. *World J Surg.* 2002 Dec 1;26(12):1468–71.

11. Efremidou EI, Papageorgiou MS, Liratzopoulos N, Manolas KJ. The efficacy and safety of total thyroidectomy in the management of benign thyroid disease: A review of 932 cases. *Can J Surg.* 2009 Feb;52(1):39.

12. Duclos A et al. Influence of experience on performance of individual surgeons in thyroid surgery: prospective cross sectional multicentre study. *BMJ.* 2012 Jan 11;344:d8041.

13. Gómez-Ramírez J, Sitges-Serra A, Moreno-Llorente P, Zambudio AR, Ortega-Serrano J. Rodríguez MT, del Moral JV. Mortality after thyroid surgery, insignificant or still an issue? *Langenbeck's Arch Surg.* 2015 May 1;400(4):517–22.

14. Singh R, Tubbs RS. Should a highly skilled surgeon be an advanced anatomist first? A view point. *Basic Sciences of Med.* 2015;4(4):53–7.

15. Palace MR. Perioperative management of thyroid dysfunction. *Health Serv Insights.* 2017 Feb 17;10:1178632916689677.

16. Mok VM, Oltmann SC, Chen H, Sippel RS. Schneider DF. Identifying predictors of a difficult thyroidectomy. *J Surg Res.* 2014 Jul 1;190(1):157–63.

17. Morais M, Capela-Costa J, Matos-Lima L, Costa-Maia J. Nonrecurrent laryngeal nerve and associated anatomical variations: The art of prediction. *Eur Thyroid J.* 2015;4(4):234–8.

18. De Filippis EA, Sabet A, Sun MR, Garber JR. Pemberton's sign: Explained nearly 70 years later. *J Clin Endocr Metab.* 2014 Jun 1;99(6):1949–54.

19. Pappalardo V, La Rosa S, Imperatori A, Rotolo N, Tanda ML, Sessa A, Dominioni L, Dionigi G. Thyroid cancer with tracheal invasion: A pathological estimation. *Gland Surgery.* 2016 Oct;5(5):541.

20. Ordookhani A, Motazedi A, Burman KD. Thrombosis in thyroid cancer. *Int J Endocrinol Metab.* 2018 Jan;16(1).

21. Malhotra S, Sodhi V. Anaesthesia for thyroid and parathyroid surgery. Continuing education in anaesthesia. *Critical Care & Pain.* 2007 Apr 1;7(2):55–8.

22. D'ORAZI V, Panunzi A, Di Lorenzo E, Ortensi AL, Cialini M, Anichini S, Ortensi A. Use of loupes magnification and microsurgical technique in thyroid surgery: Ten years experience in a single center. *G Chir.* 2016 May;37(3):101.

23. Rulli F, Ambrogi V, Dionigi G, Amirhassankhani S, Mineo TC, Ottaviani F, Buemi A, Di Stefano P, Mourad M. Meta-analysis of recurrent laryngeal nerve injury in thyroid surgery with or without intraoperative nerve monitoring. *Acta Otorhinolaryngol Ital.* 2014 Aug;34(4):223.

24. Manatakis DK, Balalis D, Soulou VN, Korkolis DP, Plataniotis G, Gontikakis E. Incidental parathyroidectomy during total thyroidectomy: Risk factors and consequences. *Int JEndocrinol.* 2016;2016, Article ID 7825305.

Chapter 9

SURGERY FOR MULTINODULAR GOITER

Madan Laxman Kapre, Sanoop Elambassery, Neeti Kapre Gupta, M. Abdul Amjad Khan, and Gauri Kapre Vaidya

CONTENTS

Evolution of MNG   75
Genesis of the Thyroid Nodule and MNG   75
Follow-Up Strategy for MNG Surgery   76
References   77

The philosophy of treatment and surgical strategies for multinodular goiter (MNG) needs to be based on the risk factors, namely discomfort due to size and cosmesis. One also needs to take into consideration the possibility of cancer phobia due to readily available reading material via health magazines and other information channels. Before we start strategizing our optimal surgical care, let us first discuss these aspects.

As the number of nodules increases, the risk of them being malignant decreases. There is no real statistical information available, but it is quoted at around 5% to 15% [1,2,14].

Discomfort due to size depends upon the location of the nodules. The posteriorly located nodule may produce dysphagia-like symptoms whereas the nodules may cause breathing discomfort when lying supine in a retrosternal location. As the nodules are benign, they push the structures around and never really invade them. In this case, symptoms such as hoarseness of voice due to involvement of the RLN are very rare. The authors have had the privilege of working in tribal areas in the hills of Melghat, India, where massively large Chikhaldara goiters were found to cause no symptoms (Figures 9.1 and 9.2).

Cosmetic issues are more prevalent in urban populations, and treatment should be assessed on the risk-benefit ratio and discussed with the patient before embarking on surgery.

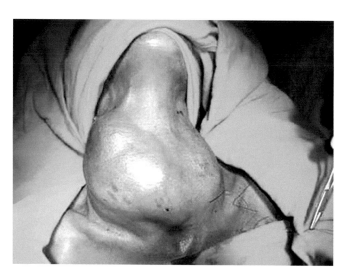

Figure 9.2 Tattooing is an ancient Voodoo way of treatment.

EVOLUTION OF MNG

It is rather relevant to understand the pathogenesis of MNG so that its malignant potential is truly understood [15]. *As the process is not "neoplastic" and it is often bilateral, it is very important to assess sudden rapid growth or pain or any symptoms pertaining to either invasion or pressure.* This information should be taken into consideration when evaluating investigative treatments and subsequent decision-making.

GENESIS OF THE THYROID NODULE AND MNG

INDICATION FOR SURGICAL TREATMENT
While there are some obvious surgical indications, such as large MNG, there are certain subtle areas, which require special mention, such as in male patients, rapid growth in size and recent appearance of pressure symptoms of malignant transformation in previously benign MNG [3,4,12,13]. The recommendation is ultrasonographically guided fine needle aspiration cytology of the suspicious nodule. Similar issues arise in patients with MNG with hyperthyroidism. It is difficult to predict which of the bilateral/unilateral MNGs are responsible for toxic symptoms. There could

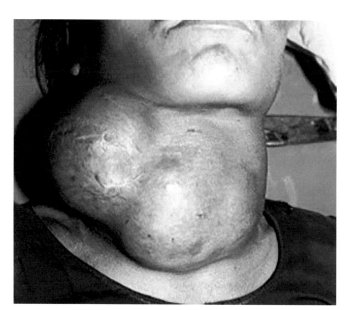

Figure 9.1 Chikhaldara multinodular goiter.

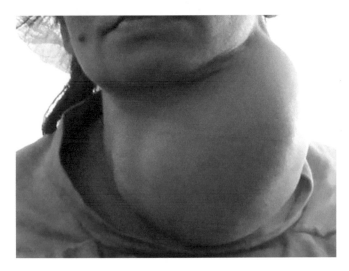

Figure 9.3   Often such massive goiters are unilateral.

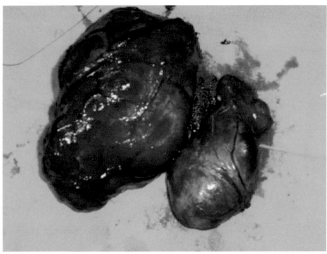

Figure 9.5   Total thyroidectomy is the surgical procedure of choice.

be an argument in favor of radionuclide imaging or Doppler along with ultrasonography (USG) for localized increased activity [5,6]. However, the authors suggest proceeding with the surgical treatment based on other parameters. All efforts should be made to stabilize the toxic symptoms and optimally achieve euthyroid status.

OPTIMIZING SURGICAL TREATMENT

There is really no great debate around treatment of unilateral multinodular goiter (Figure 9.3). The surgery of choice is excision of the ipsilateral lobe with the isthmus. The removal of the isthmus is very critical as any future hypertrophy of the isthmus will create a midline hump. Obviously, if the initial indication was cosmesis, this is rather an embarrassing situation too. The following list presents options for surgical treatments:

- Unilateral lobectomy with isthmusectomy
- Total thyroidectomy
- Sub-total thyroidectomy
- Near total thyroidectomy

There are several opinions, and the following factors should be considered in decision-making.

STRUCTURAL ISSUES

It is very difficult to find a reasonably nodule-free area during the surgical dissection (Figures 9.4 and 9.5). It is sometimes more hazardous to try to find a suitable dissecting plane and achieve

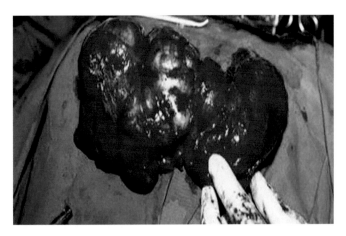

Figure 9.4   Always examine the specimen for inadvertent removal of the parathyroid.

hemostasis. Hence, in a massive Chikhaldara goiter, it is best to do total thyroidectomy. Bilateral MNG with retrosternal extension is another case where one must perform total thyroidectomy for reasons of safety.

ISSUES RELATED TO FUNCTION

It is argued that if one manages to keep some thyroid tissue, it will save the patient's dependence on exogenous thyroid support. However, it is very doubtful that the remainder of the tissue is adequate, and the patient may still require Thyroxine supplementation. The authors experienced the case of a patient requiring Thyroxin support after having been subjected to hemithyroidectomy. About a third of patients requires long term Thyroxine support and about 20% of them need it permanently [7–9].

ISSUES RELATED TO THE PARATHYROID

It may be advisable to consider lesser surgery for the safety of the parathyroids. However, experience teaches us that it is the superior set of parathyroids that are saved in all cases, and the real concern is about the inferior set of parathyroids. There is no real statistical evidence or trials to support this argument.

LOW RESOURCES, HIGH VOLUME DISEASE

The social and economic situation in Chikaldhara is really different. Oral Thyroxine is not as much of an economic burden as is the cost of calcium supplements. We have been in this situation for a number of years, and it is our considerate opinion that treatment depends greatly on available surgical skills and the need for very careful monitoring.

FOLLOW-UP STRATEGY FOR MNG SURGERY

It is worth while to discuss the specimen with the pathologist and examine all nodules after sectioning. To subject all nodules for histological examination, though ideal, is not practical. Hence, only the suspicious nodules may be subjected to histology. Should any of them prove to be malignant, they should be subjected to further treatment on their own merit.

In case of unilateral lobectomy and isthmusectomy, it is observed that they are likely to become hypothyroid and hence should be monitored [7–9]. There is no available statistical information on the incidence of MNG in the contralateral lobe. We feel that the patient should not be allowed to become hypothyroid, as a resultant high thyroid-stimulating hormone (TSH) may stimulate nodularity.

Revision surgery after earlier hemithyroidectomy for contralateral lobe is not a difficult proposition if the planes were not violated in the previous surgery. However, when the residual thyroid tissue becomes nodular and deserves surgical excision, it is a very hazardous proposition. Such surgeries must be done at tertiary high volume centers with intra-operative nerve monitoring [10]. It may also require similar localization of the parathyroid gland both pre-operatively and intra-operatively with advanced imaging studies [11].

REFERENCES

1. Gadolfi PP et al. The incidence of thyroid carcinoma in multinodular goitre: Retrospective analysis. *Acta Biomed.* 2004 Aug;75(2):114–7.

2. Bombil I et al. Incidental cancer in multinodular goitre post thyroidectomy. *S Afr J Surg.* 2014 Feb;52(1):5–9.

3. Jie Luo BS et al. Are these predictors of malignancy in patients with multinodular goitre? *J Surg Res.* 2012 May;174(2):207–10.

4. Dogan L et al. Total thyroidectomy for the surgical treatment of multinodular goitre. *Surg Today.* 2011 Mar;41(3):323–7.

5. Luster M, Verbury FA, Scheidbauer K. Diagnostic imaging work up in multinodular goitre. *Minerva Endocrinol.* 2010 Sep;35(3):153–9.

6. Sarr A et al. Toxic nodular goitre. *Daker Med.* 2007;52(2):135–40.

7. Chotigavanich C, Sureepong P, Ongard S. Hypothyroidism after hemithyroidectomy: The incidence and risk factors. *J Med Assoc Thai.* 2016 Jan;99(1): 77–83.

8. Said M, Chia V, haigh PT. Hypothyroidism after hemithyroidectomy. *World J Surg.* 2013 Dec;37(12):2839–44.

9. Vaiman M et al. Hypothyroidism following partial thyroidectomy. *Otolaryngol Head Neck Surg.* 2008 Jan;138(1):98–100.

10. Gremillion G et al. Intraoperative recurrent laryngeal nerve monitoring in thyroid surgery: Is it worth the cost? *Ochsner J.* 2012 winter;12(4):363–6.

11. Ethan F et al. Preoperative imaging for parathyroid localization in patients with concurrent disease: A systemic review. *Head Neck.* 2018;40:1577–87.

12. Kennedy JS. The pathology of dyshormonogenetic goiter. *The Journal of Patholgy.* 1969 Nov;99(3).

13. Ghosserin RA, Rosai J, Hoffes C. Dyshormonogenetic goiter: A clinicopathology study of 56 cases. *Endocr Pathol.* 1997 winter;8(4):283–92.

14. Brix TH, Hegedus L. Genetic and environmental factors in the aetiology of simple goiter. *Ann Med.* 2000 Apr;32(3):153–6.

15. Derwahl M, Studer H. Nodular goiter and goiter nodule; Where Iodine deficiency falls short of explaining the fact. *Exp Clin Endocrinol Diabetes.* 2001;109(5):250–60.

Chapter 10

MANAGEMENT OF RETROSTERNAL GOITER

Belayat Hossain Siddiquee

CONTENTS

Introduction 79
Clinical Manifestations 79
Investigation for RSG 79
Classification 80
Treatment 81
Conclusion 82
References 82

INTRODUCTION

Retrosternal goiter (RSG) was first described by Albrecht von Haller in 1749 [1] as the extension of thyroid tissue below the upper opening of the chest. When should thyroid swelling be labeled as retrosternal goiter? At least four definitions are available in the literature:

a. Candela et al. in 2007 defined the entity as any goiter that descends below the plane of the thoracic inlet or grows into the anterior mediastinum for more than 2 cm [2].

b. Shingh et al. in 1994 suggested that a retrosternal goiter existed when more than 50% of the goiter was below the plane of the thoracic inlet [3].

c. A surgical definition was used by White et al. in 2008 defining a retrosternal goiter as any goiter which required dissection in the mediastinum [4].

d. Goldenburg et al. as early as 1957 defined a retrosternal goiter as one reaching the level of the 4th thoracic vertebra [5].

All these definitions have their limitations. In the first and second definition there is nothing indicated about the total volume of the goiter and whether the retrosternal portion remains in the thorax in all postures and situations. Many goiters in erect posture sink into the thorax to some extent but in the supine position, particularly on the operating table (OT), come up to be confined only in the neck.

Every thyroid surgeon will agree that most retrosternal goiters do not require dissection in the mediastinum, as it is possible to drag them up from the neck through cervical incision.

We propose this definition: *Retrosternal goiter is one where the goiter remains in the mediastinum in any posture, entirely or partly.* The volume of the retrosternal portion is a matter of consideration, not the percentage of total goiter volume. A big goiter of less than 20% thoracic extension can give rise to symptoms of inlet obstruction.

CLINICAL MANIFESTATIONS

The retrosternal goiter is often asymptomatic, and a diagnosis is incidental during radiological investigation of a cervical goiter as part of a pre-operative check-up. But in the majority of cases they may present categorically with symptoms of retrosternal goiter, e.g., symptoms of airway obstruction (shortness of breath, dyspnea, minimal voice change), symptoms of compression of the great veins in the neck (flushing of the face, engorged veins in the neck and chest) (Figure 10.1), and symptoms of food way compression (dysphagia) [6]. Rarely, a malignant retrosternal goiter can give rise to lymph node swelling in the neck (central or lateral due to metastasis). Obstructive sleep apnea due to retrosternal goiter is also reported [7].

INVESTIGATION FOR RSG

i. Plain radiology
   Chest x-ray P/A and lateral view reveals:
   a. Superior mediastinal opacity
   b. Tracheal deviation (Figure 10.2)

ii. CT scan is indicated when the goiter is sufficiently low down in the chest to plan for a surgical approach, assess the total goiter volume, and in case of malignancy to see extrathyroid extension, adhesion, and invasion to the adjacent structures and lymphadenopathy (both cervical and mediastinal) [8] (Figures 10.3 and 10.4).

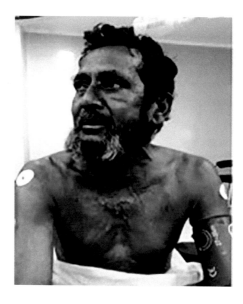

Figure 10.1   Venous engorgement and flushing of skin in neck and chest.

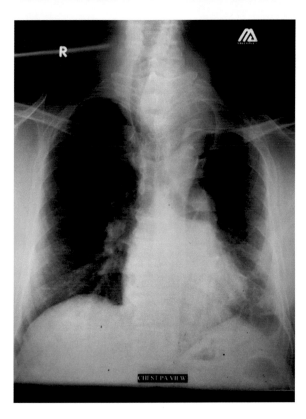

Figure 10.2　Tracheal shifting by retrosternal goiter.

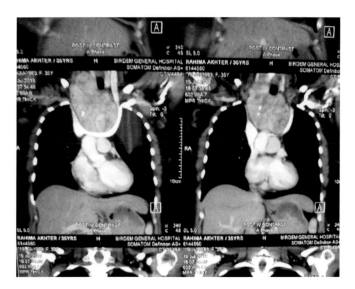

Figure 10.4　CT scan showing retrosternal goiter just above the arch of the aorta.

v.　Ultrasonographic evaluation of the retrosternal portion of the thyroid is not as good as in cervical goiter, as it is hampered by the bony structures of the thoracic cage [11].

In addition, thyroid hormone assays with TSH and other investigations for general fitness for major surgical procedures are required.

CLASSIFICATION

There are many classifications available in the literature, mainly based on anatomical location. This is a classification of retrosternal goiter from the surgical point of view.

1.　Where a significant portion of the cervical goiter persistently remains in the mediastinum but there is no adhesion with the mediastinal structures (Category 1).

2.　A goiter that is entirety in the mediastinum. These may be the goiters that wholly sink into the mediastinum from the neck or primary mediastinal thyroid, which is likely to derive blood supply from mediastinal vessels (Category 2).

3.　Any RSG with suspicion of malignancy (clinical and/or radiological) (Category 3).

The advantage of this classification is that it is possible to make a preoperative plan regarding surgical approach and anticipate probable surgical complications correlating with the clinical features.

CATEGORY 1

The goiter has a portion in the neck. The retrosternal portion derives blood supply from the neck vessels. It is usually possible to drag the retrosternal portion via a cervical collar incision without significant bleeding or any other complication like recurrent laryngeal nerve palsy or parathyroid insufficiency.

CATEGORY 2

The goiter sinks into the mediastinum. If the lower limit is not approachable digitally or if the primary mediastinum thyroid, which is developmentally located in the thorax, derives its blood supply from the mediastinal vessels, it should be removed by a sternotomy approach for complete removal to minimize complications.

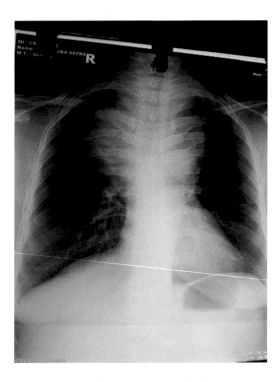

Figure 10.3　X-ray chest showing retrosternal goiter.

The high iodine content of the thyroid gives it higher attenuation in comparison to surrounding soft tissues and is more useful in identifying thyroid extension into the mediastinum.

iii.　CT-guided FNAC for perfect sampling, to ensure safety and avoid hemorrhage.

iv.　MRI is superior in more precise evaluation of the retrosternal goiter, especially its relation to extension and invasion of the adjacent structure [9,10].

CATEGORY 3

The goiter has produced pre-operative features of malignancy like vocal cord palsy and lymphadenopathy, and the CT scan features extracapsular spread and invasion of adjacent structures like trachea, esophagus, etc. These may or may not be attached to vital structures like pleura, lung, or vessels. There is a chance of massive perioperative bleeding and major complications from damage to these vital structures. There is also the possibility of clearance failure, which often remains undetected. Adequate exposure is to be ensured, and sternotomy may be required.

TREATMENT

There is a general argument that surgical removal should be performed even in the absence of clinical symptoms or signs. The widely accepted reasons for that are:

i.   Diagnosis of malignancy could be missed as FNAC from the mediastinal portion of the thyroid is difficult and potentially dangerous because of the location of the big thoracic vessels [12].

ii.   RSG gives rise to life-threatening emergencies because of sudden or rapid enlargement secondary to hemorrhage and/or malignant change.

iii. Thyroxin suppression or radio iodine ablation are rarely successful in RSG to reduce size [13].

Retrosternal goiter has some special features related to cervical goiter which indicates the surgery is obligatory in all the diagnosed cases. Clinical assessment of retrosternal goiter is not as efficient as in cervical goiter due to the inaccessibility of the intrathoracic portion, and ultrasonography images are not as good as in cervical goiter due to artifact generated by bones of the thoracic cage [14]. The retrosternal portion is difficult to approach for needle biopsy. These issues illustrate the complications to get a clear understanding about the clinico-pathological nature of retrosternal goiter. The history of retrosternal goiter shows a progressive community presenting in the fifth and sixth decade of life. Advancing age is associated with increasing comorbidity, implying that operation at an earlier stage of goiter may be associated with a reduced rate of complications [15].

The presenting symptoms, i.e., those of compression of airways, major neck vessels, or foodways in the thoracic inlet region, can only be alleviated by surgical removal of the goiter.

Although generally thought to be uncommon, acute problems may occur in 5%–11% of retrosternal goiter [16,17]. Hemorrhage in the nodule, secondary to prolonged mechanical pressure precipitate development of a laryngeal edema and congestion.

A 5-year study from July 2012 to June 2017 at the Department of Otolaryngology-Head & Neck Surgery, Bangabandhu Sheikh Mujib Medical University, Dhaka, Bangladesh, revealed that out of 1,091 patients who underwent thyroid surgery, only 26 (2.38%) were found to have retrosternal goiter and 1,065 (97.61%) were found to have cervical goiter. As per the criteria, the pre-operative categorization is shown in Table 10.1. The sex ratio between cervical goiter and retrosternal goiter was very similar (Table 10.2).

Table 10.1   Pre-operative categorization of retrosternal goiters (n = 26)

Category 1	Significant portion in the mediastinum	21 (80.77%)
Category 2	Entirely in the mediastinum	2 (7.69%)
	1 primary in the mediastinum, 1 sinks from the neck	
Category 3	Malignant, PTC (per-operative)	3 (11.54%)

Table 10.2   Sex ratio among the two groups, i.e., cervical goiter and RSG

Sex	No. of patients	Percentage	Ratio
Cervical goiter (n = 1,065)			
Female	781	73.33%	2.75:1
Male	284	26.67%	
Retrosternal goiters (n = 26)			
Female	18	69.23%	2.25:1
Male	8	30.77%	

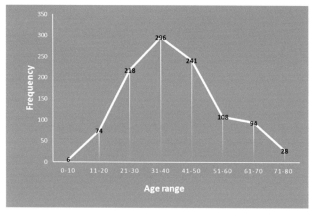

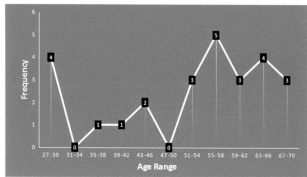

Figure 10.5   Age distribution curve of cervical and retrosternal goiter.

But the age incidence showed quite the reverse. Retrosternal goiter usually shows progressive growth commonly presenting during the fifth or sixth decade of life. In our series, among the cervical goiter, 77.84% were below the age of 50, whereas in retrosternal goiter, 69.23% were above 50 years of age. In cervical goiter, the age range was 9 to 78 years with a mean age of 40 (SD 14.33) and in retrosternal goiter the age range was 27 to 70 years with a mean age of 53 (SD 12.29). The age distribution curve of cervical and retrosternal goiter are shown in Figure 10.5.

SURGICAL MANAGEMENT

Only around 2% of retrosternal goiters require surgical access other than standard collar incision [4,18].

The surgical approach required in our series is shown in Table 10.3 and Figure 10.6.

COMPLICATIONS OF SURGERY

The main complications of thyroid surgery were compared in retrosternal goiter in contrast to cervical goiter (Tables 10.4 and 10.5).

Post-operative hemorrhage occurred in 2 cases of retrosternal goiter out of 26 (7.69%), whereas it occurred in only 5 out of 1,065 cases of cervical goiter (0.43%).

Table 10.3 Surgical approaches

Category 1 (n = 21)	Cervical (all cases)	
Category 2 (n = 2)	Cervical + sternotomy	−1
	Sternotomy	−1
Category 3 (n = 3)	Cervical	−2
	Cervical + sternotomy	−1

Note: Sternotomy required in 3 cases out of total 26 RSG (11.54%).

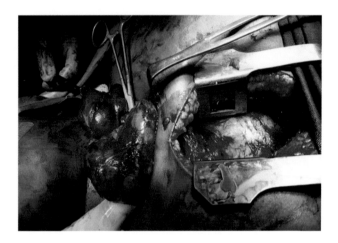

Figure 10.6 Sternotomy approach for retrosternal goiter.

Table 10.4 Recurrent laryngeal nerve palsy

	Nerve at risk	No. of palsy
Cervical goiter		
Hemi and Completion	621	24 (1.59%), 8 (0.53) permanent
Total thyroidectomy	444	
Total: 1,509		
RSG		
Hemi	8	3 (6.82%) permanent
Total thyroidectomy	18	
Total: 44		
	P = <0.001	

Table 10.5 Parathyroid insufficiency

	No. of cases	Percentage
Cervical goiter (n = 478)		
Total thyroidectomy: 444 Completion thyroidectomy: 34	Temporary: 34 Permanent: 11 Total: 45	9.41%
RSG (n = 18)		
Total thyroidectomy	Temporary: 2 Permanent: 2 Total: 4	22.22%
	P = <0.001	

CONCLUSION

The mean age of patients with retrosternal goiter is higher than cervical goiter and mostly presents in middle age and above. Sternotomy is required in selective cases of Categories 2 and 3 only. Surgery for retrosternal goiter is associated with a higher risk of complications.

REFERENCES

1. Rugiu MG. Piemonte; Surgical approach to retrosternal goiter: Do we still need sternotomy? *Acta Otorhinolaryngol Ital.* 2009 Dec;29(6):331–8.

2. Candela G et al. Surgical therapy of goiter plunged in the mediastinum. Considerations regarding our experience with 165 patients. *Chir Ital.* 2007;59(6):843–51.

3. Singh ID, Gupta V, Raina S, Goyal S, Kumar M. Large retrosternal goiter: An otolaryngological perspective-case series and review of literature. *J Otolaryngol ENT Res.* 2017;6(1):00147.

4. White ML, Doherty GM, Gauger PG. Evidence-based surgical management of substernal goiter. *World J Surg.* 2008;32:1285–300.

5. Goldenburg IS, Lindskog GE. Differential diagnosis, pathology and treatment of substernal goiter. *J Am Med Assoc.* 1957;163(7):527–9.

6. Hedayati N, McHenry CR. The clinical presentation and operative management of nodular and diffuse substernal thyroid disease. *Am Surg.* 2002;68:245–51.

7. Rodrigues J,Furtado R, Ramani A, Mitta N, Kudchadkar S, and Falari S. A rare instance of retrosternal goitre presenting with obstructive sleep apnoea in a middle-aged person. *Int J Surg Case Rep.* 2013;4(12):1064–6.

8. Makeiff M, Marlier F, Khudjadze M, Garrel R, Crampette L, Guerrier B. Substernal goiter. Report of 212cases. *Ann Chir.* 2000 Jan;125(1):18–25.

9. Buckley JA, Stark P. Intrathoracic mediastinal thyroid goiter: Imaging manifestations. *AJR Am J Roentgenol.* 1999 Aug; 173(2):471–5.

10. Belardinelli L, Gualdi G, Ceroni L, Guadalaxara A, Polettini E, Pappalardo G. Comparison between computed tomography and magnetic resonance data and pathologic findings in substernal goiters. *Int Surg.* 1995;80:65–9.

11. Bashsta B, ELLis K, Gold RP. Computed tomography of intrathoracic goiters. *AJR.*1983;140:455–60.

12. Nervi M, Iacconi P, Spinelli C, Janni A, Miccoli P. Thyroid carcinoma is intrathoracic goiter. *Langenbecks Arch Surg.* 1998;383:337–9.

13. Newman E, Shaha AR. Substernal goiter. *J Surg Oncol.* 1995;60:207–12.

14. Bonnema SJ, Andersen PB, Knudsen DU, Hegedus L. MR imaging of large multinodular goiters. Observer disagreement on dimensions of the involved trachea. *AJR Am J Roentgenol.*2002;179:259–66.

15. Hardy RG, Bliss RD, Lennard TWJ, Balasubramanian SP, Harrison BJ. Management of retrosternal goitres. *Ann R Coll Surg Engl.* 2009 Jan;91(1):8–11.

16. Mackle T, Meaney J, Timon C. Tracheoesophageal compression associated with substernal goitre. Correlation of symptoms with cross-sectional imaging findings. *J Laryngol Otol.* 2007;121:358–61.

17. Ben Nun A, Soudack M, Best LA. Retrosternal thyroid goiter: 15 years' experience. *Isr Med Assoc J.* 2006;8:106–9.

18. Mack E. Management of patients with substernal goiters. *Surg Clin North Am.* 1995;75:377–94.

Chapter 11

REMOTE ACCESS ENDOSCOPIC AND ROBOTIC THYROIDECTOMY

Kyung Tae

CONTENTS

Introduction   83
The History of Robotic/Endoscopic Thyroidectomy   83
Robotic/Endoscopic Thyroidectomy Classification   83
Author's Experience   86
Conclusions   87
References   89

INTRODUCTION

Remote access endoscopic and robotic thyroidectomies via cervical, axillary, anterior chest, breast, postauricular facelift, and transoral approaches have been developed over the past 20 years to avoid or hide visible neck scarring; such scarring is a major concern in thyroid surgery, especially in young women [1].

THE HISTORY OF ROBOTIC/ENDOSCOPIC THYROIDECTOMY

In 1997, the first endoscopic thyroidectomy was performed using a cervical approach with carbon dioxide (CO_2) insufflation [2]. Miccoli et al. developed the minimally invasive video-assisted thyroidectomy (MIVAT) technique without CO_2 insufflation, to avoid CO_2-related complications, in 1999 [3]. Since then, various remote-access thyroidectomy methods via axillary, breast, anterior chest, postauricular, and transoral routes have been developed.

Video-assisted neck surgery (VANS) without CO_2 insufflation involves a 3 to 4 cm main oblique incision in the anterior chest wall below the clavicle, and a 5 mm incision in the lateral neck that is used to insert a 5 mm endoscope. The axillary approach with CO_2 insufflation that uses three axillary incisions was developed in 2000 [4]. The gasless transaxillary approach was first developed using a 6 cm axillary incision and one small anterior chest port, but it has progressed to involve the use of a single axillary incision without an anterior chest port [5]. The gasless transaxillary approach has also been modified to create gasless unilateral axillary (GUA) and gasless unilateral axillo-breast (GUAB) approaches [6–10]. The GUAB approach involves the use of a small breast areola port in addition to the main axillary incision. The breast port provides a wide angle between the robotic or endoscopic instruments, making it easier to manipulate them and avoid collisions. However, the robotic GUAB approach has evolved into the GUA approach that does not use a breast port but offers better cosmesis [11].

The breast approach using CO_2 insufflation uses two breast ports and one parasternal port [12]. The axillo-bilateral breast approach (ABBA) uses two breast ports and an axillary port. The bilateral axillo-breast approach (BABA) requires two incisions in the areola and two incisions in each axillary area [13]. The unilateral or bilateral axillo-breast approaches with CO_2 insufflation use one breast port and two axillary ports on one or both sides, respectively.

The facelift (retroauricular) approach employs postauricular and occipital hairline incisions [15]. Also, it allows for a smaller dissection area and a shorter distance from the incision site to the thyroid gland than the transaxillary approach.

The transoral approach may include sublingual, vestibular, or combined approaches [1,15–17]. Moreover, the transoral approach is considered as a form of true natural orifice transluminal endoscopic surgery (NOTES) and is less invasive in terms of working space than other types of remote access thyroidectomy.

ROBOTIC/ENDOSCOPIC THYROIDECTOMY CLASSIFICATION

Remote access robotic and endoscopic thyroidectomy can be classified according to the use of CO_2 gas insufflation and the site of the incision (Table 11.1) [1]. Carbon dioxide insufflation methods include the cervical, axillary, breast, anterior chest, and transoral approaches, as well as various axillo-breast approaches such as the ABBA, BABA, and unilateral or bilateral axillo-breast approaches. Gasless methods include the MIVAT, anterior chest, axillary, postauricular facelift, and transoral approaches. There are also various modifications and combinations of these approaches.

OPERATIVE PROCEDURES

Of the various remote access thyroidectomy procedures, the gasless transaxillary approach, BABA, gasless postauricular facelift approach, and transoral vestibular approach are commonly used today. The operative procedures of these four approaches are as follows.

THE GASLESS UNILATERAL AXILLARY (GUA) APPROACH

A 5- to 6-cm skin incision is made in the axillary fossa (Figure 11.1a) [1,6–10], and a skin flap is elevated under direct vision in the plane of the subplatysmal layer over the pectoralis major muscle from the axilla to the anterior neck area. The dissection encompasses the space between the two heads of the sternocleidomastoid (SCM)

Table 11.1 Classification of robotic and endoscopic thyroidectomies

Carbon dioxide (CO_2) insufflation methods
Cervical approach
Anterior chest approach
Axillary approach
Breast approach with parasternal port
Axillo-breast approach
Axillo-bilateral breast approach (ABBA)
Bilateral axillo-breast approach (BABA)
Unilateral/bilateral axillo-breast approach
Transoral approach
Gasless methods
Minimally invasive video-assisted thyroidectomy (MIVAT)
Anterior chest approach
Video-assisted neck surgery (VANS)
Axillary approach
Axillary approach with anterior chest port
Single incision axillary approach
Gasless unilateral axillo-breast (GUAB) or axillary (GUA) approach
Facelift (retroauricular) approach
Transoral approach

Source: Reproduced from Tae et al. *Clin Exp Otorhinolaryngol* 2019;12:1–11.

muscle and progresses below the sternothyroid and sternohyoid muscles to expose the thyroid gland. An external retractor is used to maintain an adequate working space without CO_2 insufflation (Figure 11.1b). A second 0.5-cm (endoscopic procedure) or 0.8-cm (robotic procedure) skin incision is made just inferior to the axillary incision to insert a trocar. The purpose of this second axillary incision is to minimize the length of the main axillary incision. Three robotic arms including a 30° face-down robotic endoscope, Prograsp forceps, and a Maryland dissector are then inserted through the main axillary incision port. The Harmonic curved shears (dominant hand side) are placed at the second axillary incision port in a right-side approach (Figure 11.1c). In an endoscopic procedure, a 30° face-down endoscope and other endoscopic instruments are placed at the main axillary incision, and the energy-based devices or endoscopic instruments are inserted through the second axillary incision port and the main axillary incision.

The superior thyroid vessels are cut individually close to the thyroid gland, using the Harmonic curved shears, to preserve the external branch of the superior laryngeal nerve (Figure 11.1d). The superior parathyroid gland is identified and carefully preserved with an intact blood supply. The thyroid gland is then retracted medially, and the paratracheal lymph nodes and perithyroidal soft tissue are dissected while preserving the entire recurrent laryngeal nerve (RLN) (Figure 11.1e). The isthmus is divided, and the ipsilateral total lobectomy with a central neck dissection is completed (Figure 11.1f). Finally, a suction drain is inserted and the wound closed.

THE BILATERAL AXILLO-BREAST APPROACH (BABA)
After making incisions on both upper circumareolar areas, the working space is elevated to the level of the thyroid cartilage superiorly and to the medial border of the SCM muscle laterally. An endoscope is placed through the right breast port, and the left breast port is used for the endoscopic or robotic instruments. Two axillary cannulas are inserted, and the working space is maintained using CO_2 insufflation at a pressure of 5 to 6 mmHg (Figure 11.2) [1]. The midline fascia between the strap muscles and the isthmus is divided. The thyroid gland is dissected while preserving the parathyroid glands and RLNs. Then, the resected specimen is removed and

placed in a plastic bag through the 12 mm breast port. The midline of the strap muscles is re-approximated, a suction drain is placed, and the skin is closed.

THE GASLESS POSTAURICULAR FACELIFT APPROACH
A skin incision is made in the postauricular sulcus, curved posteriorly at the upper third of the auricle, and continued along the occipital hairline (Figure 11.3a) [1,14,18]. The skin flap is elevated in the plane of the subplatysma over the SCM muscle under direct vision, posteriorly to the posterior border of the SCM muscle, superiorly to the lower border of the mandible, and inferiorly to the sternal notch. The great auricular nerve and the external jugular vein are identified and preserved. The sternohyoid and sternothyroid muscles are dissected and retracted upwards to expose the thyroid gland, after which an external retractor is placed to maintain the working space (Figure 11.3b). A 30° face-down endoscope and three robotic instruments including Maryland dissectors, Prograsp forceps, and Harmonic curved shears are inserted through the postauricular incision (Figure 11.3c). The parathyroid glands are identified and preserved, and the RLN is identified in the tracheoesophageal groove and preserved (Figure 11.3d). Berry's ligament and the thyroid isthmus are dissected, and the lobectomy with isthmusectomy is completed (Figure 11.3e). Afterwards, a suction drain is placed and the wound is closed layer by layer.

THE TRANSORAL VESTIBULAR APPROACH
A 1.5- to 2-cm horizontal incision is made at the end of the lower lip frenulum, and two lateral incisions are made close to the oral commissure to avoid a mental nerve injury (Figure 11.4a) [1]. Epinephrine diluted in normal saline is injected into the submental area for hydrodissection. Blunt dissection of the submental area is performed using a dilator. A 30° rigid endoscope is placed in the center, and 5- or 8 mm trocars are inserted on either side of the endoscope for two endoscopic dissectors or monopolar electrocautery. The CO_2 insufflation pressure is set at 5 to 6 mmHg. A working space is usually created in the plane of the subplatysmal layer by endoscopy without a surgical robot. The skin flap is widened to the level of the sternal notch inferiorly and the SCM muscle laterally (Figure 11.4b). After creating the working space, a 30° robotic endoscope and robotic instruments such as bipolar Maryland forceps or monopolar scissors are placed on either side of the endoscope. If necessary, a third robotic instrument, such as Cardinal forceps, is inserted through the right axillary port (Figure 11.4c). The midline fascia between the strap muscles is divided and the sternohyoid and sternothyroid muscles are dissected to expose the thyroid gland (Figure 11.4d). Next, the isthmus is dissected and divided, and a thyroidectomy is performed while preserving the RLN and parathyroid glands (Figure 11.4e). Special care must be taken to preserve the RLN when dissecting the Berry's ligament area. The lobectomy with isthmusectomy is completed (Figure 11.4f), and the specimen is removed using a plastic bag via the central oral incision or the axillary port. The divided strap muscles are re-approximated and the surgical wound in the oral vestibule is closed with absorbable sutures; usually no drain is required.

ADVANTAGES AND LIMITATIONS OF REMOTE ACCESS THYROIDECTOMY
Remote access endoscopic and robotic thyroidectomy has many advantages. It provides excellent cosmesis and a magnified surgical view [1,19]. Notably, robotic procedures using the da Vinci Surgical System (Intuitive Surgical, Sunnyvale, California) can provide a 3-dimensional 10–12-fold magnified view, making it easy to identify the parathyroid glands and RLN. It also provides the ability

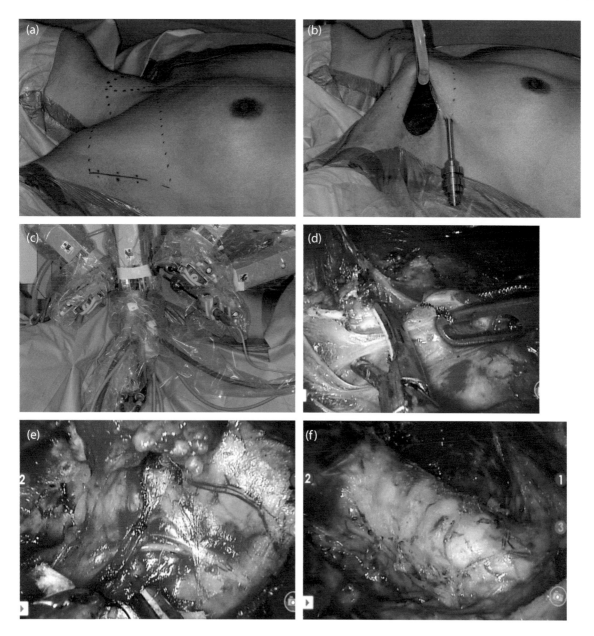

Figure 11.1 The gasless unilateral axillary (GUA) approach. (a) A 5 to 6 cm main skin incision is made in the axillary fossa, and a second 0.5 or 0.8 cm skin incision is made just inferior to the main axillary incision to insert a trocar. (b) After creating a working space, an external retractor is placed to maintain an adequate working space without carbon dioxide (CO_2) insufflation. (c) Three robotic arms including a 30° face-down robotic endoscope, Prograsp forceps, and a Maryland dissector are then inserted through the main axillary incision port, and the Harmonic curved shears are placed at the second axillary incision port in a right-side approach. (d) The superior thyroid vessels are cut individually close to the thyroid gland, using Harmonic curved shears, to preserve the external branch of the superior laryngeal nerve. (e) The thyroid gland is then retracted medially, and the paratracheal lymph nodes and perithyroidal soft tissue are dissected while preserving the whole course of the recurrent laryngeal nerve. (f) The surgical view after the thyroid lobectomy is shown.

to use three robotic instruments simultaneously and enables fine motion scaling, hand-tremor filtering, innovative instrumentation with extended freedom of motion, and surgical education [1]. The use of a third robotic instrument is very important for obtaining counter-traction that can facilitate dissection and improve surgical dexterity.

However, remote access thyroidectomy also has several disadvantages. It is not a minimally invasive surgery in terms of skin flap elevation for creating a working space, nor is it a maximally invasive surgery, but it requires a wide dissection area to reach the thyroid gland. Nonetheless, the thyroidectomy procedure itself is as refined as the conventional method [1]. Also, some patients have complained of asymmetric and band-like contractures of the neck, anterior chest, and axillary areas that might be caused by fibrotic contractures of soft tissue and muscles [20,21].

Bilateral and total thyroidectomies are rather difficult via unilateral facelift and transaxillary approaches, although lobectomy can be done easily using these approaches [1]. However, lobectomy is currently recommended for small, low-risk thyroid cancers; hence, this could provide a rationale for surgeons to consider facelift and transaxillary approaches [22].

The high cost of robotic thyroid surgery is another major drawback. Also, it is a technically difficult procedure with a steep learning curve that presents an issue in terms of patient safety. Moreover,

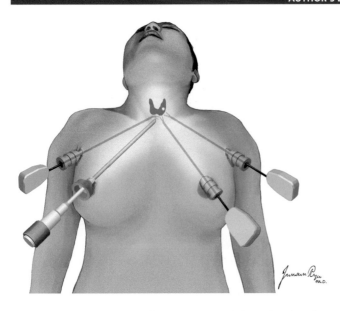

Figure 11.2 The bilateral axillo-breast approach (BABA) with carbon dioxide (CO_2) insufflation. Four skin incisions are made: two in the areola and one in each of the two axillary areas. (Reproduced from Tae et al. *Clin Exp Otorhinolaryngol* 2019;12:1–11.)

the operative time of a robotic thyroidectomy is significantly longer than that of a conventional thyroidectomy due to the longer flap dissection time and the time needed for robot docking [23–26].

SALIENT POINTS

- Of remote access robotic and endoscopic thyroidectomy techniques, transaxillary, BABA, postauricular facelift, and transoral approaches are commonly used today.
- The various approaches have their own advantages and disadvantages. Therefore, we need to understand the advantages and limitations of each.
- Remote access thyroidectomy is feasible and comparable to conventional thyroidectomy in highly selective patients.
- Strict patient selection criteria are important for the patient's safety and the success of the surgery.
- The most important advantage of remote access thyroidectomy is its excellent cosmesis.
- Disadvantages of remote access thyroidectomy include the invasiveness needed to create the working space, longer operative time, higher cost, and technical difficulty.

AUTHOR'S EXPERIENCE

Of the four common remote access thyroidectomy techniques (the gasless transaxillary approach, BABA, the gasless postauricular facelift approach, and the transoral vestibular approach), the author has used the gasless transaxillary, postauricular, and transoral approaches for thyroidectomies since 2005 [6–11,18,19,27]. Each of the four most common remote access thyroidectomy procedures has its own advantages and disadvantages as shown in Table 11.2 [1]. Therefore, it is difficult to conclude which approach is best.

Generally, CO_2 insufflation methods have the advantage of exposing and maintaining the working space following a small skin incision made in a remote access site beyond the neck [1]. Therefore, post-operative cosmesis may be better, potentially, than when using gasless methods that require long skin incisions at a remote site. However, CO_2 insufflation can result in CO_2-related complications such as subcutaneous emphysema, hypercapnia, respiratory acidosis, cerebral edema, and CO_2 embolisms although there is a low risk of an adverse event if pressure levels of 4 to 6 mmHg are used [28]. Gasless methods have the advantage of maintaining a clear surgical view without gas fumes and the absence of complications related to CO_2 insufflation. They also enable surgeons to use instruments employed in a conventional thyroidectomy to dissect skin flaps and control bleeding [1]. Also, surgical view clarity is greater with gasless methods, such as the gasless transaxillary and facelift approaches, than in the BABA and transoral approaches [1].

Surgical invasiveness related to skin flap elevation is greatest in the BABA and transaxillary approach, and least in the transoral approach. However, the working space is widest in the transaxillary approach, making it easy to place and manipulate three robotic or endoscopic instruments. Meanwhile, the BABA and transoral approach make it easier to perform total thyroidectomy than the transaxillary and facelift approaches. Especially, the working space of the facelift approach is narrow, and it is very difficult to approach the contralateral thyroid lobe via the unilateral incision [18]. The latter permits one to perform a selective lateral neck dissection; a central neck dissection can be performed in all four approaches. However, this is relatively difficult in the BABA due to an inadequate angle of approach. Post-operative cosmesis is very good in all the procedures.

Although there are many reports of the feasibility and safety of remote access thyroidectomy, complication rates are potentially higher, especially during the learning curve and when performed by low-volume surgeons, because of the challenging surgical techniques. In meta-analyses, rates of complications such as RLN paralysis and hypoparathyroidism were not significantly different in robotic and conventional thyroidectomies [23–26]. However, in subgroup analyses, transient RLN paralysis was higher in the robotic procedure than in the conventional procedure [24]. Also, there can be serious complications such as injury to the esophagus and trachea, compromised airways due to hematomas, and, in rare instances, serious CO_2 embolisms [28].

Unusual complications can also occur. For instance, a transient brachial plexus injury has been reported in the robotic transaxillary approach. Also, the marginal branch of the facial nerve can be injured in the postauricular facelift approach, possibly as a result of a robotic instrument compressing the nerve at the narrow postauricular port [18]. Mental nerve injuries can also occur in the transoral approach.

Therefore, strict patient selection criteria are needed for successful surgical outcomes. The safety of patients must be the first priority, especially during the steep learning curve. Also, an appropriate training program for surgeons is required [29]. Furthermore, the possibility of converting to an open procedure should always be discussed with patients before surgery.

Cosmetic excellence is the main reason patients and surgeons choose robotic and endoscopic thyroidectomy approaches. Cosmetic outcomes are indeed superior in robotic and endoscopic thyroidectomies than in conventional surgeries [7,26]. Long-term cosmetic satisfaction after scar maturation is also significantly greater in the transaxillary approach than in a conventional thyroidectomy [19].

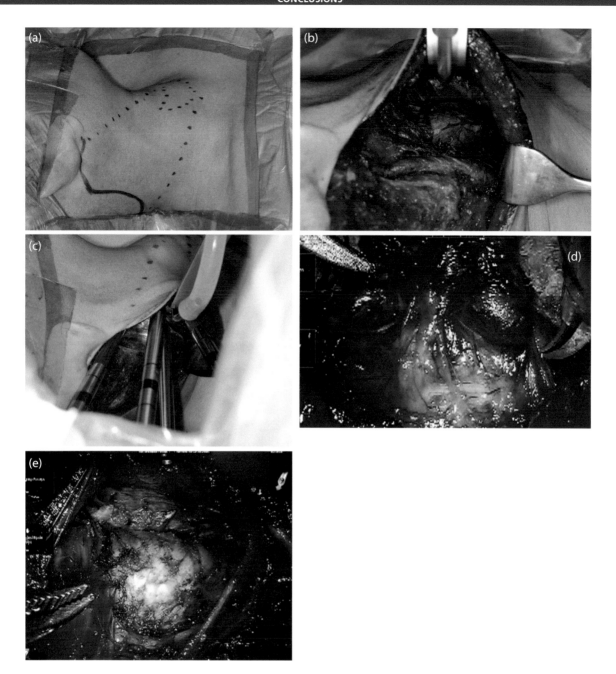

Figure 11.3 The postauricular facelift approach. (a) A skin incision is made in the postauricular sulcus, curved posteriorly at the upper third of the auricle, and continued along the occipital hairline. (b) The skin flap is elevated in the sub-platysmal plane over the sternocleidomastoid (SCM) muscle under direct vision to expose the thyroid glands. (c) A 30° endoscope and three robotic instruments including Maryland dissectors, Prograsp forceps, and Harmonic curved shears are inserted through the postauricular incision. (d) The recurrent laryngeal nerve (RLN) is identified in the tracheoesophageal groove and preserved. (e) Thyroid lobectomy with isthmusectomy is complete.

The oncologic outcome is an important issue in the treatment of thyroid cancer and should not be neglected or overlooked in favor of cosmesis or functional outcomes. However, the literature on oncologic outcomes, such as locoregional recurrences and disease survival after robotic or endoscopic thyroidectomy, is very limited. In some studies, oncologic outcomes, including disease-specific survival and recurrence rates, were not significantly different in robotic transaxillary or conventional thyroidectomies, although the follow-up periods were rather short [30,31]. Further studies with long-term follow-ups and large patient samples are needed to assess the ultimate long-term oncologic outcomes of remote access robotic and endoscopic thyroidectomy.

CONCLUSIONS

A robotic and endoscopic thyroidectomy using a remote access approach is feasible and offers a comparable outcome to a conventional transcervical thyroidectomy in highly selective patients; it also yields excellent cosmesis. However, it has disadvantages in terms of surgical invasiveness for the working space, longer operative times, higher costs, and technical difficulties. Strict patient selection criteria are very important. We also need to understand the advantages and limitations of various types of remote access thyroidectomies.

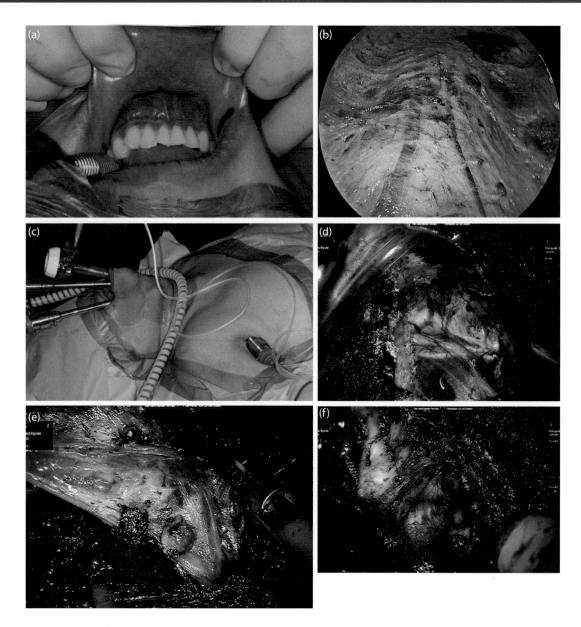

Figure 11.4 The transoral vestibular approach with carbon dioxide (CO_2) insufflation. (a) A 1.5 to 2 cm horizontal incision is made at the end of the lower lip frenulum, and two lateral incisions are made close to the oral commissure to avoid mental nerve injury. (b) A working space is created in the plane of the sub-platysmal layer by endoscopy without a surgical robot to the level of the sternal notch inferiorly and the SCM muscle laterally. (c) After creating a working space, a 30° robotic endoscope and two robotic instruments, such as bipolar Maryland forceps and monopolar scissors, are placed on either side of the endoscope, and Cardinal forceps are inserted through the right axillary port. (d) The midline fascia between the strap muscles is divided and the sternohyoid and sternothyroid muscles are dissected to expose the thyroid gland. (e) The dissection of the superior pole is performed while preserving the superior parathyroid gland. (f) Thyroid lobectomy with isthmusectomy is complete while preserving the recurrent laryngeal nerve (RLN).

Table 11.2 Comparison of remote access thyroidectomies

	Gasless axillary	BABA	Gasless facelift	Transoral
Invasiveness needed for working space	++++	++++	+++	++
Manipulability of instruments in working space	++++	+++	+++	+++
Operative time	+++	++++	+++	+++
Clarity of surgical view	++++	+++	++++	+++
Applicability of total thyroidectomy	++	+++	+	+++
Applicability of central neck dissection	+++	++	+++	+++
Applicability of lateral neck dissection	++++	++	++++	+/−
Cosmetic satisfaction	+++	++++	+++	++++
Complication rate	+	+	+	+

Source: Reproduced from Tae et al. *Clin Exp Otorhinolaryngol* 2019;12:1–11.
Abbreviation: BABA; Bilateral axillo-breast approach.

REFERENCES

1. Tae K, Ji YB, Song CM, Ryu JS. Robotic and endoscopic thyroid surgery: Evolution and advances. *Clin Exp Otorhinolaryngol.* 2019;12:1–11.

2. Huscher CS, Chiodini S, Napolitano C, Recher A. Endoscopic right thyroid lobectomy. *Surg Endosc.* 1997;11:877.

3. Miccoli P, Berti P, Conte M, Bendinelli C, Marcocci C. Minimally invasive surgery for thyroid small nodules: Preliminary report. *J Endocrinol Invest.* 1999;22:849–51.

4. Ikeda Y, Takami H, Sasaki Y, Kan S, Niimi M. Endoscopic neck surgery by the axillary approach. *J Am Coll Surg.* 2000;191:336–40.

5. Yoon JH, Park CH, Chung WY. Gasless endoscopic thyroidectomy via an axillary approach: Experience of 30 cases. *Surg Laparosc Endosc Percutan Tech.* 2006;16:226–31.

6. Tae K, Ji YB, Cho SH, Kim KR, Kim DW, Kim DS. Initial experience with a gasless unilateral axillo-breast or axillary approach endoscopic thyroidectomy for papillary thyroid microcarcinoma: Comparison with conventional open thyroidectomy. *Surg Laparosc Endosc Percutan Tech.* 2011;21:162–9.

7. Tae K, Ji YB, Jeong JH, Lee SH, Jeong MA, Park CW. Robotic thyroidectomy by a gasless unilateral axillo-breast or axillary approach: Our early experiences. *Surg Endosc.* 2011;25:221–8.

8. Tae K, Ji YB, Cho SH, Lee SH, Kim DS, Kim TW. Early surgical outcomes of robotic thyroidectomy by a gasless unilateral axillo-breast or axillary approach for papillary thyroid carcinoma: 2 years' experience. *Head Neck.* 2012;34:617–25.

9. Tae K, Song CM, Ji YB, Kim KR, Kim JY, Choi YY. Comparison of surgical completeness between robotic total thyroidectomy versus open thyroidectomy. *Laryngoscope.* 2014 Apr;124(4):1042–7.

10. Tae K et al. Functional voice and swallowing outcomes after robotic thyroidectomy by a gasless unilateral axillo-breast approach: Comparison with open thyroidectomy. *Surg Endosc.* 2012;26:1871–7.

11. Song CM, Cho YH, Ji YB, Jeong JH, Kim DS, Tae K. Comparison of a gasless unilateral axillo-breast and axillary approach in robotic thyroidectomy. *Surg Endosc.* 2013 Oct;27(10):3769–75.

12. Ohgami M et al. Scarless endoscopic thyroidectomy: Breast approach for better cosmesis. *Surg Laparosc Endosc Percutan Tech.* 2000;10:1–4.

13. Choe JH et al. Endoscopic thyroidectomy using a new bilateral axillo-breast approach. *World J Surg.* 2007;31:601–6.

14. Terris DJ, Singer MC, Seybt MW. Robotic facelift thyroidectomy: II. Clinical feasibility and safety. *Laryngoscope.* 2011;121:1636–41.

15. Wilhelm T, Metzig A. Endoscopic minimally invasive thyroidectomy (eMIT): A prospective proof-of-concept study in humans. *World J Surg.* 2011;35(3):543–51.

16. Wang C et al. Thyroidectomy: A novel endoscopic oral vestibular approach. *Surgery.* 2014;155:33–8.

17. Anuwong A. Transoral endoscopic thyroidectomy vestibular approach: A series of the first 60 human cases. *World J Surg.* 2016;40(3):491–7.

18. Sung ES, Ji YB, Song CM, Yun BR, Chung WS, Tae K. Robotic thyroidectomy: Comparison of a postauricular facelift approach with a gasless unilateral axillary approach. *Otolaryngol Head Neck Surg.* 2016;154:997–1004.

19. Ji YB, Song CM, Bang HS, Lee SH, Park YS, Tae K. Long-term cosmetic outcomes after robotic/endoscopic thyroidectomy by a gasless unilateral axillo-breast or axillary approach. *J Laparoendosc Adv Surg Tech A.* 2014;24:248–53.

20. Kwak DH, Kim WS, Kim HK, Bae TH. A band-like neck scar contracture after bilateral axillo-breast approach robotic thyroidectomy. *Arch Plast Surg.* 2016 Nov;43(6):614–5.

21. Kim JH, Park JW, Gong HS. Axillary web syndrome after transaxillary robotic thyroidectomy. *J Robot Surg.* 2014 Sep;8(3):281–3.

22. Berber E et al. American Thyroid Association statement on remote-access thyroid surgery. *Thyroid.* 2016;26:331–7.

23. Jackson NR, Yao L, Tufano RP, Kandil EH. Safety of robotic thyroidectomy approaches: Meta-analysis and systematic review. *Head Neck.* 2014;36:137–43.

24. Lang BH, Wong CK, Tsang JS, Wong KP, Wan KY. A systematic review and meta-analysis comparing surgically-related complications between robotic-assisted thyroidectomy and conventional open thyroidectomy. *Ann Surg Oncol.* 2014 Mar;21(3):850–61.

25. Kandil E et al. Robotic thyroidectomy versus nonrobotic approaches: A meta-analysis examining surgical outcomes. *Surg Innov.* 2016 Jun;23(3):317–25.

26. Sun GH, Peress L, Pynnonen MA. Systematic review and meta-analysis of robotic vs conventional thyroidectomy approaches for thyroid disease. *Otolaryngol Head Neck Surg.* 2014 Apr;150(4):520–32.

27. Tae K et al. Early experience of transoral thyroidectomy: Comparison of robotic and endoscopic procedures. *Head Neck.* 2019 Mar;41(3):730–8.

28. Kim KN, Lee DW, Kim JY, Han KH, Tae K. Carbon dioxide embolism during transoral robotic thyroidectomy: A case report. *Head Neck.* 2018 Mar;40(3):E25–8.

29. Perrier ND, Randolph GW, Inabnet WB, Marple BF, VanHeerden J, Kuppersmith RB. Robotic thyroidectomy: A framework for new technology assessment and safe implementation. *Thyroid.* 2010 Dec;20(12):1327–32.

30. Tae K, Song CM, Ji YB, Sung ES, Jeong JH, Kim DS. Oncologic outcomes of robotic thyroidectomy: 5-year experience with propensity score matching. *Surg Endosc.* 2016 Nov;30(11):4785–92.

31. Lee SG et al. Long-term oncologic outcome of robotic versus open total thyroidectomy in PTC: A case-matched retrospective study. *Surg Endosc.* 2016 Aug;30(8):3474–9.

Chapter 12

ROBOTIC THYROIDECTOMY

Neil S. Tolley and Christian Camenzuli

CONTENTS

Introduction   91
Indications and Contraindications   91
Concluding Remarks   95
Authors' Experience and Pearls of Wisdom   95
References   95

INTRODUCTION

Minimally invasive access thyroid surgery has been around for more than a decade. Initially this took the form of endoscopic procedures that were reported as early as 1997 [1]. These procedures offered a magnified view for safer dissection and also moved the incision away from the neck developing the concept of remote-access thyroid surgery in an attempt to improve cosmetic results. Endoscopic thyroidectomy was, however, a challenging operation offering significant limitations in terms of hand-to-eye coordination because of the 2D nature of the image, unstable image due to assistant-held endoscopes, unsuitable instrumentation (often using laparoscopic instruments), limited range of motion, and line of site access. All of these made fine dissection difficult. Most endoscopic techniques also require the need for carbon dioxide insufflation to keep the working space opened. This has been associated with a number of adverse outcomes including air embolism, hypercapnia, and respiratory acidosis.

The robotic approach to thyroid surgery was pioneered by Chung and colleagues in 2007 using the da Vinci® Surgical System robot platform (Intuitive Surgical, Sunnyvale, California) [2]. The introduction of the robotic system has provided solutions to the limitations inherent with endoscopic techniques. The robot offers a stable magnified 3D image and offers the surgeon seven degrees of freedom by virtue of using endowristed instrumentation. Most of the present robotic techniques also eliminate the need for carbon dioxide insufflation. These advantages make robotic thyroidectomy a favorable option for patients concerned about their scar or those patients that have an inherent biological predisposition to keloid and hypertrophic scarring.

INDICATIONS AND CONTRAINDICATIONS

Robotic thyroidectomy can be performed using several established and developing techniques that will be discussed in the next section. Common to all techniques are a set of selection criteria that should be followed to ensure best possible outcomes.

Patients who are either very concerned about having a visible scar in the neck or else who have a history of adverse healing (e.g., keloids) could be considered. The ideal candidate for a robotic procedure is not obese since this presents increased difficulty and is associated with longer operative time. However, this is only a relative contraindication. Increasingly, patients with high body mass index (BMI) are being accepted owing to improved instrumentation and surgical expertise. Another anatomical consideration is having good neck mobility, which is important for positioning. Patients with a history of previous surgery or radiotherapy to the neck should not be offered this surgery.

Tumors that are small (≤ 4 cm) and do not extend beyond the thyroid capsule are ideal for a robotic approach. With increasing experience this has, however, become a relative contraindication since robotic thyroidectomy can be extended to include neck dissection for nodal metastases [3]. Anaplastic thyroid cancer and cancers that are invading surrounding structures are not appropriate for this procedure. The presence of thyroiditis around the tumor increases the difficulty of dissection and therefore is considered a relative contraindication.

Thyroid surgery in Graves' disease is challenging and robotic thyroidectomy was not initially considered a suitable treatment. This view has largely changed over the years with most surgeons accepting this indication for the robotic approach. Caution needs to be applied when embarking on robotic surgery in patients with advanced Graves' disease, especially in the hands of the inexperienced [4]. Substernal extension of the goiter is considered an absolute contraindication.

TECHNIQUE

Throughout the years several different approaches have been used to perform robotic thyroidectomy. This section will review the principle operative steps of the commonly used techniques and discuss the advantages and limitations of each.

TRANS-AXILLARY APPROACH

This was the first approach used for robotic thyroidectomy. After general anesthesia is achieved, the patient is placed in a supine position with the neck extended. The contralateral arm is tucked on the side of the patient. The ipsilateral upper limb is elevated with the shoulder internally rotated. The elbow is then flexed with the back of the hand resting on the central forehead (the salute position), making sure there is appropriate support and padding. Improper positioning of the arm can lead to nerve injury, and therefore some groups routinely use peripheral nerve monitors in an attempt to avoid this complication. It is strongly recommended that the arm is not placed in forced extension due to brachial plexus tension.

The incision line is then marked. A line is drawn from the thyroid cartilage to the anterior axillary line and from the sternal notch to the anterior axillary line. An incision of around 5 cm will take place between these markings on the lateral border of pectoralis major. It is important that the patient is marked prior to surgery so that an optimal site for the incision is chosen; otherwise the incision can extend onto the upper arm.

After the incision, dissection is carried out subcutaneously and a flap superficial to the pectoralis major fascia is developed. This dissection continues until the anterior aspect of the sternocleidomastoid muscle is encountered as far as the sternal notch. At this point the avascular plane between the sternal and clavicular heads of the sternocleidomastoid is identified and dissected leading to the separation of the two heads and exposure of the thyroid lobe. Dissection should proceed at least to the external jugular vein and often posterior to this. This permits less tension on the superior flap which might otherwise interfere with the optimal function of the robotic instruments. This occurs as a consequence of lateral pressure on the trocars that is transmitted to the cogs of the robotic arm which control the unique motion to the endowristed instruments. The omohyoid, which is a landmark for the superior pole of the thyroid lobe, is retracted cranially but usually divided. The strap muscles are dissected off the thyroid lobe. It is important to divide the inferior and superior attachments of the sternothyroid muscle. If a hemithyroidectomy is being performed, the strap muscles are raised to the contralateral third of the thyroid lobe. A self-retaining retracting device with integrated suction (Modena or Chung) is then introduced. The authors' preference is for the Modena, which is far better engineered. This device should be assembled from the contralateral side and placed below the sternal head of the sternocleidomastoid and strap muscles to keep the operating space exposed. The robot is then docked. The camera arm and instrument arms should be positioned to allow maximum mobility without clashing of the other robotic arms. The camera arm should be placed first at an angle of 220°. The camera endoscope should be inserted to its maximum travel before insertion into the space. The 8- or 12-mm 30°-down endoscope should be placed low laterally and high medially at the site of the thyroid. The two operator arms are then inserted low and laterally for similar reasons and technique. Finally, the fourth retractor arm is placed superiorly along the camera endoscope (Figure 12.1). Space does not permit a large degree of movement when using this arm. As dissection proceeds it can often be removed altogether to facilitate a greater operating space. In terms of robotic instrumentation, the 5 mm Maryland dissector is loaded on the non-dominant hand and an energy-sealing device (e.g., Harmonic® Ethicon Endo-surgery, Cincinnati, Ohio) on the dominant hand. The 8 mm bipolar forceps have been found to be gentler and more versatile than the Prograsp forceps. The author prefers to conduct dissection with the 5 mm DeBakey and 5 mm Maryland instruments before using the 5 mm Harmonic instrument (Figure 12.1). This allows precise delineation of the recurrent laryngeal nerve (RLN) and parathyroid glands. Intra-operative neural monitoring is used as a standard of care. The Harmonic instrument employs old C14 harmonic technology that can safely seal vessels up to 3 mm. It has the disadvantage of not being endowristed—a significant handicap. A Ligasure® 8 mm instrument, which is endowristed, is available but it can only seal and not cut. It is bulky and inferior to the Harmonic instrument in the authors' opinion. The operating table assistant has the role of supplying the console surgeon with cotton pledgets during dissection, changing these as appropriate, and providing compression of structures such as the internal jugular vein. The assistant is also tasked with providing arm-resets if clashes occur and ensuring that the instruments or arms are not harming patient structures out of the console operative field of the surgeon. Furthermore, the assistant is utilized to troubleshoot problems that may occur with the robotic instruments and employ the nerve stimulator probe where required.

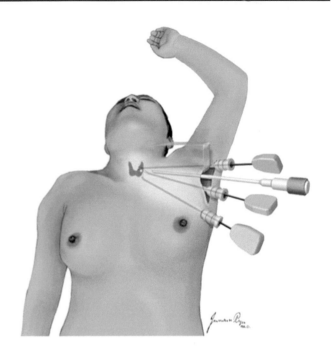

Figure 12.1 Positions of robotic arms, camera, and retractor in transaxillary approach. (Reproduced with permission from Tae K et al. *Clin Exp Otorhinolaryngol.* 2019 Feb;12(1):1–11.)

After identifying the RLN and parathyroid glands, the superior pole vessels are identified and divided. The same approach and care is taken to identify and preserve the external laryngeal nerve as in any standard lateral approach thyroidectomy.

The superior thyroid pole is approached by using the 8 mm bipolar forceps to retract the pole caudally and medially. The Maryland and Harmonic devices are used to dissect, seal, and divide the superior thyroid vessels. The nerve stimulator probe is used to make sure there is a safe distance between the external branch of the superior laryngeal nerve and the vessels before sealing. The superior parathyroid should be identified and dissected and the upper pole separated from the cricothyroid muscle. The bipolar forceps is now adjusted to provide more medial retraction of the thyroid lobe. The RLN is followed superiorly to the laryngeal entry point. Nerve stimulation is regularly employed during dissection, and attention needs to be paid with regard to heat generation by the Harmonic instruments and traction of the RLN if it should pass through Berry's ligament. The inferior parathyroid is identified and dissected off the thyroid. The inferior thyroid vessels are dissected, sealed, and transected as intracapsular dissection of the thyroid lobe proceeds. Dissection progresses medial to the nerve using the Maryland dissector and sealing device to dissect the thyroid off the trachea. The isthmus is then divided using the sealing device, and the thyroid is retrieved. If the operation performed is a total thyroidectomy (TT), the strap muscles have to be fully dissected off, the thyroid lobe. Where indicated, it is the authors' preference to approach thyroidectomy from the right side due to the more oblique and vertical course of the RLNs on the right and left side respectively. The superior pole vessels are divided in addition to the inferior and middle thyroid veins. The assistant retracts the trachea medially to facilitate this. Dissection of the contralateral lobe off the trachea then proceeds to mobilize this lobe. Dissection continues between the trachea and thyroid until the contralateral tracheoesophageal groove is reached. The RLN is then identified and confirmed with the nerve stimulator and dissection continues until the thyroid is free and retrieved. After meticulous hemostasis, all instrumentation is removed. A drain is not necessary and the authors' preference is not to use one. Some surgeons routinely drain after this procedure as the amount of subcutaneous dissection amounts to three times that compared to a traditional cervical approach. Skin is closed with subcuticular absorbable sutures and dermabond [5].

Specific complications associated with this approach include chest wall paresthesia due the extensive dissection to develop the flap, pressure from the retractor, and brachial plexus neuropathy. This approach is relatively contraindicated for patients with a history of chest wall or axillary surgery and patients who suffer from conditions that limit their shoulder mobility such as arthritis or rotator cuff injury [6].

AXILLO-BREAST APPROACH

The site and size of the axillary wound used in the transaxillary approach have received criticism because despite being an improvement from a cervical incision, an axillary wound cannot always be covered with clothing and therefore still leads to a visible scar. The axillo-bilateral breast approach (ABBA) was the original procedure developed to try to decrease the size of axillary wound. This has now been largely superseded by a further modification known as bilateral axillo-breast approach (BABA). These approaches minimize the axillary scar, and the peri-areolar scars typically heal nicely and are easily covered by clothing.

In the BABA approach, after general anesthesia, the patient is placed in the supine position with a pillow under the shoulders. The arms are kept by the patient's side. Guidelines are then drawn marking the thyroid cartilage notch, cricoid cartilage, suprasternal notch, midline, the anterior border of the sternocleidomastoid muscle bilaterally, superior border of the clavicle, and 2 cm below the border. The incisions of around 8 mm in length are also marked in both axillae and peri-areolar lines. Trajectory lines are then marked from the incision sites to the cricoid cartilage. These guides are important to direct the operating space, which should be limited to the thyroid cartilage cranially, sternocleidomastoid muscles laterally, and 2 cm below the clavicles caudally. The operating space is then injected with diluted adrenaline (1:200,000) below the platysma, which helps to hydrodissect the area and facilitate raising of the flap. A 12 mm circumareolar incision is carried out on the right nipple. A mixture of diathermy and blunt dissection (using a vascular tunneler) is used to develop a subcutaneous narrow tunnel to the working zone. An 8 mm circumareolar incision is made in the left nipple and similar dissection is carried out. Ports are inserted and a low pressure (5 to 6 mmHg) carbon dioxide insufflation is temporarily instituted. The remaining space is dissected using an energy sealing device under endoscopic view (camera inserted through the 12 mm port). An 8 mm incision is carried out in each axilla at this point. The robot is then docked inserting the camera through the right areola and an energy sealing device arm through the left areola. Prograsp forceps and Maryland dissector are inserted through the axillary ports and the remainder of the operating space is developed (Figure 12.2).

The linea alba cervicalis is divided at this point which separates the strap muscles. The isthmus is divided centrally along its whole length using the energy sealing device exposing the trachea. The lobe being dissected is at this point retracted medially with the Prograsp forceps whilst the straps are retracted laterally with the Maryland dissector. Lateral dissection is carried out to expose the thyroid lobe in its entirety.

The dissection then continues infero-laterally. The identification of the inferior thyroid artery is an important landmark to the identification of the RLN. The use of blunt dissection helps to avoid damage to the nerve while developing the plane. Intra-operative neuromonitoring is also possible with this robotic approach. The inferior parathyroid gland is identified and dissected away from the thyroid lobe. The inferior vessels are dissected, sealed, and divided. The dissection continues

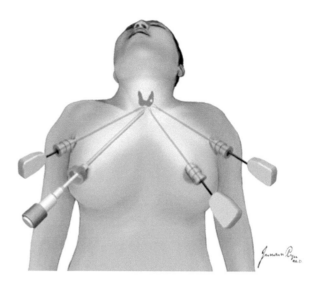

Figure 12.2 Positions of robotic arms and camera in BABA. (Reproduced with permission from Tae K et al. *Clin Exp Otorhinolaryngol.* 2019 Feb;12(1):1–11.)

superficially to the RLN and cranially releasing Berry's ligament. The superior pole is then dissected using one of the following three approaches: lateral, antero-medial, or postero-medial. Care should be given to leave the cricothyroid fascia intact and therefore protect the external laryngeal nerve. The superior parathyroid gland should also be dissected and preserved. When the specimen is free, it is put in an endobag and extracted through the left axillary port which might need to be extended. In a total thyroidectomy, dissection continues in a similar fashion on the other side.

At completion, the operative field is washed with warm saline and hemostasis is achieved. The midline raphe is closed with an absorbable continuous suture. If drains are required they are inserted through the axillary ports. The skin is closed with absorbable subcuticular sutures [7].

RETROAURICULAR APPROACH

This was described in 2011 by Terris and colleagues using the standard incision used for facelift and parotid surgery [8]. After general anesthesia, the patient is positioned supine with the head slightly tilted to the opposite side. The incision site is marked in the retroauricular space extending from the posterior auricular sulcus down to the mastoid along the hairline. After the incision, a subcutaneous dissection is performed exposing the sternocleidomastoid. During this part of the dissection care is taken to avoid damage to the greater auricular nerve and the marginal branch of the facial nerve. Dissection continues subplatysmally, exposing the strap muscles down to the sternal notch. The dissection should continue by opening the strap muscles and clearing the connective tissue to expose the thyroid gland. A self-retaining retractor is fixed in a position that retracts the strap muscles. The robot is docked with the Maryland dissector and energy sealing device controlled by the non-dominant and dominant hand respectively (Figure 12.3).

The superior thyroid pole is retracted antero-inferiorly using the Prograsp forceps arm and the superior thyroid vessels are identified, sealed, and transected. The superior parathyroid should then be identified and dissected off the thyroid gland in order to preserve it. The lobe is now retracted medially and the RLN identified through careful dissection. The nerve needs to be dissected up to the laryngeal insertion point. A safe space needs to be created between the nerve and the thyroid gland. The inferior parathyroid should be identified and dissected away from the thyroid gland. The inferior

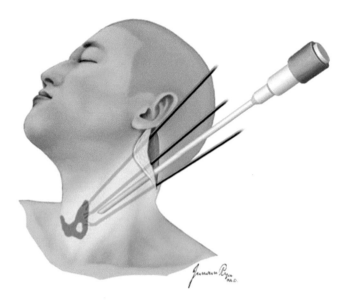

Figure 12.3 Positions of robotic arms and camera in retroauricular approach. (Reproduced with permission from Tae K et al. *Clin Exp Otorhinolaryngol.* 2019 Feb;12(1):1–11.)

thyroid vessels are identified, sealed, and transected. The thyroid lobe is then dissected off the trachea and the isthmus divided. Once free, the thyroid is delivered through the retroauricular incision. If required, a drain can be inserted. The subcutaneous tissue is closed with interrupted absorbable sutures and the skin is closed with subcutaneous absorbable suture.

The main disadvantage of this approach is that only a unilateral lobectomy can be performed. The approach itself is more comfortable for ENT surgeons who are trained in parotid surgery and are familiar with the relevant anatomy. Compared to the transaxillary and BABA approaches, subcutaneous dissection is significantly less in this approach. This may reduce operation time and infection risk [9].

TRANSORAL APPROACH

Transoral robotic thyroidectomy is the latest reported technique. The transoral endoscopic thyroidectomy through a vestibular approach (TOETVA) was pioneered by Anuwong in 2016 [10]. The anesthetized patient is placed in the supine position with slight neck extension. Three incisions are carried out in the gingival-buccal sulcus of the lower lip: a 2 cm incision in the midline around 1 cm above the frenulum and two 6 mm incision lateral and anterior to the inferior canines. Blunt dissection is used through the central incision until the periosteum of the chin is reached. Diluted adrenaline (1:500,000) is injected subplatysmally for hydro-dissection. Blunt development of the subplatysmal plane is carried out down to the sternal notch. Similar dissection is carried out through the lateral incisions. The robot is docked at this point with the camera in the midline, the Maryland dissector on the left, and energy sealing device on the right. Carbon dioxide insufflation at a low pressure (5 to 6 mmHg) is used to maintain the operative space (Figure 12.4).

The linea alba cervicalis is opened and the strap muscles are dissected off the thyroid lobe. The isthmus is divided centrally. The superior pole is dissected carefully with identification, sealing, and transection of the superior thyroid vessels. The superior parathyroid gland is identified and dissected off the thyroid lobe. The lobe is subsequently retracted inferiorly and the RLN identified. Nerve stimulator devices can be used to confirm nerve integrity. The nerve is dissected up to its insertion into the larynx. Berry's ligament is then divided with the dissection continuing caudally. The inferior parathyroid should be identified and dissected off. The

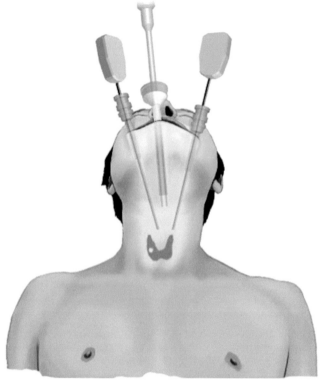

Figure 12.4 Positions of robotic arms and camera in TOETVA. (Reproduced with permission from Tae K et al. *Clin Exp Otorhinolaryngol.* 2019 Feb;12(1):1–11.)

inferior thyroid vessels are identified, sealed, and transected. If the operation is a total thyroidectomy, identical dissection takes place on the contralateral side. When the thyroid is free, it is extracted in an endobag through the central port. The strap muscles are closed with a continuous absorbable suture. The buccal mucosa is closed with an interrupted absorbable suture [11].

This technique is being hailed by some as the ultimate solution for minimally invasive thyroid surgery. It promises a scarless technique and limits the dissecting space due to the close proximity to the thyroid gland [12]. The use of robotic equipment has overcome the main obstacle of a restricted working space. The procedure has been associated with chin hypoesthesia due to mental nerve damage and flap perforation. It also utilizes gas insufflation to maintain the operating space open with well-documented complications.

SALIENT POINTS

- Strict inclusion and exclusion criteria are important to ensure favorable patient outcomes.
- There are different approaches to robotic thyroidectomy having advantages and disadvantages.
- Robotic thyroidectomy is safe for low risk and favorable prognosis cancer.
- It offers superior cosmetic results when compared to the conventional cervical approach.

OUTCOMES

Any surgical procedure on the thyroid gland must be compared with the gold standard of conventional open thyroidectomy for safety, completeness of resection in oncological cases, and patient satisfaction.

The evidence accumulated so far has shown that robotic thyroidectomy is safe with similar complication rates to conventional surgery. Robotic procedures take longer than open procedures and have a significant increased cost compared to conventional surgery [13]. Excellent outcomes have also been replicated in patients undergoing robotic thyroidectomy for Graves' disease [14].

The value of robotic thyroidectomy has also been evaluated in low-risk excellent prognosis thyroid cancer. Studies reveal that robotic thyroidectomy is as safe as conventional thyroid surgery for thyroid cancer with similar rates of R0 resections and recurrence rates [15].

The advantage of robotic thyroidectomy is purely cosmetic, which is closely related to patient satisfaction. While all the other outcomes are comparable between the two techniques, the scale is heavily tipped toward robotic techniques when it comes to cosmetic outcome [13,16].

CONCLUDING REMARKS

Robotic surgery, despite its current controversial status, has nonetheless existed in standard surgical practice for more than 10 years, being used in thousands of patients worldwide. Robotic techniques will continue to evolve and the Lindy effect supports the premise that it is now firmly established within the surgical armamentarium. Advances in technology and competition will make it safer, easier, and cheaper to use, which will lead to a larger number of surgeons and institutions adopting robotic techniques—the Rogers adoption phenomenon. It is very likely that the indications and procedures amenable for a robotic approach will expand in the future. Single port robotic platforms launched in 2019 offer exciting potential for the robotic thyroid surgeon.

AUTHORS' EXPERIENCE AND PEARLS OF WISDOM

As a cautionary note, robotic thyroid surgery is not suitable for every surgeon or institution. It should only be undertaken by surgeons with a high-volume practice to provide a suitable case load to maintain skills, expertise, and justify the time and cost involved. Its adoption should only be considered after a surgeon has attained expert status in conventional thyroid surgery.

Mandatory training, proctorship, audit, appraisal, and credentialing are required to ensure that this technology is introduced into their practice carefully, responsibly, and for the right reasons.

Neil Tolley pioneered robotic thyroid and parathyroid surgery in the U.K. using the transaxillary robotic approach.

REFERENCES

1. Hüscher CS, Chiodini S, Napolitano C, Recher A. Endoscopic right thyroid lobectomy. *Surg Endosc*. 1997;11(8):877.

2. Kang S et al. Robot-assisted endoscopic surgery for thyroid cancer: Experience with the first 100 patients. *Surg Endosc*. 2009;23(11):2399–2406.

3. Paek SH, Kang KH, Park SJ. Expanding indications of robotic thyroidectomy. *Surg Endosc*. 2018;32(8):3480–3485.

4. Aidan P, Pickburn H, Monpeyssen H, Boccara G. Indications for the gasless transaxillary robotic approach to thyroid surgery: Experience of forty-seven procedures at the American Hospital of Paris. *Eur Thyroid J*. 2013;2(2):102–109.

5. Alzahrani HA, Mohsin K, Ali DB, Murad F, Kandil E. Gasless trans-axillary robotic thyroidectomy: The technique and evidence. *Gland Surg*. 2017;6(3):236–242.

6. Patel D, Kebebew E. Pros and cons of robotic transaxillary thyroidectomy. *Thyroid*. 2012;22(10):984–985.

7. Koo DH, Bae DS, Choi JY. Bilateral axillo-breast approach robotic thyroidectomy: Introduction and update. *Surgical Robotics*. 2017: doi:10.5772/intechopen.68951.

8. Terris DJ, Singer MC, Seybt MW. Robotic facelift thyroidectomy: II. Clinical feasibility and safety. *Laryngoscope*. 2011;121(8):1636–1641.

9. Alabbas H, Bu Ali D, Kandil E. Robotic retroauricular thyroid surgery. *Gland Surg*. 2016;5(6):603–606.

10. Anuwong A. Transoral endoscopic thyroidectomy vestibular approach: A series of the first 60 human cases. *World J Surg*. 2016;40:491–497.

11. Richmon JD, Kim HY. Transoral robotic thyroidectomy (TORT): Procedures and outcomes. *Gland Surg*. 2017;6(3):285–289.

12. Sun H, Dionigi G. Applicability of transoral robotic thyroidectomy: Is it the final solution? *J Surg Oncol*. 2019;119(4):541–542.

13. Sun GH, Peress L, Pynnonen MA. Systematic review and meta-analysis of robotic vs conventional thyroidectomy approaches for thyroid disease. *Otolaryngol Head Neck Surg*. 2014;150(4):520–532.

14. Kwon H et al. Comparison of bilateral axillo-breast approach robotic thyroidectomy with open thyroidectomy for Graves' disease. *World J Surg*. 2016;40(3):498–504.

15. Pan J et al. Robotic thyroidectomy versus conventional open thyroidectomy for thyroid cancer: A systematic review and meta-analysis. *Surg Endosc*. 2017;31(10):3985–4001.

16. Jackson NR, Yao L, Tufano RP, Kandil EH. Safety of robotic thyroidectomy approaches: Meta-analysis and systematic review. *Head Neck*. 2014;36(1):137–143.

Chapter 13

INTRA-OPERATIVE NEURAL MONITORING

Rahul Modi

CONTENTS

How Common Is RLN Paralysis?   97
Importance of a Laryngeal Exam—Pre-Operative and Post-Operative Assessment   97
Intra-Operative Neural Monitoring—Utility and Applications   98
Standards for Intra-Operative Nerve Monitoring   98
New Horizons in IONM   100
References   103

The importance of preserving the integrity of the laryngeal nerves in thyroid and parathyroid surgery cannot be overemphasized. Both the superior and the recurrent laryngeal nerves (RLN) play a very important role in ensuring a robust voice and the dynamic nature of the glottis. The famous Greek physician and anatomist Galen (2nd century AD), identified and named the recurrent laryngeal nerves. However, since human dissections were considered a taboo during the middle ages, it was only in the 16th century that Vesalius provided detailed anatomic drawings of both the superior and recurrent laryngeal nerves in his famous textbook *De humani corporis fabrica* [1].

As understanding of the surgical anatomy improved over the years, the treatment outcomes became better. In the late 19th century, Kocher pioneered safe thyroid surgery in Europe whereas the same was practiced in the United States by Halsted based upon his observation with Kocher. Identification of the RLN during surgery slowly became the gold standard in preserving the structural integrity of the nerve over several decades, however, there were some initial reservations. It was Lahey in the 1930s who pioneered routine identification and dissection of the nerve during thyroid surgery to ensure structural integrity [2]. With focus on improving surgical outcomes by reducing nerve palsy rates, intra-operative nerve monitoring (IONM) has been developed over the years as a useful adjunct to visual identification.

The need for additional monitoring during surgery rests upon the insight that a visually preserved nerve may not be functional as physical injuries such as stretch or compression and thermal injuries due to electro-cautery may remain unnoticed during surgery. IONM has emerged as a reliable tool in predicting a functioning nerve at the end of a lobectomy. Studies have repeatedly shown a high negative predictive value (NPV) >95% in prognosticating nerve functioning at the end of surgery [3–5].

Thyroid surgery is unique in that one routinely performs bilateral neural dissection, hence putting both the nerves at risk. Thus, a bilateral vocal cord paralysis is a realistic possibility with adverse impact on quality of life.

This chapter aims to provide an overview of the technical considerations both in terms of application and utility of IONM of the RLN and SLN during thyroid and parathyroid surgery.

HOW COMMON IS RLN PARALYSIS?

RLN paralysis rates during thyroid and parathyroid surgery have possibly been underreported in the past. Earlier studies have quoted figures in the range of 1%–2% for permanent paralysis in expert hands; however, this number was found to increase substantially when routine post-operative laryngoscopy was done to assess vocal cord function [6]. More broad based studies have found the incidence of nerve paralysis to vary from 2.3% to as high as 26% [7]. A review of more than 25,000 patients found the average rate of RLN paralysis to be around 9.8%. Unilateral vocal paralysis can cause significant voice change severe enough to demand a change in vocation, especially for professional voice users, along with possible aspiration and dysphagia, whereas bilateral vocal cord paralysis can become a life-altering complication requiring tracheostomy tube dependence, gastrostomy to avoid aspiration, and grave impact on overall quality of life.

IMPORTANCE OF A LARYNGEAL EXAM— PRE-OPERATIVE AND POST-OPERATIVE ASSESSMENT

Ipsilateral vocal cord paralysis is an important predictor of invasiveness in thyroid malignancy. Up to 70% of cases of invasive thyroid cancer may have unilateral vocal cord paralysis [8]. Voice change is present in only a third of the patients with vocal cord paralysis, hence making a pre-operative laryngeal exam imperative for accurate diagnosis of vocal cord paralysis. The knowledge of vocal cord function in the pre-operative setting also helps the surgeon in surgical planning, patient counseling, and prevents significant medicolegal problems due to wrongful accusation. IONM is also more accurate and reliable with the knowledge of pre-operative vocal cord function. A laryngeal examination is important in the post-operative setting as well, as patients with vocal cord paralysis may not have voice change and voice change may arise with vocal cord paralysis [8]. Various international guidelines including those recommended by the German Association of Endocrine Surgeons [9], the British Association of Endocrine and Thyroid Surgeons (BAETS) [10], and the International Neural Monitoring Study Group (INMSG) recommend routine use of pre-operative and post-operative laryngeal examinations for all thyroidectomies [11]. The National Comprehensive Cancer Network (NCCN) [12] and the American Thyroid Association (ATA) [13] recommend the same for all thyroid malignancies. The American Academy of Otolaryngology—Head and Neck Surgery (AAO-HNS) recommends routine voice assessment both in the pre-operative and post-operative setting [14]. Use of pre-operative laryngeal examination is recommended in patients with suspicion of invasive thyroid disease, history of previous neck surgery, or any evidence of voice change. Post-operative laryngeal examination is a must in patients with any change in voice after thyroid surgery. Intra-operative nerve monitoring plays a valuable role in predicting post-operative vocal cord function.

INTRA-OPERATIVE NEURAL MONITORING—UTILITY AND APPLICATIONS

A recent systematic review published in the Cochrane database [15] failed to show any advantage of using IONM over visual examination in preventing temporary or permanent paralysis of the recurrent laryngeal nerve. Although there was a trend toward better outcomes in the IONM section, it was not found to be statistically significant. This could probably be because of paucity of well-designed and executed trials with a large number of participants and diligent follow up to come to an effective conclusion. Given the overall low rates of permanent RLN paralysis this might be a difficult task. What is, however, interesting to note is that despite the lack of published evidence in favor of use of IONM, there is a general trend toward increased usage/acceptance. A recently published survey [16] of more than 1,000 thyroid surgeons noted that surgeons <45 years of age and those with <15 years of experience tend to use it more frequently than others. Also, the use of IONM was found to be more common in North America (70.4%) than elsewhere (27.4%), and the majority (>80%) of users routinely performed it in all their thyroid surgeries. Also, smaller case studies have shown better outcomes in revision cases, retrosternal goiters, and surgeries for invasive thyroid cancer [17].

IONM has been found to be useful mainly in these scenarios:

1. Neural mapping, especially in complex thyroid surgeries
2. Discerning different pathologic states of RLN
3. Surgical management in the event of intra-operative RLN injuries (prognostication)

The utility of IONM is best realized when the electric stimulation of the nerve complements visual identification. IONM can be performed in various ways. Invasive and non-invasive modalities exist. The most commonly used modalities include use of surface electrodes either prefixed to a special endotracheal tube or electrodes that can be applied over regular ET tubes. Conventional IONM involves intermittent neural stimulation, whereas newer methods are utilizing continuous neural stimulation. The monitoring systems may relay an audio signal alone or in combination with an electromyographic (EMG) waveform. These waveforms provide useful information such as the amplitude and latency of the signal which are further helpful in prognostication of neural function and predicting outcomes.

1. *Neural Mapping Using IONM*: For surgeries where one can expect an abnormal course of the RLN secondary to history of previous neck or thyroid surgery, invasive disease, or inherent anomalous course of the nerve, such as a non-recurrent laryngeal nerve, the use of IONM can provide critical information. Linear, paratracheal stimulation of the nerve using a 2 mA current along the expected course of the nerve can be utilized to chart the course of the nerve prior to actual visualization. This is especially useful while operating in revision surgeries where the thick scar tissue may obviate accurate visual identification, and electrical stimulation can guide the surgeon to perform the surgery safely. Routine use of IONM is recommended to enable the surgeon as well as the operating room team to be familiar with the system and interpret the recorded signal critically.

2. *Utility of IONM in Different Pathologic States of IONM*: In the presence of a vocal cord paralysis in the pre-operative setting, residual EMG signal may still be recorded from an invaded

nerve [18]. This information is important as resection of such a nerve may possibly worsen the aspiration or dysphagia by disabling the residual functional nerve fibers. IONM can thus provide a unique insight into the functional status of the nerve compared to visual inspection alone.

3. *Surgical Management in the Event of Intra-operative RLN Injuries*: One of the most important advantages of using the IONM system is the ability to accurately predict the post-operative function of the nerve during surgery. This is of immense importance to the surgeon, especially during bilateral thyroid surgery or total thyroidectomy. Visual identification alone of the RLN, the hitherto gold standard, is fraught with inaccuracies and may adversely impact surgical decision-making. Unrecognized RLN palsy is not uncommon, and only about 10% of the neural injuries were identified accurately intra-operatively [6,7,19]. This is due to the fact that neural injuries secondary to blunt trauma or thermal injury may have been missed. Thus, visual confirmation alone as an indicator for structural integrity of the nerve is not accurate in predicting a functional outcome. In contrast, multiple studies have suggested a high negative predictive value close to 95% for IONM, especially when used in accordance with established standards [3–5,20–23]. A surgeon thus can proceed for surgery on the contralateral side with great confidence that the ipsilateral nerve is not only structurally intact but also functionally preserved. In the event of an injury, IONM can also help the surgeon in tracing the site of the injury, thus simultaneously acting as a learning tool and allowing to take any remedial action. IONM systems, however, have a lower positive predictive value [11,23,24]. This arises partly from the way a loss of signal (LOS) event is recorded and subsequent troubleshooting is done to differentiate equipment malfunction from a true neural injury. Studies have suggested that a standardized definition of LOS with a universally accepted troubleshooting algorithm along with knowledge of normative range of neural parameters will significantly help in providing more accurate neural prognostication [25]. The INMSG has done pioneering work in defining a true LOS and suggested a detailed algorithm to standardize troubleshooting during surgery. This has been described in greater detail in a later section on interpretation of loss of signal during IONM.

STANDARDS FOR INTRA-OPERATIVE NERVE MONITORING

INTRODUCTION

Considerable heterogeneity exists in the usage of IONM across various centers. This may arise due to multiple reasons ranging from usage of different monitoring methods, use of different stimulators, or use of different recording techniques. These technical differences make uniform applicability of IONM a challenge. It is therefore important to define certain monitoring standards for ensuring optimum wide-scale usability of IONM. Standards also help in reducing common setup-related errors by following certain predefined algorithms. The INMSG has developed guidelines with the goal of achieving the aforementioned objectives.

TECHNIQUE—IONM

A basic setup of the neural monitoring equipment is shown in Figure 13.1a and b.

The most preferred neural monitoring equipment is an endotracheal tube-based system that includes a graphic monitor documentation of

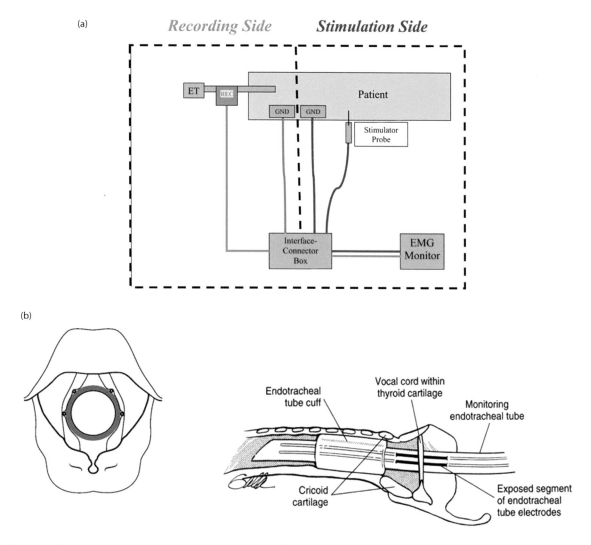

(a) *Recording Side* *Stimulation Side*

(b)

Figure 13.1   (a and b) Basic monitoring equipment set-up (Adapted from Jeannon JP et al. *Int J Clin Pract.* 2009 Apr;63(4):624–9.) (Abbreviations: ET = endotracheal tube; REC = recording electrodes; GND = ground electrodes).

the EMG waveform. It consists of a recording side and a stimulation side. Both needle-based electrodes or surface electrodes may be used for recording EMG data from the thyroarytenoid or vocalis muscle. Prefabricated endotracheal tubes with paired stainless steel electrodes exposed at the level of the glottis are available for this procedure. Alternatively, adhesive pads with thin electrodes which can be placed over a standard tube can be used. Additional (attachment) electrodes to record posterior cricoarytenoid (PCA) muscle twitch are available, however, they add very little to the sensitivity of the system [26]. Monopolar or bipolar stimulating electrodes may be used for stimulation, monopolar electrodes being preferable for mapping whereas bipolar electrodes are used for focal stimulation.

THE SETUP

Adherence to a standard setup algorithm reduces the monitoring related problems faced intra-operatively. While the IONM equipment is being setup, it is important to keep the electrocautery unit more than 10 feet away from the neural monitoring unit to avoid electrical interference. This setup is compatible with both Harmonic® and Ligasure® technologies. After the equipment is setup, care is taken to ensure that the recording side and the stimulation side circuitry is complete. The setup also requires implanting ground electrodes over the shoulder or the sternum area. Poor grounding can lead to a noisy baseline, making it difficult to interpret the EMG data.

Similar to any other task in the OR, IONM is teamwork, with the major participants being the surgeons, anesthesiologist, and the monitoring technician. IONM requires a clear understanding of the entire process by all its participants. A key member of the team is the anesthesiologist, who should understand that there are some special considerations for administering anesthesia during IONM.

It has been shown that use of muscle relaxants during anesthesia may attenuate EMG response and may make it difficult to perform quantitative analysis during IONM. The central guiding principle for the anesthesiologist during IONM for thyroid and parathyroid surgery is the avoidance of prolonged muscle relaxation and preservation of spontaneous muscular activity. Hence, use of muscle relaxants or paralytic agents to maintain anesthesia should be avoided. A combination of inhalational anesthesia with intravenous agents such as Propofol provides sufficient depth to avoid any inadvertent movement at the level of the cords.

Use of short acting muscle relaxants is acceptable at the time of induction. The endotracheal tube should be inserted without the use of any lubricant jelly or any other coating. Excessive salivation may also obscure the EMG signals, therefore it is recommended to use suction and possibly a drying agent.

As discussed previously, special endotracheal tubes are available which have the recording electrodes embedded over the surface. Alternatively, adhesive pads can be used over standard electrodes.

It is critical that these electrodes should abut closely to the vocal cords, hence selection of the largest possible size tube for intubation is important to ensure low impedance. Tube selection gains additional importance during SLN monitoring. Darr et al. [27] found that use of a special tube can also improve the monitoring responses.

It is prudent to check proper placement of the tube once it is secured, as this is the first and foremost step in ensuring an optimum monitoring setup. As the tube can move in or out appreciably after positioning the patient, it is imperative that proper tube placement checks are performed once the patient is in the final position. Endotracheal tube movement up to 6 cm has been documented and can lead to poor electrode contact with the vocal cords [28].

The one commonly followed method by our group that has proved to be consistently reliable is presence of respiratory variations. Respiratory variations are small waveforms with amplitudes between 30 and 70 uV which cause coarsening of the baseline EMG that is seen during a small window of time when the effect of the muscle relaxant given at the time of induction wears off and the patient is in a lighter plane of anesthesia just before the patient starts to move spontaneously or "buck." In absence of respiratory variation, a repeat direct laryngoscopy preferably by the surgeon to confirm tube placement is essential. A recently published study by our unit found that identification of respiratory variation was possible in 91% of their patients, whereas the remaining 9% required a repeat laryngoscopy [29]. It was also found that presence of respiratory variations independently predicted a good intra-operative evoked vagus and RLN response obviating a need for a repeat laryngoscopy in all patients. At final positioning, the impedance of the electrodes should be <5 ohms and that the imbalance between the two sides should be less than 1 ohm. Higher impedance imbalance may suggest inappropriate tube placement requiring repositioning whereas if the overall impedance is high then the ground electrodes require a check or replacement.

INTRA-OPERATIVE SETUP

Once the setup is complete, it is important to set the monitor event threshold at 100 uV and the stimulator probe to a pulsatile output of 4 per second. At the initiation of surgery, the absence of paralytic agents can be checked by stimulation of the strap muscles. This results in a gross muscle twitch which also confirms a functional stimulation side.

Pre-dissection suprathreshold vagal nerve stimulation is key in establishing the functionality of the system. It is only after this is verified that one can truly accept any tissue as not being the RLN. A suprathreshold current of 2 mA is useful for neural mapping; once the nerve has been identified, the current can be reduced to 1 mA for further testing and end of surgery prognostication. Caragacianu et al. [30] found no statistically significant difference exists between the amplitude when stimulated by suprathreshold levels at 1 or 2 mA. Normative values were thus defined at 1 mA. Amplitude of >250 uV was found to be highly predictive of a functioning RLN. Other factors such as latency and shape of the waveform were not found to have a significant predictive value [30]. Repetitive stimulation of the RLN at levels of 1 and 2 mA has been reported to be extremely safe and no detrimental effects have been reported [30]. It should be noted that any negative response is not termed as true negative unless a true positive has been established.

LOSS OF SIGNAL (LOS) DURING IONM: PROBLEM-SOLVING AND TRUE LOS

Loss of signal during IONM could be encountered due to various reasons during a surgery. The surgeon should first rule out equipment/setup-related LOS before labeling it as a true LOS.

As soon as a LOS is encountered, assessment of the laryngeal twitch response to ipsilateral and contralateral vagal stimulation should be performed to evaluate the integrity of the IONM setup. Presence of laryngeal twitch establishes that the stimulating side of the equipment is functioning adequately. A common recording equipment issue faced is a displaced or a malpositioned ET, hence this should also be checked by the anesthesiologist and readjusted if required. Other issues related to adequacy of current and use of paralytic agents should also be considered. A detailed algorithm depicting steps for identification of a true LOS from a false positive LOS is shown in Figure 13.2. Aggressive adherence to the algorithm outlined previously improves positive predictive value in the setting of a loss of signal. To be called a true LOS, the event must satisfy three conditions:

1. Presence of a satisfactory EMG (amplitude >100 uV) prior to the event
2. No or low response (i.e., 100 uV or lower) with stimulation at 1–2 mA in a dry field
3. Absence of laryngeal twitch and/or a glottic twitch on ipsilateral vagal stimulation

A true LOS should prompt the surgeon to identify the site of the injury. This provides an opportunity to treat the nerve injury if possible and also acts a learning exercise. This may impact the surgical plan and the surgeon may consider postponing surgery on the contralateral side. IONM guided staging of thyroid surgery is discussed in greater detail in a later section.

PASSIVE EMG ACTIVITY DURING IONM

Any passive EMG activity occurring frequently may signify mechanical nerve injury or a thermal stress secondary to cautery usage. This should prompt an urgent evaluation by the surgeon. One needs to ascertain that the cautery muting device is attached to both the monopolar and bipolar cautery cables to avoid interference artifacts.

MONITORING SAFETY

Multiple studies have established safety of repetitive stimulation of the facial nerve in otological and neuro-otological surgery, and various workers have reported that application of IONM for RLN during thyroid and parathyroid surgery as safe [11]. Based on literature review as well as their cumulative experience, the International Neural Monitoring Study Group has specified that repetitive stimulation of the RLN or vagus is not associated with neural injury. IONM has been safely employed in children and adults assuming proper patient isolation and grounding [11].

NEW HORIZONS IN IONM

NEURAL MONITORING AND STAGED THYROIDECTOMY IN THYROID CANCER SURGERY—AN EMERGING CONCEPT

Presence of bilateral nodal metastases are frequently seen in thyroid cancers. Surgeries in these patients typically involve a total thyroidectomy, central neck dissection, along with bilateral lateral neck dissection. Apart from being extensive, these surgeries carry a high risk of complications. In the lateral neck these include cranial nerve injuries, chyle leak, post-operative bleeding, and possible internal jugular vein sacrifice, whereas in the central compartment/neck these include bilateral RLN palsy and hypoparathyroidism. It is thus challenging to ensure both safety and efficacy while performing surgery in patients with bulky nodal disease.

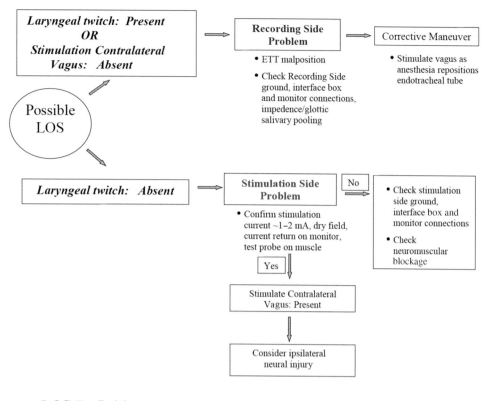

LOS Definition:

1 -EMG change from initial satisfactory EMG
2 -No or low response (i.e.,100 μV or less)with stimulation @ 1–2 mA, dry field
3-No laryngeal twitch and/or observed glottic twitch

With LOS:

1-Map lesion and determine Type I(Segmental) or Type II (Global) injury
2-Consider contralateral surgery timing

Figure 13.2   Intra-operative LOS evaluation standard.

Staging of surgery may offset some of these complications, especially those which are temporary in nature. An RLN with neuropraxia may recover between the two stages of surgery reducing the risk of bilateral vocal cord palsy (VCP). Similarly, parathyroid glands may recover functionally in the intervening period. Merchavy et al. [31] have reported significantly lower incidence of transient hypocalcemia in patients undergoing completion thyroidectomy when compared to patients undergoing total thyroidectomy. Benefits of staging bilateral radical neck dissection have been documented earlier. It was Frazzell, in 1961 [32], who proposed a planned staging of surgeries where ligation of bilateral internal jugular veins was anticipated. Staging of thyroidectomy was suggested first by Luigi Porta in 1811.

Routine use of IONM makes it possible for surgeons to make an informed decision with regards to staging of surgery. Evidence suggesting utility of LOS as a decision-making tool during surgery is slowly accumulating. Goretski et al. [33] have reported that incidence of bilateral VCP drops to zero from 17% in bilateral surgery where LOS is incorporated in the surgical strategy.

It is the policy in our practice to offer staging of surgery upfront to patients with extensive bilateral nodal disease. Apart from reducing the incidence of complications as described previously, we have found that it also prevents/reduces surgical fatigue thus ensuring better outcomes. Similar practices have also been reported by other tertiary care referral centers. Dralle et al. [34] found that 94% of surgeons in Germany would stage a total thyroidectomy if they encountered an LOS during the surgery This is especially true for centers with a higher case load. However, a detailed pre-operative consent process is imperative when staging of surgery is being contemplated as a possibility [35].

Management of recurrent laryngeal nerve depends upon the pre-operative vocal cord function (Figure 13.3).

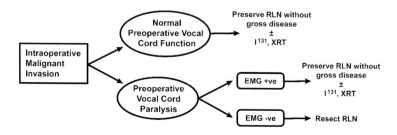

Figure 13.3   Management algorithm for the recurrent laryngeal nerve with preoperative vocal cord paralysis [50].

SUPERIOR LARYNGEAL NERVE MONITORING

Recently published guidelines on SLN monitoring by the International Neural Monitoring Study Group [36] have highlighted the fact that neural monitoring of the SLN is associated with higher rates of nerve identification than through visual identification. The laryngeal head of the sternothyroid serves as a useful landmark for identification of the external branch of the superior laryngeal nerve (EBSLN). A twitch in the cricothyroid muscle seen upon stimulation is currently the most accurate measure of nerve localization. A specially designed electrode array incorporated on an endotracheal tube can also record EMG activity from glottis in 100% of the patients [27]. For a detailed discussion on the technique and utility of SLN monitoring, the reader is requested to refer to the guidelines published by the INMSG [36].

CONTINUOUS VAGAL MONITORING AND NEURAL INJURY PREVENTION

One of the biggest drawbacks of the existing IONM formats is that it only allows the surgeon to intermittently stimulate and evaluate the functional integrity of the RLN. Although immensely useful in resolving a surgeon's dilemma, the nerve remains at risk for injuries in between stimulations [22,37]. This could possibly explain the suggestion that in its present format, IONM may have limited ability to prevent neural injury [9,22,38–43]. An ideal IONM format would be the one that provides real time EMG data which can alert the surgeon before irreversible neural damage sets in. Early studies have shown that continuous IONM or CIONM can provide that information. It is important, however, that the accepted format differentiates true events from electrical artifacts. Combining reduction in amplitude with increase in latency, our group has defined mild and severe combined events (Table 13.1), which when identified, can prevent irreversible neural damage. Modification of a surgical maneuver when such an event occurs can prevent development of a complete LOS and subsequent VCP. It is evident that given the nature of IONM overall, these systems are more useful for preventing impeding neural damage secondary to a stretch or compression [44] than an inadvertent transection of the nerve by the surgeon.

INTRA-OPERATIVE IDENTIFICATION OF NON-RECURRENT LARYNGEAL NERVE

The non-recurrent laryngeal nerve (NRLN) is an anatomical variant of the RLN with no functional impact, the only consequence being increased susceptibility to intra-operative injury by a surgeon unaware of its presence. The presence of right NRLN is reported as 0.5%–1% of all RLNs and left NRLN being reported as only 0.04% [45,46]. Our series on NRLN monitoring recommends an electrophysiologic algorithm where presence of positive EMG response to proximal stimulation of the vagus nerve at the superior border of thyroid cartilage and absence of EMG response to distal stimulation of the vagus nerve below the inferior border of fourth tracheal ring reliably identifies an NRLN [47] (Figure 13.4). Currently, no dependable technique of pre-operative acknowledgement or exclusion of NRLN is available. The aforementioned electrophysiologic algorithm reliably alerts a surgeon regarding the presence of NRLN prior to the dissection in the related cervical region. This vagal stimulation technique for NRLN identification is supported by Brauckhoff et al. [48]. Anatomically, three types of NRLN are described in the literature (Figure 13.5). Essentially, the right NRLN behaves similarly to the right RLN, in terms of amplitude, threshold, and latency. Some workers have suggested that a latency of less than 3.5 ms strongly suggests a NRLN [49]. However, further studies are warranted before it is considered a definitive indication of NRLN.

Table 13.1 Mild and severe combined amplitude

Mild Combined Event (mCE): Amplitude decrease of >50%–70% with a concordant latency increase of 5%–10%
Severe Combined Event (sCE): Amplitude decrease of >70% with a concordant latency increase of >10%

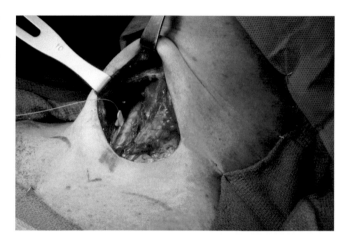

Figure 13.4 APS electrode on vagus nerve.

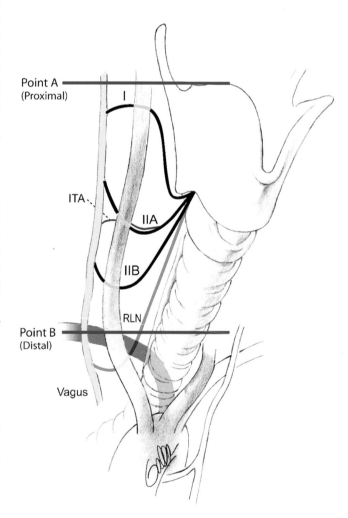

Figure 13.5 Non-recurrent laryngeal nerve with its variants.

REFERENCES

1. Dedo HH. The paralyzed larynx: An electromyographic study in dogs and humans. *Laryngoscope.* 1970 Oct;80(10):1455–517.

2. Lahey FH, Hoover WB. Injuries to the recurrent laryngeal nerve in thyroid operations: Their management and avoidance. *Ann Surg.* 1938 Oct;108(4):545–62.

3. Dralle H, Sekulla C, Lorenz K, Brauckhoff M, Machens A. Intraoperative monitoring of the recurrent laryngeal nerve in thyroid surgery. *World J Surg.* 2008 Jul;32(7):1358–66.

4. Thomusch O, Sekulla C, Machens A, Neumann HJ, Timmermann W, Dralle H. Validity of intra-operative neuromonitoring signals in thyroid surgery. *Langenbecks Arch Surg.* 2004 Nov;389(6):499–503.

5. Tomoda C et al. Sensitivity and specificity of intraoperative recurrent laryngeal nerve stimulation test for predicting vocal cord palsy after thyroid surgery. *World J Surg.* 2006 Jul;30(7):1230–3.

6. Bergenfelz A et al. Scandinavian Quality Register for Thyroid and Parathyroid Surgery: Audit of surgery for primary hyperparathyroidism. *Langenbecks Arch Surg.* 2007 Jul;392(4):445–51.

7. Jeannon JP, Orabi AA, Bruch GA, Abdalsalam HA, Simo R. Diagnosis of recurrent laryngeal nerve palsy after thyroidectomy: A systematic review. *Int J Clin Pract.* 2009 Apr;63(4):624–9.

8. Randolph GW, Kamani D. The importance of preoperative laryngoscopy in patients undergoing thyroidectomy: Voice, vocal cord function, and the preoperative detection of invasive thyroid malignancy. *Surgery.* 2006 Mar;139(3):357–62.

9. Musholt TJ et al. German Association of Endocrine Surgeons practice guidelines for the surgical treatment of benign thyroid disease. *Langenbecks Arch Surg.* 2011 Jun;396(5):639–49.

10. *The British Association of Endocrine and Thyroid Surgeons.* Third National Audit Report 2009. 2009.

11. Randolph GW et al. Electrophysiologic recurrent laryngeal nerve monitoring during thyroid and parathyroid surgery: International standards guideline statement. *Laryngoscope.* 2011 Jan;121(Suppl 1):S1–16.

12. Sherman SI et al. Thyroid carcinoma. *J Natl Compr Canc Netw.* 2005 May;3(3):404–57.

13. Haugen BR et al. 2015 American Thyroid Association Management Guidelines for adult patients with thyroid nodules and differentiated thyroid cancer: The American Thyroid Association Guidelines task force on thyroid nodules and differentiated thyroid cancer. *Thyroid.* 2015 Jan;26(1):1–133.

14. Chandrasekhar SRG et al. American academy of otolaryngology head and neck surgery clinical practice guidelines: Improving voice outcomes after thyroid surgery. *Otolaryngol Head Neck Surg.* 2013;148(6S):S1–37.

15. Cirocchi R et al. Intraoperative neuromonitoring versus visual nerve identification for prevention of recurrent laryngeal nerve injury in adults undergoing thyroid surgery. *Cochrane Database Syst Rev.* 2019 Jan 19;1:CD012483.

16. Feng AL, Puram SV, Singer MC, Modi R, Kamani D, Randolph GW. Increased prevalence of neural monitoring during thyroidectomy: Global surgical survey. *Laryngoscope.* 2019 Jul 30;00:1–8.

17. Patow CA, Norton JA, Brennan MF. Vocal cord paralysis and reoperative parathyroidectomy. A prospective study. *Ann Surg.* 1986 Mar;203(3):282–5.

18. Kamani D, Randolph G, Potenza A, cernea C. Electrophysiologic monitoring characteristics of the recurrent laryngeal nerve preoperatively paralyzed or invaded with malignancy. *Otolaryngol Head Neck Surg.* 2013;149(5).

19. Hamelmann WH, Meyer T, Timm S, Timmermann W. A Critical Estimation of Intraoperative Neuromonitoring (IONM) in thyroid surgery. *Zentralbl Chir.* 2002 May;127(5):409–13.

20. Chan WF, Lo CY. Pitfalls of intraoperative neuromonitoring for predicting postoperative recurrent laryngeal nerve function during thyroidectomy. *World J Surg.* 2006 May;30(5):806–12.

21. Beldi G, Kinsbergen T, Schlumpf R. Evaluation of intraoperative recurrent nerve monitoring in thyroid surgery. *World J Surg.* 2004 Jun;28(6):589–91.

22. Hermann M, Hellebart C, Freissmuth M. Neuromonitoring in thyroid surgery: Prospective evaluation of intraoperative electrophysiological responses for the prediction of recurrent laryngeal nerve injury. *Ann Surg.* 2004 Jul;240(1):9–17.

23. Lorenz K, Sekulla C, Schelle J, Schmeiss B, Brauckhoff M, Dralle H. What are normal quantitative parameters of intraoperative neuromonitoring (IONM) in thyroid surgery? *Langenbecks Arch Surg.* 2010 Sep;395(7):901–9.

24. Phelan E, Kamani D, Shin J, Randolph GW. Neural monitored revision thyroid cancer surgery: Surgical safety and thyroglobulin response. *Otolaryngol Head Neck Surg.* 2013 Jul;149(1):47–52.

25. Chan WF, Lang BH, Lo CY. The role of intraoperative neuromonitoring of recurrent laryngeal nerve during thyroidectomy: A comparative study on 1,000 nerves at risk. *Surgery.* 2006 Dec;140(6):866–72; discussion 72-3.

26. Marcus B et al. Recurrent laryngeal nerve monitoring in thyroid and parathyroid surgery: The University of Michigan experience. *Laryngoscope.* 2003 Feb;113(2):356–61.

27. Darr AE, Tufano R, Ozdemir S, Kamani D, Hurwitz S, Randolph GW. Superior laryngeal nerve quantitative intraoperative monitoring is possible in all thyroid surgeries. *Laryngoscope.* 2013;124(4).

28. Yap SJ, Morris RW, Pybus DA. Alterations in endotracheal tube position during general anaesthesia. *Anaesth Intensive Care.* 1994 Oct;22(5):586–8.

29. Chambers KJ et al. Respiratory variation predicts optimal endotracheal tube placement for intra-operative nerve monitoring in thyroid and parathyroid surgery. *World J Surg.* 2014 Oct 9;39(2):393–9.

30. Caragacianu D, Kamani D, Randolph GW. Intraoperative monitoring: Normative range associated with normal postoperative glottic function. *Laryngoscope.* 2013 May;123(12):3026–31.

31. Merchavy S et al. Comparison of the incidence of postoperative hypocalcemia following total thyroidectomy vs completion thyroidectomy. *Otolaryngol Head Neck Surg.* 2015 Jan;152(1):53–56.

32. Frazell EL, Moore OS. Bilateral radical neck dissection performed in stages. Experience with 467 patients. *Am J Surg.* 1961 Dec;102:809–14.

33. Goretzki PE, Schwarz K, Brinkmann J, Wirowski D, Lammers BJ. The impact of intraoperative neuromonitoring (IONM) on surgical strategy in bilateral thyroid diseases: Is it worth the effort? *World J Surg.* 2010 Jun;34(6):1274–84.

34. Dralle H, Sekulla C, Lorenz K, Nguyen Thanh P, Schneider R, Machens A. Loss of the nerve monitoring signal during bilateral thyroid surgery. *Br J Surg.* 2012 Aug;99(8):1089–95.

35. Dionigi G, Frattini F. Staged thyroidectomy: Time to consider intraoperative neuromonitoring as standard of care. *Thyroid.* 2013 Jul;23(7):906–8.

36. Barczynski M et al. External branch of the superior laryngeal nerve monitoring during thyroid and parathyroid surgery: International neural monitoring study group standards guideline statement. *Laryngoscope.* 2013 Jul 6;123(S4).

37. Scott AR, Chong PS, Hartnick CJ, Randolph GW. Spontaneous and evoked laryngeal electromyography of the thyroarytenoid muscles: A canine model for intraoperative recurrent laryngeal nerve monitoring. *Ann Otol Rhinol Laryngol.* 2010 Jan;119(1):54–63.

38. Dralle H et al. Risk factors of paralysis and functional outcome after recurrent laryngeal nerve monitoring in thyroid surgery. *Surgery.* 2004 Dec;136(6):1310–22.

39. Randolph GW, Kobler JB, Wilkins J. Recurrent laryngeal nerve identification and assessment during thyroid surgery: Laryngeal palpation. *World J Surg.* 2004 Aug;28(8):755–60.

40. Chiang FY, Lu IC, Kuo WR, Lee KW, Chang NC, Wu CW. The mechanism of recurrent laryngeal nerve injury during thyroid surgery—the application of intraoperative neuromonitoring. *Surgery.* 2008 Jun;143(6):743–9.

41. Dionigi G et al. Why monitor the recurrent laryngeal nerve in thyroid surgery? *J Endocrinol Invest.* 2010 Dec;33(11):819–22.

42. Higgins TS, Gupta R, Ketcham AS, Sataloff RT, Wadsworth JT, Sinacori JT. Recurrent laryngeal nerve monitoring versus identification alone on post-thyroidectomy true vocal fold palsy: A meta-analysis. *Laryngoscope.* 2011 May; 121(5):1009–17.

43. Angelos P. Ethical and medicolegal issues in neuromonitoring during thyroid and parathyroid surgery: A review of the recent literature. *Curr Opin Oncol.* 2012 Jan;24(1):16–21.

44. Phelan E, Potenza A, Slough C, Zurakowski D, Kamani D, Randolph G. Recurrent laryngeal nerve monitoring during thyroid surgery: Normative vagal and recurrent laryngeal nerve electrophysiological data. *Otolaryngol Head Neck Surg.* 2012 Oct;147(4):640–6.

45. Henry JF, Audiffret J, Denizot A, Plan M. The nonrecurrent inferior laryngeal nerve: Review of 33 cases, including two on the left side. *Surgery.* 1988 Dec;104(6):977–84.

46. Fellmer PT, Bohner H, Wolf A, Roher HD, Goretzki PE. A left nonrecurrent inferior laryngeal nerve in a patient with right-sided aorta, truncus arteriosus communis, and an aberrant left innominate artery. *Thyroid.* 2008 Jun;18(6):647–9.

47. Kamani D, Potenza AS, Cernea CR, Kamani YV, Randolph GW. The nonrecurrent laryngeal nerve: Anatomic and electrophysiologic algorithm for reliable identification. *Laryngoscope.* 2014 Jul 9;125(2).

48. Brauckhoff M, Walls G, Brauckhoff K, Thanh PN, Thomusch O, Dralle H. Identification of the non-recurrent inferior laryngeal nerve using intraoperative neurostimulation. *Langenbecks Arch Surg.* 2002 Jan;386(7):482–7.

49. Brauckhoff M, Machens A, Sekulla C, Lorenz K, Dralle H. Latencies shorter than 3.5 ms after vagus nerve stimulation signify a nonrecurrent inferior laryngeal nerve before dissection. *Ann Surg.* 2011 Jun;253(6):1172–7.

50. Randolph GW, Kamani D. Intraoperative nerve monitoring. *Ent and audiology news.* 2017 July/August;26(3).

Chapter 14

SURGICAL MANAGEMENT OF DIFFERENTIATED THYROID CANCERS

Anil D'cruz and Richa Vaish

CONTENTS

Introduction 105
Active Surveillance as an Alternative to Surgery 105
Completion Thyroidectomy 106
Debate of Hemi- versus Total Thyroidectomy 107
Surgical Tips and Tricks 108
References 109

INTRODUCTION

There is a reported thyroid cancer epidemic worldwide attributed to liberal and widespread use of imaging [1]. The age standardized incidence of thyroid cancer in females has risen from 1.5/100 000 to 7.5/100 000 between 1953 and 2002 [2]. This change in trend is seen in many countries across the globe including the USA, France, and Italy, but is most marked in Korea as a result of an active screening program in that country [3,4]. The majority of these cancers are small when detected—less than 2 cm in diameter—and treatment has not translated into an overall reduction in mortality from thyroid cancer [5]. The most plausible explanation for this phenomenon is overdiagnosis of these indolent cancers, many of which would otherwise not have manifested clinically during the life span of the individual. This is corroborated by the fact that thyroid cancer is identified incidentally at autopsy in 8%–65% of individuals who died of other causes [6].

ACTIVE SURVEILLANCE AS AN ALTERNATIVE TO SURGERY

Active surveillance has been advocated for small cancers <1 cm, referred to as micropapillary thyroid cancers. The biological rationale for this approach is that these cancers are detected due to the widespread use of imaging, and many of them would probably have remained dormant through the life span of the individual. There is a school of thought that suggests observation of these select cases of papillary microcarcinoma and active intervention only in the event of disease progression. This strategy is proposed for papillary microcarcinoma that are deemed low risk with localized disease, non-aggressive histology, and no evidence of metastasis or local invasion. The data supporting this philosophy is predominantly from Japan. In a study, Ito et al. observed 1,235 patients with low-risk papillary thyroid microcarcinoma (PTMC) followed up periodically with neck ultrasonography [7]. The patients were monitored for tumor enlargement, development of neck node metastasis, and progression to clinical disease. At 10 years, the incidence rates of these parameters were 8.0%, 3.8%, and 6.8% respectively. In all 191 patients who underwent surgery for various reasons, there was no reported

mortality. In another study by Oda et al., of 2,153 low-risk PTMC, 1,179 patients chose observation and 974 immediate surgery [8]. The authors concluded that the oncological outcomes in the groups were similar but unfavorable events (vocal cord palsy, hypoparathyroidism, hematoma, and surgical scar) were more prevalent in the immediate surgery group. There was no PTMC-related death in either group. Haser et al. reviewed the existing literature and suggested active surveillance as a safe and viable option with the potential to be a long-term management strategy for low-risk PTMC [9]. However, there is a need to select the patients carefully and strictly adhere to the follow-up protocol. Brito et al. proposed a clinical framework to facilitate risk stratification in these patients classifying PTMC patients as ideal, appropriate, or inappropriate for active surveillance based on three domains, namely tumor/neck ultrasound features (e.g., size of the primary tumor and location within the thyroid gland); patient features (e.g., age, comorbidities, willingness to accept observation); and medical team features (e.g., availability and experience of the multidisciplinary team) [10]. The patients should be counseled in detail about the pros and cons of the procedure and the awareness, impact on the psychology, and quality of life should be factored into the decision algorithm.

SURGERY FOR DTC

Thyroid cancers are a disease with surgery being the mainstay of treatment. The need, as well as the extent of surgery, must be balanced taking into account the indolent nature of the majority of these cancers against the potential morbidity of treatment. The thyroid is in close proximity to the recurrent laryngeal nerve (RLN) and the parathyroids, placing them at risk during surgery. The reported incidence for temporary and permanent RLN palsy is 2.1%–8.3% and 0.3%–1.7%, while temporary and permanent hypocalcemia ranges between 3.3%–34% and 1.1%–10%, respectively [11]. The morbidity varies with the extent of surgery performed for the primary, experience of the surgeon, and volume of work at the treating center. The morbidity of surgery, therefore, is unacceptable given that 99% of patients are alive at 20 years in the vast majority of cases [12]. The extent of the surgery needs to be carefully weighed against this potential morbidity.

The main goal at surgery is complete clearance of the disease to reduce the risk of recurrence. The minimum surgery for thyroid cancer is an ipsilateral complete extracapsular lobectomy. Nodulectomy or partial thyroidectomy is to be deprecated. The logical reason is that should completion thyroidectomy be warranted for any reason, reoperation in a violated thyroid bed carries an increased risk of nerve and parathyroid damage. The isthmus is usually a part of a lobectomy procedure making the hemithyroidectomy the procedure of choice when indicated (see the following section). For a similar reason, subtotal thyroidectomy, leaving behind significant residual thyroid tissue in both tracheoesophageal grooves, is condemned as it is associated with higher chance of recurrence as well as increased risk of complications at repeat surgery. Total thyroidectomy is therefore to be performed when indicated with an attempt to remove all apparent thyroid disease. However, given the fact that these cancers have an excellent prognosis, surgical enthusiasm must be tempered against potential morbidity and a bit of thyroid tissue (typically described as less than 1 gm) if left back in the region of Berry's ligament to safeguard the point of entry of the recurrent laryngeal nerve or the blood supply to the parathyroids is prudent. Such a procedure is called near total thyroidectomy. It must, however, be kept in mind that lack of surgical expertise must not be used as a cover when performing a near total thyroidectomy. Meticulous clearance of all thyroid tissue and disease is important as it decreases loco regional recurrence as well as facilitates the radioiodine treatment for microscopic residual disease and metastasis.

EXTENT OF SURGERY

The surgery of primary thyroid gland disease is either total or hemithyroidectomy, as mentioned previously. Hemithyroidectomy is advocated for low risk cancers occurring in young patients, usually females, with the classical variant of well differentiated thyroid cancers, with tumors less than 4 cm in diameter, predominantly unifocal and intraparenchymal, and without evidence of regional or distant metastasis (Table 14.1) [35]. Proponents of hemithyroidectomy cite similar survival to total thyroidectomy in this group of patients across many large series with tens of thousands of patients [13]. There is logically a low incidence of associated morbidity as only one-side nerve and parathyroid glands are at risk. Any recurrence can be treated as and when it occurs in the relatively untouched field on the opposite side with no determinant to outcomes [14]. However, serum thyroglobulin cannot be used as an accurate marker for detecting recurrence with an intact thyroid lobe in situ. Conversely, total thyroidectomy, which entails removal of both the lobes of the thyroid along with the isthmus, is advocated in cases with large tumors, aggressive histology, multifocal disease, and in the presence of regional or distant metastasis (Table 14.1). While theoretically it is associated with higher morbidity as both sides' nerves and parathyroids are at risk, the procedure is safe in the hands of an experienced surgeon. Total thyroidectomy is recommended in all cases where adjuvant radioiodine therapy is considered. In addition, since there is no residual thyroid tissue after this procedure, serum thyroglobulin becomes a reliable marker for follow-up and to detect disease recurrence [15]. The Hartley Dunhill procedure, which

entails hemithyroidectomy on one side plus subtotal resection on the other side and subtotal thyroidectomy bilaterally, was popular at one time but is now obsolete and not recommended for reasons cited previously [16]. In a quarter to half of patients presenting with a solitary nodule, fine needle aspiration cytology (FNAC) is inconclusive and reported indeterminate (Bethesda III, IV & V) with a rate of malignancy on final histology ranging from 5%–6.5% [17–19]. While molecular markers have been extensively researched to help resolve this conundrum by either ruling in or ruling out cancer, these tests are not yet the standard of care due to prohibitive costs, as well as the lack of a single comprehensive test with sufficient positive and negative predictive values to be cost effective [20]. Surgery is often considered in these patients on the perceived risk of malignancy based on high risk clinical factors (age, gender, family history, prior radiotherapy), size of the nodule, and high-risk sonographic features (macrocalcification, hypoechogenicity, etc.). Lobectomy is the optimal initial and definitive therapeutic surgical procedure for the majority of these cancer patients and termed a diagnostic lobectomy [21,22]. Such patients should be counseled that the final histology may reveal malignancy and if they fall into high risk, completion thyroidectomy may be warranted as a second procedure.

COMPLETION THYROIDECTOMY

Resurgery in form of completion thyroidectomy is warranted in cases that required total thyroidectomy upfront but were offered a lesser procedure. Such surgery should be contemplated either immediately after initial surgery (within the first few days) or after 2–3 months, once the inflammation/fibrosis and adhesions settle to make surgery simpler and decrease potential morbidity [23]. Intra-operative nerve monitoring (IONM) should be considered in thyroid resurgeries to protect the RLN. In a study of 854 cases of resurgery in benign and malignant conditions, the transient nerve palsy was significantly less with IONM compared to nerve visualization alone. There was also a trend of lesser permanent palsy with the use of IONM which, however, was not statistically significant [24]. Various meta-analysis and systemic reviews have been performed to assess the effect of IONM; however, results are conflicting [25]. A review addressing the methodological quality assessment of these meta-analyses concludes that the quality is critically low [26]. A well-powered large randomized controlled trial is needed to produce more robust evidence. However, given the potential benefit it is prudent and medico-legally safer to use IONM in this setting.

Surgery for PTC Aggressive Variants: Tall cell variant, columnar variant, solid/trabecular variant, hobnail variant, and diffuse sclerosing are aggressive histological variants of PTC. These tumors are associated with biologically more aggressive cancers manifested by higher stage, larger T-size, vascular invasion, distant metastasis, and extrathyroidal extension [27]. These cancers should be treated with total thyroidectomy upfront followed by radioiodine ablation [28].

Radiation Exposure/Fallout: These cancers occur as a result of radiation exposure during childhood or adolescence. The risk of developing cancer varies with the dose of radiation and the age at the time of exposure. Younger age and mean dose more than 0.05–0.1 Gy are associated with an increased risk [29]. The usual latent period from exposure to manifestation of thyroid cancers is 5–10 years. PTC is the most commonly associated thyroid cancer. Radiation induced cancers are typically multifocal with extrathyroidal extension. Many of these cancers also present with advanced disease and distant metastasis [30]. Hence, total thyroidectomy is recommended as the initial surgical procedure in this situation.

Table 14.1 Low risk versus high risk thyroid cancers

Factors	Low risk (lobectomy)	High risk (total thyroidectomy)
Age [34]	<55 years	>55 years
Size	<1 cm	>4 cm
Extent of disease	Intrathyroid	Gross extrathyroid
Histology	Differentiated papillary Minimally invasive follicular carcinoma	Aggressive variants of papillary Widely invasive follicular carcinoma
Focality	Unifocal	Multifocal
Nodal metastasis (regional/distant)	Absent	Present

Source: Adapted from Thyroid Cancer: ASCO tumor board.

Familial Well-Differentiated Thyroid Cancers: Approximately 5% of well-differentiated thyroid cancers are familial. These are commonly associated with syndromes like Familial Adenomatous Polyposis, Gardner's syndrome, Carney's complex, Werner's syndrome, Cowden's disease, etc. These cancers are more aggressive than sporadic cancers and are more often associated with extrathyroidal extension, multifocality, regional metastasis, and a higher incidence of recurrence [31–33]. Such cases should be offered total thyroidectomy for the reasons cited. The cribriform morular histological variant should alert the clinician to the possibility of familial adenomatous polyposis, and the patient should be screened for colonic polyps.

DEBATE OF HEMI- VERSUS TOTAL THYROIDECTOMY

Despite most guidelines suggesting that a hemithyroidectomy is an adequate surgical procedure for nodules less than 4 cms in the absence of other adverse features, there has been considerable debate for more than two decades on the adequacy of this procedure for nodules between 1–4 cm in size.

The widely followed ATA guidelines (2015) are not very definitive on this issue and state:

> "For patients with thyroid cancer >1 cm and <4 cm without extrathyroidal extension, and without clinical evidence of any lymph node metastases (cN0), the initial surgical procedure can be either a bilateral procedure (near total or total thyroidectomy) or a unilateral procedure (lobectomy). Thyroid lobectomy alone may be sufficient initial treatment for low-risk papillary and follicular carcinomas; however, the treatment team may choose total thyroidectomy to enable RAI therapy or to enhance follow up based upon disease features and/or patient preferences" [36].

This ambiguity stems from conflicting results across large published series in the literature. The evidence in favor of total thyroidectomy in nodules >1 cm comes from various studies. From the National Cancer Database (NCDB), Bilimoria et al. reported 52,173 patients who underwent thyroid surgery between 1985–1998, of which 43,227 (82.9%) had total thyroidectomy and 8,946 (17.1%) had lobectomy [37]. Of these, 23.9% were tumors <1 cm, 29.8% were 1–2 cm, and 46.3% were tumors >2 cm. The study results showed that the extent of surgery impacted the recurrence and survival significantly in patients with tumors >1 cm after making adjustments for tumor, treatment, and hospital characteristics. Similar results were obtained for tumors sized between 1–2 cm after omitting the potential confounding effect of larger tumors. The limitation of the study, however, was that the details of disease characteristics and patient factors that could have influenced the results were not defined by the authors. Hay et al. published six decades of temporal trends in initial therapy and long-term outcomes in the management of thyroid cancers including 2,444 patients [38]. For the patients with MACIS (distant **M**etastasis, patient **A**ge, **C**ompleteness of resection, local **I**nvasion, and tumor **S**ize) score <6 (low risk), between 1940 and 1949, lobectomy as the initial procedure that was performed in 70%, and during 1950–1959 in 22% of cases. Total thyroidectomy accounted for 91% of the initial procedure between 1960 and 1999. Radioactive ablation was performed in 3% of cases after total thyroidectomy between 1950 and 1969, which increased to 18%, 57%, and 46% in successive decades. The 40-year rates for cause specific mortality and tumor recurrence was significantly higher between 1940 and 1949 compared to between 1950 and 1999. The

study results also showed that use of radioiodine remnant ablation did not improve the excellent outcomes (achieved before 1970) further in this group of patients. Mazzaferri et al. in a study of 1,355 patients looked at the long-term impact of the surgical and medical therapy in papillary and follicular thyroid cancers [39]. The authors concluded that for tumors >1.5 cm with no distant metastasis, near total thyroidectomy followed by radioactive iodine ablation reduces tumor recurrence and mortality. Recently published meta-analysis addressed this issue for tumors ≤1 cm, which included six studies (1980–2014) with 2,939 patients, of which 72.6% underwent total thyroidectomy and 27.5% lobectomy [40]. The recurrence rates were significantly higher in lobectomy compared to total the thyroidectomy group. However, the mortality rates in the two groups were similar. Another meta-analysis of 13 studies with 7,048 patients concluded that the gender male, extra thyroid extension, lymph node metastasis, tumor size more than 2 cm, distance metastasis, and subtotal thyroidectomy were the risk factors influencing recurrence [41]. In another recently published study from Korea, the authors analyzed 16,057 patients with 5,266 having a tumor size between 1 and 4 cm [42]. The mean tumor size was 1.84 ± 0.74 cm. Of all, 4,292 (81.5%) total thyroidectomy and 974 (18.5%) lobectomies were performed. Recurrence rates following total thyroidectomy were 5.7% compared to 9.4% following lobectomy (Table 14.2). The lobectomy has lower disease-free survival (DFS) and higher disease-specific survival (DSS) compared to total thyroidectomy. The extent of surgery was an independent risk factor for DFS but not for DSS.

In contrast, there are studies to support the role of lobectomy in cancers up to 4 cms in diameter. Adam et al. performed updated analysis of NCDB thyroidectomies with tumor size of 1–4 cm. The study included 61,775 patients of which 54,926 underwent total thyroidectomy and 6,849 lobectomies. After making adjustments for patient demographic and clinical factors, including comorbidities, extrathyroidal extension, multifocality, nodal and distant metastases, and radioiodine treatment, the overall survival (OS) was similar in the two groups for tumor size of 1–4 cm and also after stratifying according to the tumor sizes 1–2 and 2.1–4 cm (Table 14.3).

Haigh et al. identified 5,432 thyroidectomies in Surveillance, Epidemiology, and End Results (SEER) database. According to AMES classification (age, metastasis, extrathyroidal spread, size), 4,402 (81%) were categorized as low-risk and 1,030 (19%) as high-risk, 92.5% of tumors were smaller than 5 cm, and 85.4% were intrathyroidal. Total thyroidectomy was performed in 83.2% of the low-risk cancers and 92.1% of the high-risk tumors. The 10-year survival rate in the low-risk group was 89% after total thyroidectomy compared to 91% after partial thyroidectomy (P = 0.07). Whereas in high-risk patients, the 10-year survival rate was 72% after total thyroidectomy compared to 78% after partial thyroidectomy

Table 14.2 Studies comparing hemi- versus total thyroidectomy: Recurrence rates

Study	End point	HT	TT	Results
Hay et al. (1940–1991)	20-year local recurrence	14%	2%	Significant
	20-year regional nodal metastasis	19%	6%	Significant
Bilimoria et al. (1985–1998)	10-year recurrence rate	9.8%	7.7%	Significant
Nixon et al. (1986–2005)	10-year local recurrence	0%	0%	NS
	10-year regional recurrence	0%	0.8%	NS

Table 14.3   Studies comparing hemi- versus total thyroidectomy: Survival outcomes

Study	Patient population	Sample size total/lobectomy	Endpoints	Result	Recommendations
Hay et al. (1940–1991)	Low-risk (AMES) papillary thyroid cancer (PTC), Mayo clinic	1,663 Total thyroidectomy (TT): 1,468 (88.2%) Hashimoto's thyroiditis (HT): 195 (11.73%)	Cause specific mortality (CSM), recurrence rate	Not significant (NS) for CSM and distant metastasis, significant for nodal and local recurrence	Seven-fold difference in local recurrence, optimal surgery is total thyroidectomy
Mendelsohn et al. (1998–2001)	PTCs T1–4N0-1, SEER database	22,724 TT: 16,760 (73.7%) HT: 5,964 (26.2%)	Disease specific survival, overall survival (OS)	NS	Benefit of total thyroidectomy is not uniform across all populations
Bilimoria et al. (1985–1998)	PTC T1–4N0-1 NCBS	52,173 TT: 43,227 (82.85%) HT: 8,946 (17.15%)	Ten-year recurrence and survival	Improved for total thyroidectomy, significantly	Total thyroidectomy for PTC ≥ 1 cm
Nixon et al. (1986-2005)	WDTC T1/2N0 MSKCC	889 TT: 528 (59.39%) HT: 361 (40.61%)	Ten-year OS, disease specific survival, recurrence free survival	NS	Lobectomy is safe option for intrathyroidal malignancy
Adam et al. (1998–2006)	PTC, T1/2N0-1 NCDB	61,775 TT: 54,926 (88.91%) HT: 6,849 (11.09%)	OS (adjusted)	NS	Tumor size alone questionable indication for total thyroidectomy

(P = 0.66). The authors concluded that the extent of thyroidectomy had no significant impact on survival in these patients. In another SEER database study, Barney et al. included 23,605 patients between 1983 and 2002. Results showed that 10-year OS and cause-specific survival (CSS) were similar in total thyroidectomy when compared to hemithyroidectomy both on univariate and multivariate analysis. Mendelson et al. studied 22,724 patients from the SEER database, of which 5,964 underwent lobectomy. There was no survival difference between patients who underwent total thyroidectomy versus lobectomy. In a study from MSKCC, 899 patients with pT1T2N0 were analyzed, and 59% of patients underwent total thyroidectomy and 41% lobectomy. The results of the study showed that extent of surgery did not impact OS, local recurrence, or regional recurrence. Song et al. performed propensity score matched paired analysis on recurrence in a cohort of 2,345 patients to compare the outcomes of lobectomy versus total thyroidectomy. Of all patients, 83.7% underwent total thyroidectomy and 16.3% lobectomy. There was no significant difference in DFS between the two groups. Extent of surgery was not an independent factor affecting persistent or recurrent disease.

Interpretation of these Results: These studies are large but mainly retrospective and therefore have limitations and a selection bias. It is pertinent to note that even in studies advocating lobectomy for nodule size up to 4 cm, the majority of patients underwent a total thyroidectomy in upwards of 60% of patients. Details regarding patient characteristics, tumor characteristics, and completeness of surgery are missing in many studies. These studies are heterogenous in terms of aims and end points. The end points in these studies are very varied and include overall survival, cause specific survival, disease free survival, locoregional recurrence, need for radioiodine ablation, and morbidity. A randomized trial would be ideal to provide convincing results but is implausible due to the very large sample size required, given an excellent outcome, few events, and the need for prolonged follow-up.

In clinical practice and in the real-world scenario there is no debate that lesions <1 cm that are intrathyroidal are treated with a hemithyroidectomy while a total thyroidectomy is recommended for lesions greater than 4 cms. While survival is similar in lesions between 1 and 4 cm and recommended in the ATA guidelines, the patient and family must be taken into confidence and the pros and cons of the procedures discussed.

SURGICAL TIPS AND TRICKS

Samuel Gross once stated of thyroid surgery: "Can the thyroid in the state of enlargement be removed? Emphatically, experience answers 'NO'. Should the surgeon be so foolhardy to undertake it, every stroke of the knife will be followed by a torrent of blood and lucky it would be if his victim lived long enough for him to finish his horrid butchery. No honest and sensible surgeon would ever engage in it." It was Kocher who standardized the procedure of thyroidectomy and was awarded the Nobel Prize in 1909 for his work on thyroid surgeries. Thyroid surgery has come a long way since then, and today thyroidectomy is a safe procedure. A detailed description of thyroidectomy is out of scope of this chapter. While there is no substitute to a thorough knowledge of thyroid anatomy and meticulous surgery, a few tips and tricks that the authors find useful in reducing the morbidity of thyroidectomy from literature and personal experience are mentioned in the following section. There is a recent interest in minimally invasive and remote access surgery which are covered elsewhere in this book.

1. *Incision:* For open access surgery, the incision must be adequate in length balancing proper exposure against cosmesis. Small incisions result in inadequate exposure and excessive traction leading to necrosis of the skin edges and poor cosmesis on healing. An incision is best placed in a natural skin crease extending from anterior border of one sternocleidomastoid to the other two fingers' breadth above the suprasternal notch. Placing it too low will drag the incision into the chest and result in a hypertrophic scar. For similar reasons the incision should be placed slightly higher in patients with large pendulous breasts. It is prudent to mark the incision in the sitting position prior to induction for easier identification of the best suited skin crease rather than when the neck is in extension.

2. The incision should be symmetrically equal on both sides of the midline even if the procedure is performed on one side as it is esthetically more acceptable.

3. The external branch of the superior laryngeal nerve (EBSLN) is classically described to be located in Joll's triangle (midline, superior pole of the thyroid and the superior pedicle laterally and the insertion of the straps superiorly). However, it is easier to consider the relationship of the nerve to the superior pedicle of the thyroid. In the majority of patients, the nerve is a centimeter away from the junction of the superior pole with the thyroid and ligating the superior pedicle close to the gland will safeguard the nerve. Similarly, induvial ligation of the branches on the superior pole helps identify and preserve a low-lying nerve. Overzealous attempts at demonstrating the nerve should be avoided as it can result in troublesome bleeding from small vessels, which places the nerve at risk.

4. *Parathyroids*: The parathyroids are variable in location but in the vast majority of patients the superior parathyroid is located close to the nodule of Zuckerkandl in the middle third of the lobe of the thyroid gland in relation to its posterior border. The inferior parathyroid which can be more variable in position is typically located within a centimeter from the inferior pole. The superior parathyroid is always dorsal to the recurrent laryngeal nerve and the inferior ventral to it. This plane of the recurrent laryngeal nerve to the parathyroids is often referred to as the plane of Payne and Pyrtec. If the parathyroids are not found in their usual location they should be searched dorsal or ventral to the nerve depending on which gland is being searched. The glands are symmetrically placed on both sides in 70%–80% of cases and this helps making contralateral identification easier. Despite locating the gland, hypoparathyroidism results due to disruption to its blood supply. This is safeguarded by performing capsular dissection which is literally hugging the thyroid gland and ligating the tertiary branches of the inferior thyroid artery beyond the parathyroid and close to the thyroid capsule. This also minimizes the risk to the recurrent laryngeal nerve.

5. Parathyroids are identified, dissected off the thyroid gland, and reflected laterally to preserve the blood supply to these glands which traverses lateral to medially. A Ligaclip® is used to tag the parathyroids, which helps to achieve hemostasis, avoid the use of diathermy close to the parathyroid, as well as serve as an identification marker should a central compartmental nodal clearance be necessary (Figure 14.1).

6. Parathyroids are differentiated from fat tissue lymph nodes by their tan color, soft consistency, and a characteristic elliptical or kidney shape with the presence of a vascular hilum.

7. If the parathyroid is devascularized inadvertently during the surgery, it should be autotransplanted, which is usually into the ipsilateral sternocleidomastoid muscle. A dusky parathyroid with an intact blood supply is due to venous engorgement or a subcapsular hematoma. A fine 24/25 G needle is used to puncture the capsule that often results in a return of normal color prior to autotransplantation.

8. Meticulous clearance along the isthmus and pyramidal lobe if present is dissected in its entirety along with the gland. It can harbor disease, especially in multicentric PTC as borne out by our study where PL contained disease deposits in 10.53% of the cases [43].

9. *Ensuring completeness of thyroidectomy*: Areas prone to incomplete clearance and that have residual thyroid tissue or disease left behind are the superior pole, pyramidal lobe, delphian nodes, tissue in relation to Berry's ligament, and embryonal thyroid rest cells. Meticulous dissection in these areas prevents this happening. The pyramidal lobe is usually located in approximately 1–2/3rd of patients on the left in relation to the isthmus and can extend as high as the hyoid. If not found on the left it should be searched for on the right.

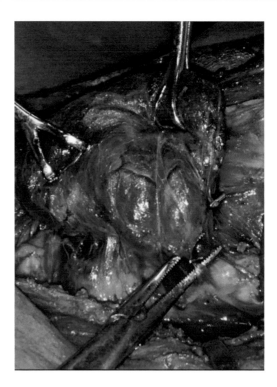

Figure 14.1 Capsular dissection of thyroid lobe with ligation of tertiary branches of inferior thyroid artery: Ligaclip® to mark the parathyroid.

Embryonal rests are in relationship to the inferior pole usually in continuity but can occasionally be isolated and at a distance away. The surgeon should ensure meticulous clearance of disease in these areas.

10. *Recurrent laryngeal nerve*: The RLN is classically located where it forms one of the boundaries of Beahr's triangle, the other two being the carotid and the inferior thyroid artery. The recurrent laryngeal nerve may have branches, and awareness and identification are imperative to prevent damage. Branching may be present in up to 60% of patients and are usually motor when cephalad the inferior thyroid artery. In cases of resurgery where it is difficult to identify the nerve amidst the fibrosis, it is prudent to identify the nerve below the scar of the last surgery in a relatively virgin area. Such cases can be located in Lore's triangle which is lower down in the neck, formed by the trachea or the esophagus in the midline, carotid artery laterally, and the surface of the lower pole of the thyroid superiorly.

11. *Aids at thyroidectomy*: Various aids such as magnification, hemostasis instruments (Harmonic scalpel), IONM, and Fluoptics for parathyroid localization have been described and propagated by various authors with some cited benefits. However, there is no conclusive proof to advocate their routine use. In cases of resurgery, one may consider using intra-operative nerve monitoring. There is no substitute to meticulous surgical technique and thorough understanding of the anatomy.

REFERENCES

1. Brito JP, Davies L. Is there really an increased incidence of thyroid cancer? *Curr Opin Endocrinol Diabetes Obes.* 2014 Oct;21(5):405–408.

2. Ferlay J et al. Cancer incidence in five continents. Vol I to IX: IARC CancerBase No 9. http://ci5.iarc.fr

3. Vaccarella S, Franceschi S, Bray F, Wild CP, Plummer M, Dal Maso L. Worldwide thyroid-cancer epidemic? The increasing impact of overdiagnosis. *N Engl J Med.* 2016 Aug;375(7):614–617.

4. Ahn HS, Kim HJ, Welch HG. Korea's thyroid-cancer "epidemic"—screening and overdiagnosis. *N Engl J Med.* 2014 Nov;371(19):1765–1767.

5. Brito JP, Morris JC, Montori VM. Thyroid cancer: Zealous imaging has increased detection and treatment of low risk tumours. *BMJ.* 2013 Aug;347:f4706.

6. Dean DS, Gharib H. Epidemiology of thyroid nodules. *Best Pract Res Clin Endocrinol Metab.* 2008 Dec;22(6):901–911.

7. Ito Y, Miyauchi A, Kihara M, Higashiyama T, Kobayashi K, Miya A. Patient age is significantly related to the progression of papillary microcarcinoma of the thyroid under observation. *Thyroid.* 2014;24:27–34.

8. Oda H et al. Incidences of unfavorable events in the management of low-risk papillary microcarcinoma of the thyroid by active surveillance versus immediate surgery. *Thyroid.* 2016 Jan;26(1):150–155.

9. Haser GC et al. Active surveillance for papillary thyroid microcarcinoma: New challenges and opportunities for the health care system. *Endocr Pract.* 2016 May;22(5):602–611.

10. Brito JP, Ito Y, Miyauchi A, Tuttle RM. A clinical framework to facilitate risk stratification when considering an active surveillance alternative to immediate biopsy and surgery in papillary microcarcinoma. *Thyroid.* 2016 Jan; 26(1):144–149.

11. Bergamaschi R, Becouarn G, Ronceray J, Arnaud JP. Morbidity of thyroid surgery. *Am J Surg.* 1998 Jul;176(1):71–75.

12. Davies L, Welch HG. Thyroid cancer survival in the United States: Observational data from 1973 to 2005. *Arch Otolaryngol Head Neck Surg.* 2010 May;136(5):440–444.

13. Adam MA et al. Extent of surgery for papillary thyroid cancer is not associated with survival: an analysis of 61 775 patients. *Ann Surg.* 2014 Oct;260(4):601–605; discussion 605–7.

14. Haigh PI, Urbach DR, Rotstein LE. Extent of thyroidectomy is not a major determinant of survival in low- or high-risk papillary thyroid cancer. *Ann Surg Oncol.* 2005 Jan; 12(1):81–89.

15. Barney BM, Hitchcock YJ, Sharma P, Shrieve DC, Tward JD. Overall and cause-specific survival for patients undergoing lobectomy, near-total, or total thyroidectomy for differentiated thyroid cancer. *Head Neck.* 2011 May;33(5):645–649.

16. Mendelsohn AH, Elashoff DA, Abemayor E, St John MA. Surgery for papillary thyroid carcinoma: Is lobectomy enough? *Arch Otolaryngol Head Neck Surg.* 2010 Nov;136(11):1055–1061.

17. Song E et al. Lobectomy is feasible for 1–4 cm papillary thyroid carcinomas: A 10-year propensity score matched-pair analysis on recurrence. *Thyroid.* 2019 Jan;29(1):64–70.

18. Wang C-CC et al. A large multicentre correlation study of thyroid nodule cytopathology and histopathology. *Thyroid.* 2011;21(3):243–251.

19. Cibas ES, Ali SZ. The 2017 Bethesda system for reporting thyroid cytopathology. *Thyroid.* 2017;27(11):1341–1346.

20. D'Cruz AK et al. Molecular markers in well-differentiated thyroid cancer. *Eur Arch Orhinolaryngol.* 2018 Jun; 275(6):1375–1384.

21. Schneider DF et al. Gauging the extent of thyroidectomy for indeterminate thyroid nodules: An oncologic perspective. *Endocr Pract.* 2017 Apr;23(4):442–450.

22. Chiu CG et al. Hemithyroidectomy is the preferred initial operative approach for an indeterminate fine needle aspiration biopsy diagnosis. *Can J Surg.* 2012 Jun;55(3):191–198.

23. Glockzin G et al. Completion thyroidectomy: Effect of timing on clinical complications and oncologic outcome in patients with differentiated thyroid cancer.

24. Barczyński M, Konturek A, Pragacz K, Papier A, Stopa M, Nowak W. Intraoperative nerve monitoring can reduce prevalence of recurrent laryngeal nerve injury in thyroid reoperations: Results of a retrospective cohort study. *World J Surg.* 2014 Mar;38(3):599–606.

25. Cirocchi R et al. Intraoperative neuromonitoring versus visual nerve identification for prevention of recurrent laryngeal nerve injury in adults undergoing thyroid surgery. *Cochrane Database Syst Rev.* 2019;1:CD012483. World J Surg. 2012 May;36(5):1168–73.

26. Sanabria A et al. Methodological quality of systematic reviews of intraoperative neuromonitoring in thyroidectomy: A systematic review. *JAMA Otolaryngol Head Neck Surg.* 2019 Jun;145(6):563–573.

27. Nath MC, Erickson LA. Aggressive variants of papillary thyroid carcinoma: Hobnail, tall cell, columnar, and solid. *Adv Anat Pathol.* 2018 May;25(3):172–179.

28. Silver CE, Owen RP, Rodrigo JP, Rinaldo A, Devaney KO, Ferlito A. Aggressive variants of papillary thyroid carcinoma. *Head Neck.* 2011 Jul;33(7):1052–1059.

29. Iglesias ML et al. Radiation exposure and thyroid cancer: A review. *Arch Endocrinol Metab.* 2017 Mar-Apr;61(2):180–187.

30. Seaberg RM, Eski S, Freeman JL. Influence of previous radiation exposure on pathologic features and clinical outcome in patients with thyroid cancer. *Arch Otolaryngol Head Neck Surg.* 2009 Apr;135(4):355–359.

31. Uchino S et al. Familial nonmedullary thyroid carcinoma characterized by multifocality and a high recurrence rate in a large study population. *World J Surg.* 2002 Aug;26(8):897–902.

32. Nose V. Familial thyroid cancer: A review. *Modern Pathol.* 2011;24:S19–33.

33. Uchino S et al. Detection of asymptomatic differentiated thyroid carcinoma by neck ultrasonographic screening for familial nonmedullary thyroid carcinoma. *World J Surg.* 2004 Nov;28(11):1099–1102.

34. Nixon IJ et al. Defining a valid age cutoff in staging of well-differentiated thyroid cancer. *Ann Surg Oncol.* 2016 Feb; 23(2):410–415.

35. https://connection.asco.org/discussion/thyroid-cancer-asco-tumor-boards.

36. Haugen BR et al. 2015 American Thyroid Association management guidelines for adult patients with thyroid nodules and differentiated thyroid cancer: The American Thyroid Association guidelines task force on thyroid nodules and differentiated thyroid cancer. *Thyroid.* 2016 Jan;26(1):1–133.

37. Bilimoria KY et al. Extent of surgery affects survival for papillary thyroid cancer. *Ann Surg.* 2007;246(3):375–381.

38. Hay ID et al. Papillary thyroid carcinoma managed at the Mayo Clinic during six decades (1940–1999): Temporal trends in initial therapy and long-term outcome in 2,444 consecutively treated patients. *World J Surg.* 2002 Aug;26(8):879–885.

39. Mazzaferri EL, Jhiang SM. Long-term impact of initial surgical and medical therapy on papillary and follicular thyroid cancer. *Am J Med.* 1994 Nov;97(5):418–428.

40. Macedo FI, Mittal VK. Total thyroidectomy versus lobectomy as initial operation for small unilateral papillary thyroid carcinoma: A meta-analysis. *Surg Oncol.* 2015 Jun; 24(2):117–122.

41. Guo K, Wang Z. Risk factors influencing the recurrence of papillary thyroid carcinoma: A systematic review and meta-analysis. *Int J Clin Exp Pathol.* 2014 Aug;7(9):5393–5403.

42. Choi JB et al. Oncologic outcomes in patients with 1-cm to 4-cm differentiated thyroid carcinoma according to extent of thyroidectomy. *Head Neck.* 2019 Jan;41(1):56–63.

43. Irawati N, Vaish R, Chaukar D, Deshmukh A, D'Cruz A. Surgical anatomy of the pyramidal lobe in cancer patients: A prospective cohort in a tertiary centre. *Int J Surg.* 2016 Jun; 30:166–168.

Chapter 15

MANAGEMENT OF NODAL METASTASIS IN THYROID CANCER

Neeti Kapre Gupta, Ashok Shaha, Madan Laxman Kapre, Nirmala Thakkar, and Harsh Karan Gupta

CONTENTS

Quantification of the Problem   113
Diagnosis   113
Conclusions   116
References   116

QUANTIFICATION OF THE PROBLEM

Depending upon tumor factors, patient factors, and the imaging modality employed, reported prevalence of neck nodes in differentiated thyroid cancers is approximately 50%–80% [1–4]. At the first instance, DTC lymphatic spreads to the level VI or central compartment. Later, they may metastasize to superior mediastinal (level VII) lymph nodes and lateral compartment (level I–V). However, levels II–IV are most commonly involved. The skip metastasis to level II lymph nodes in the absence of level VI nodes, which is in fact the first echelon for differentiated thyroid cancers, is uncommon. Generally, superior pole nodules follow such a pattern [5].

Nodal disease does increase the risk of recurrence, especially when lymph node metastases are macroscopic, although it does not impact significantly on survival. It is less clear how the microscopic lymph node metastases impact recurrence and survival [6–10] (Table 15.1).

DIAGNOSIS

It is mandatory that all patients undergo operative neck ultrasonography for cervical lymph nodes undergoing thyroidectomy for malignancy or suspicion for malignancy. Ultrasound-guided FNB of sonographically suspicious lymph nodes 8–10 mm in the smallest diameter should be performed to confirm malignancy. A positive result would obviously change management (Recommendation 33, ATA Guidelines 2015) [14]. There is enough literature to support the superiority of CT scan in diagnosis of metastatic nodes [15]. Contrast-enhanced CT scan has incremental value over ultrasound in diagnosing level VI nodes, especially with the presence of the thyroid gland. It also helps in delineating lateral compartment nodes and their relationship to jugular veins and carotid arteries better. There is a myth regarding contraindication for use of

Table 15.1 Prognosticators for increased risk of nodal metastases

Prognosticators of nodal metastasis [11]
1. Under the age of 15 years [12]
2. Male sex
3. Extra thyroidal extension
4. Aggressive pathological variants such as tall cell, columnar cell, diffuse sclerosing, or insular
5. BRAF/TERT mutation positivity [13]

iodinated contrast in thyroid cancer imaging. This is largely due to better understanding of the wash out time of the contrast media. Therefore, there is no harm in using contrast-enhanced CT scans to provide more anatomical information on nodal metastasis. Generally, the presence of bulky nodal disease is also associated with locally extensive disease and occasionally the presence of distant metastasis. Therefore, contrast CT scans provide a good one-time imaging opportunity to screen neck nodes, lung nodules, and mediastinal nodes, along with precise information on local extension of the disease. It also gives us an assessment of the disease extension into the strap muscles or the laryngotracheal framework. MRI should be reserved for cases where extensive vascular or esophageal involvement is suspected.

There is currently no recommendation for PET scan as an upfront imaging modality to assess nodal disease in thyroid cancers (Recommendation 33, ATA Guidelines, 2015) [14].

Thus, the CT scan offers the following advantages:

- Improved nodal diagnosis, particularly nodes in the central compartment
- Detection of extrathyroidal extension, including aerodigestive tract involvement
- Imaging of mediastinal nodes and metastatic lung nodules
- Iodinated contrast is no longer contraindicated

FNB is an important diagnostic test to be performed pre-operatively to document metastatic nodal involvement. Additionally, FNB-Tg wash out in the evaluation of suspicious cervical lymph nodes is appropriate in selected patients; however, its interpretation may be difficult in patients with a normally functioning thyroid gland [16]. Frozen sections provide a very reliable diagnostic tool intra-operatively. The authors have their own experience with crush imprint cytology as a surrogate to frozen section examination. This method of intra-operative pathology has an accuracy of approximately 97%.

SURGICAL MANAGEMENT OF METASTASES NECK NODES IN DIFFERENTIATED THYROID CANCERS

Management is broadly classified into central compartment neck dissection and lateral compartment neck dissection.

Central compartment neck dissection (CCND) in presence of documented metastatic nodes in a pre-operative setting is referred to as therapeutic CCND. Nodal dissection done in the absence of clinical, radiologically proven disease is referred to as prophylactic CCND.

Therapeutic CCND is no longer an issue of debate (Recommendation 36, ATA Guidelines 2015) and is performed in the following scenarios:

1. Clinically and radiologically manifested or pathologically proven central compartment nodal disease.

2. Documented lateral compartment nodal diseases.

Prophylactic central compartment neck dissection, however, attracts great controversy. Even in the presence of several meta-analyses, there is still no consensus statement [17–20].

Arguments in support of prophylactic central compartment neck dissection are:

1. No imaging or pathology exam is absolute for detection of central compartment nodes prior to surgery [21].

2. Intra-operative surgeon assessment is not reliable [22].

3. Occult central compartment metastasis are present in up to 80% of cases.

4. Accurate staging helps in better planning of adjuvant treatment [23].

5. Revision surgery in central compartment has significantly higher incidence of recurrent laryngeal nerve palsy and hypocalcemia [24,25].

Arguments opposing prophylactic central compartment neck dissection are:

1. Significantly higher incidence of hypoparathyroidism, especially in low volume centers [26].

2. No significant detriment to survival outcomes [17,18].

The American Thyroid Association Consensus Statement on central compartment neck dissection clearly defines anatomical boundaries, indications, and terminologies for surgical procedures [27]. The central compartment extends between the carotid arteries laterally on either side, superiorly from hyoid bone and inferiorly up to the innominate artery. This includes the pre-laryngeal (delphian), pre-tracheal, and paratracheal lymph nodes. Level VII lymph nodes are the superior mediastinal lymph nodes.

All surgeons will minimally differ in philosophies on central compartment neck dissection (CCND) surgery. The following surgical procedures are commonly practiced:

● *Exploration of central compartment*: Minimal dissection is done to identify presence of metastatic nodes in central compartment.

   In absence of clinically identifiable node, procedure is terminated.

   If nodes are identified, a formal CCND is performed.

● *Sampling of central compartment*: Clinically suspicious nodes are subjected to intra-operative pathology assessment (frozen section or crush imprint cytology)

   If reported positive, formal CCND clearance is performed.

● *Central compartment nodal clearance*: This is often referred to as therapeutic CCND. This entails clearance of all lymphatic tissue and fibro fatty tissue from carotid arteries on either side bilaterally and from hyoid to innominate artery above downwards.

   Quite a few surgeons perform ipsilateral CCND only in an attempt to preserve contralateral parathyroids and their vasculature. This entails clearance of pre-laryngeal, pre-tracheal, and para-tracheal (between carotid and trachea) on the ipsilateral side; bilateral CCND would encompass clearance of all pre-laryngeal, pre-tracheal, and bilateral para-tracheal nodes.

SURGICAL TIPS

Dissection in central compartment often commences after the total thyroidectomy is performed. The key step is actually taken during the initial ligating of the terminal branch of the inferior thyroid

artery and to trace and identify the terminal branch or end artery to the inferior parathyroid gland. This can be marked or clipped with a Ligaclip® to ease identification of the parathyroids with their supplying vessels during further dissection. Some surgeons prefer the clearance of para-tracheal nodes only medial to the RLN, i.e., between the RLN and trachea. The presumption is that this results in lowering the rate of hypoparathyroidism as the majority of parathyroid blood supply comes laterally. Also, there is an adequate oncological clearance as most of the metastatic nodes are medial to the RLN. The authors, however, believe in thorough ipsilateral CCND. The operating surgeon stands at the head end of the table, and an assistant applies gentle traction over the cricothyroid joint anteriorly. This maneuver allows the surgeon to work better along the RLN clearing all nodes on either side of it (Figures 15.1 and 15.2). One must also constantly bear in mind variations in the course of the nerve on either side. Being more angulated to the tracheoesophageal groove, the right RLN may be at more risk of injury. It is better to keep the nerve in its prevertebral fascia coverings and avoid handling to prevent neuropraxic and vascular damage. Magnification by the way of optical loops is preferred by some surgeons for allowing adequate clearance of disease and preservation of the RLN and the parathyroids with their vasculature. Use of intra-operative nerve monitoring during central compartment neck dissection is also recommended for reducing chances of RLN injuries, particularly in revision surgery.

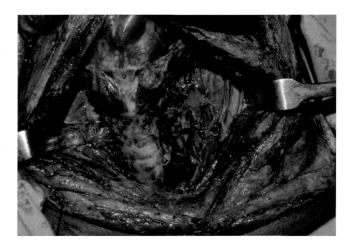

Figure 15.1 Completed level 2 to 4 with thyroidectomy.

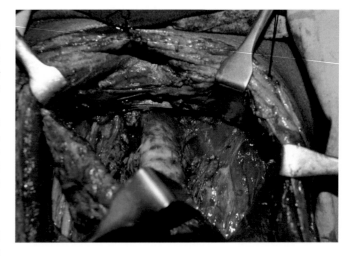

Figure 15.2 Complete central neck dissection from head end.

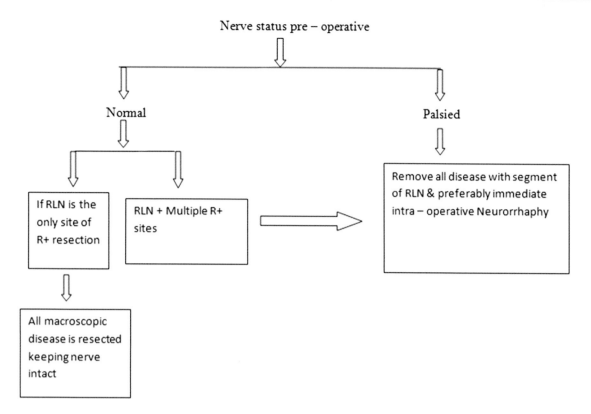

Figure 15.3 Nerve status pre-operative.

In case of nodal disease severely engulfing or involving the RLN, the following algorithm may prove useful (Figure 15.3).

The reasoning for primary nerve repair is the return of function in approximately 50% of patients [28]. This enables maintenance of the bulk of the vocal cord muscles and aids voice rehabilitation.

In the event of accidental parathyroidectomy along with CCND, auto-transplantation of the concerned gland must be transplanted in the strap or the SCM muscles. It is important to mark the transplantation site and to have a small bit of tissue for histopathological confirmation. If at the end of the procedure the parathyroid gland appears dusky, one should suspect hematoma in the parathyroid capsule. A small nick with a scalpel or needle may help to relieve this hematoma and the gland may partially or completely regain its color. In this case nothing is required to be done. For a devascularized gland, however, auto-transplantation may still yield a more successful outcome.

LATERAL COMPARTMENT

Following are the indications for Neck Dissection:

1. Extensive nodal disease in central compartment
2. Documented nodes in lateral compartment

There is no indication for performing prophylactic lateral compartment neck dissection (Recommendation 37, ATA Guidelines 2015) [14].

Several philosophies are in practice for managing the lateral neck in DTC, such as elective nodal sampling, ultrasound directed compartmental resections, and super selective nodal dissection [29].

Historically, Berry picking or selective sampling and removal of nodes is condemned. A selective neck dissection clearing all lymph nodes and fibrofatty tissue from levels II–IV is generally practiced preserving the sternocleidomastoid muscle, internal jugular vein, and the spinal accessory nerve. Sacrificing any of these structures should be considered only in the presence of gross disease with obvious involvement of the structures. Lymph nodes at the levels of I and V should ideally be cleared only in the presence of obvious involvement by disease. Some authors recommend the dictum of

clearing level V in case level II nodes are involved (Figure 15.4). There is always a debate about clearance of level IIb in view of scant metastases at this nodal station and increased risk of traction injuries to the spinal accessory nerve during this dissection [30]. The level IIb clearance should be mandatory in case of positive nodes at level IIa.

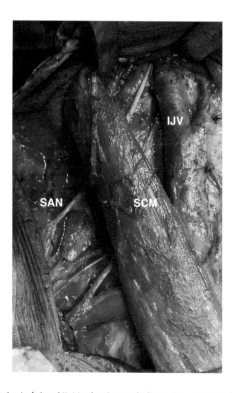

Figure 15.4 Left level II–V selective neck dissection, sparing the internal jugular vein (IJV), sternocleidomastoid (SCM), and spinal accessory nerve (SAN).

Table 15.2   Risk of nodal recurrence in differentiated thyroid cancers

	Risk of recurrence–avg (range)
Clinically N0, pN0	4% (0%–9%)
Clinically N0, microscopic pN1	6% (4%–11.5%)
No. of nodes ≤5	4% (3%–8%)
No. of nodes >5	19% (7%–21%)
Nodes with extranodal extension	24% (15%–32%)

A very interesting study by Dr. Randolph et al. [31] estimates the chances of nodal recurrence in node positive patients. Number of nodes, nodal dimensions, evidence of extranodal extension, and lymph node ratios are important prognostic factors. Patients with small volume nodal disease, <5 nodes, microscopic metastases, and without extranodal extension have lower chances of recurrence (approximately 5%), whereas patients with high volume nodal disease, >5 nodes, >5 mm nodal diameter, and extranodal extension have a higher chance (approximately 20%) of nodal recurrence (Table 15.2).

Revision surgery for nodal recurrence: Revising lateral neck is a relatively simpler proposition. Revision surgery for central compartment neck dissection has decidedly higher morbidity. The physician needs to seek balance between the fact that surgical resection of gross nodal disease is the best treatment on one hand and that unnecessary surgery stands the risk of increased chances of nerve injuries and hypocalcemia on the other. Therefore, patient selection remains the key. Generally, a size threshold criterion is advocated (central compartment node ≥8 mm, lateral compartment node ≥10 mm). Only such nodes should be subjected to FNAC. Low volume neck disease can be safely kept under observation since the risk of revision surgery is far higher than the benefit awarded. However, sometimes, the following factors influence the decision to proceed with surgery:

1. Aggressive histology
2. Previous nodal burden
3. Thyroglobulin doubling time
4. Proximity to delicate visceral structures
5. Patient anxiety

Such surgeries should ideally be undertaken at high volume centers by experienced surgeons. Precise pre-operative cross sectional imaging as needed, supplemented by functional scans such as PET-CT, is a prerequisite. Use of magnification, and accurate localization of the nodes, including employment of intra-operative sonology, are important prerequisites for reducing the incidence of post-operative hypoparathyroidism. Intra-operative nerve monitoring will ensure physiology integrity and identification of the RLN.

Percutaneous ethanol injection has been tried specifically for patients who are poor surgical candidates. Up to 80% resolution of structural nodal disease and lowering of Tg to acceptable range (<3 ng/mL) has been observed. However, multiple sessions are often required and this technique is not very effective for larger nodes (>2 cm) [32].

CONCLUSIONS

Nodal metastasis in well-differentiated thyroid cancers is an entirely surgical disease. One of the important prognostic factors in the various scoring systems is completeness of resection. Now the concept of dynamic risk stratification is universally accepted, and it is the surgeon's responsibility to resect all the disease.

No structural disease should be left behind. As there are very reasonable survival outcomes in differentiated thyroid cancers it is the surgeons' responsibility to procure disease free status with minimum morbidity in the form of hypoparathyroidism or RLN injury.

REFERENCES

1. Kim E, Park JS, Son KR, Kim JH, Jeon SJ, Na DG. Preoperative diagnosis of cervical metastatic lymph nodes in papillary thyroid carcinoma: Comparison of ultrasound, computed tomography, and combined ultrasound with computed tomography. *Thyroid*. 2008;18:411–8.
2. Noguchi S, Noguchi A, Murakami N. Papillary carcinoma of the thyroid. I. Developing pattern of metastasis. *Cancer*. 1970;26:1053–60.
3. Stulak JM, Grant CS, Farley DR, Thompson GB, van Heerden JA, Hay ID, Reading CC, Charboneau JW. Value of preoperative ultrasonography in the surgical management of initial and reoperative papillary thyroid cancer. *Arch Surg*. 2006;141:489–94.
4. Arturi F et al. Early diagnosis by genetic analysis of differentiated thyroid cancer metastases in small lymph nodes. *Endocrinol Metab*. 1997;82:1638–41.
5. Lei J, Zhong J, Jiang K, Li Z, Gong R, Zhu J. Skip lateral lymph node metastasis leaping over the central neck compartment in papillary thyroid carcinoma. *Oncotarget*. 2017 Apr;8910:27022–33.
6. Bardet S et al. Macroscopic lymph-node involvement and neck dissection predict lymph-node recurrence in papillary thyroid carcinoma. *Eur J Endocrinol*. 2008;158:551–60.
7. Lundgren CI, Hall P, Dickman PW, Zedenius J. Clinically significant prognostic factors for differentiated thyroid carcinoma: A population-based, nested case-control study. *Cancer*. 2006;106:524–31.
8. Podnos YD, Smith D, Wagman LD, Ellenhorn JD. The implication of lymph node metastasis on survival in patients with well-differentiated thyroid cancer. *Am Surg*. 2005;71:731–4.
9. Lebouleux S et al. Prognostic factors for persistent or recurrent disease of papillary thyroid carcinoma with neck lymph node metastases and/or tumor extension beyond the thyroid capsule at initial diagnosis. *Endocrinol Metab*. 2005;90:5723–9.
10. Mazzaferri EL, Young RL. Papillary thyroid carcinoma: A 10 year follow-up report of the impact of therapy in 576 patients. *Am J Med*. 1981;70:511–8.
11. Stack BC Jr. (Chair) et al.; American Thyroid Association Surgical Affairs Committee. American Thyroid Association Consensus Review and Statement Regarding the Anatomy, Terminology, and Rationale for Lateral Neck Dissection in Differentiated Thyroid Cancer.
12. Choi YJ, Yun JS, Kook SH, Jung EC, Park YL. Clinical and imaging assessment of cervical lymph node metastasis in papillary thyroid carcinomas. *World J Surg*. 2010;34:1494–9.
13. Xing M et al. BRAF mutation predicts a poorer clinical prognosis for papillary thyroid cancer. *J Clin Endocrinol Metab*. 2005;90:6373–9.
14. Cooper DS et al. Revised American Thyroid Association management guidelines for patients with thyroid nodules and differentiated thyroid cancer. *Thyroid*. 2009;19:1167–214.

15. Lesnik D et al. Papillary thyroid carcinoma nodal surgery directed by a preoperative radiographic map utilizing CT scan and ultrasound in all primary and reoperative patients. *Head Neck.* 2014;36:191–202.

16. Salmaslıoğlu A et al. Diagnostic value of thyroglobulin measurement in fine needle aspiration biopsy for detecting metastatic lymph nodes in patients with papillary thyroid carcinoma. *Langenbecks Arch Surg.* 2011;396:77–81.

17. Zhao WJ, Luo H, Zhou YM, Dai WY, Zhu JQ. Evaluating the effectiveness of prophylactic central neck dissection with total thyroidectomy for cN0 papillary thyroid carcinoma: An updated meta-analysis. *Eur J Surg Oncol.* 2017 Nov;43(11):1989–2000.

18. Zhao W et al. The effect of prophylactic central neck dissection on locoregional recurrence in papillary thyroid cancer after total thyroidectomy: A systematic review and meta-analysis: pCND for the locoregional recurrence of papillary thyroid cancer. *Ann Surg Oncol.* 2017 Aug;24(8):2189–98.

19. Wang TS, Cheung K, Farrokhyar F, Roman SA, Sosa JA. A meta-analysis of the effect of prophylactic central compartment neck dissection on locoregional recurrence rates in patients with papillary thyroid cancer. *Ann Surg Oncol.* 2013 Oct;20(11):3477–83.

20. Zetoune T et al. Prophylactic central neck dissection and local recurrence in papillary thyroid cancer: A meta-analysis. *Ann Surg Oncol.* 2010 Dec;17(12):3287–93.

21. Khokhar MT et al. Preoperative high-resolution ultrasound for the assessment of malignant central compartment lymph nodes in papillary thyroid cancer. *Thyroid.* 2015 Dec;25(12):1351–4.

22. Scherl S. et al. The effect of surgeon experience on the detection of metastatic lymph nodes in the central compartment and the pathologic features of clinically unapparent metastatic lymph nodes: What are we missing when we don't perform a prophylactic dissection of central compartment lymph nodes in papillary thyroid cancer? *Thyroid.* 2014;24(8):1282–8.

23. Wang TS, Evans DB, Fareau GG, Carroll T, Yen TW. Effect of prophylactic central compartment neck dissection on serum thyroglobulin and recommendations for adjuvant radioactive iodine in patients with differentiated thyroid cancer. *Ann Surg Oncol.* 2012 Dec;19(13):4217–22.

24. Lang BH, Lee GC, Ng CP, Wong KP, Wan KY, Lo CY. Evaluating the morbidity and efficacy of reoperative surgery in the central compartment for persistent/recurrent papillary thyroid carcinoma. *World J Surg.* 2013 Dec;37(12):2853–9.

25. Tufano RP, Bishop J, Wu G. Reoperative central compartment dissection for patients with recurrent/persistent papillary thyroid cancer: Efficacy, safety, and the association of the BRAF mutation. *Laryngoscope.* 2012 Jul;122(7):1634–40.

26. Sosa JA, Bowman HM, Tielsch JM, Powe NR, Gordon TA, Udelsman R. The importance of surgeon experience for clinical and economic outcomes from thyroidectomy. *Ann Surg.* 1998;228:320–30.

27. Carty SE, Cooper DS, Doherty GM, Duh QY, Kloos RT, Mandel SJ, Randolph R. Consensus statement on the terminology and classification of central neck dissection for thyroid cancer. *Thyroid.* 2009;19:1153–8.

28. Nishida T, Nakao K, Hamaji M, Kamiike W, Kurozumi K, Matsuda H. Preservation of recurrent laryngeal nerve invaded by differentiated thyroid cancer. *Ann Surg.* 1997 Jul;226(1):85–91.

29. Roh JL, Kim JM, Park CI. Lateral cervical lymph node metastases from papillary thyroid carcinoma: Pattern of nodal metastases and optimal strategy for neck dissection. *Ann Surg Oncol.* 2008;15:1177–82.

30. Farrag T, Lin F, Brownlee N, Kim M, Sheth S, Tufano RP. Is routine dissection of level II-B and V-A necessary in patients with papillary thyroid cancer undergoing lateral neck dissection for FNA-confirmed metastases in other levels. *World J Surg.* 2009;33:1680–83.

31. Randolph GW et al. American Thyroid Association Surgical Affairs Committee's Taskforce on Thyroid Cancer Nodal Surgery. The prognostic significance of nodal metastases from papillary thyroid carcinoma can be stratified based on the size and number of metastatic lymph nodes, as well as the presence of extranodal extension. *Thyroid.* 2012 Nov;22(11):1144–52.

32. Fontenot TE, Deniwar A, Bhatia P, Al-Qurayshi Z, Randolph GW, Kandil E. Percutaneous ethanol injection vs reoperation for locally recurrent papillary thyroid cancer: A systematic review and pooled analysis. *JAMA Otolaryngol Head Neck Surg.* 2015 Jun;141(6):512–8.

Chapter 16

COMPLICATIONS OF THYROID SURGERY

Gregory W. Randolph, Dipti Kamani, Cristian Slough, and Selen Soylu

CONTENTS

Introduction 119
Seroma 119
Infection 119
Hematoma 119
Hypertrophic or Keloid Scar 120
Aerodigestive Injury 120
Airway Concerns 120
Salient Points 123
Authors' Experience/Pearls of Wisdom 123
Concluding Remarks 123
References 123

INTRODUCTION

"Measure twice, cut once" is a famous carpentry proverb aptly extrapolated to the surgical world and is of particular relevance when discussing surgical complications. Up until the 19th century, thyroidectomy was associated with high mortality rate and was recommended to be performed only to save lives. With pioneering work from Kocher, the modern day thyroidectomy is a safe and elegant procedure. Presently, complications in thyroid surgery are infrequent but have the potential for high morbidity and possibly mortality. The avoidance of surgical complications and adequate management of complications is best achieved through pre-operative and intra-operative diligence. Pre-operative communication with patients and their families is also very important. An informed patient or caregiver can pick up early signs of an evolving complication and can at times be the difference between a minor setback and a major complication. Finally, meticulous surgical technique and sound anatomical and physiological knowledge are critical.

SEROMA

The incidence of seroma following thyroid surgery varies from 1.3% to 7% [1]. Seroma is more likely to occur following surgery for large goiters, total thyroidectomies, those with extensive sub-platysmal dissections, and patients with a thick sub-dermal layer. The symptoms include neck swelling and increased pain, and seroma can lead to infection, flap necrosis, and potential wound healing issues with resulting cosmetic complications. The etiology of seroma is not well understood, but risk factors include old age, higher body mass index, and hypocalcemia that may lead to seroma formation [1]. There is some evidence to suggest that new vessel sealing devices when compared to conventional techniques resulted in fewer post-operative seromas, likely related to less extensive surgical site dissection and decreased manipulation [1]. Smaller seromas may be managed conservatively with reassurance as the majority are resorbed spontaneously in 6–8 weeks. Larger and more uncomfortable seromas can be managed with sterile serial percutaneous aspirations often requiring more than one aspiration. The aspirated fluid can be sent for culture if there are concerns for infection. Placement of a drain at the time of surgery, particularly for large goiters, may help reduce the rate of seroma formation, although there is no clear evidence of their efficacy for this [2,3]. Seromas should not be confused with hematomas, which present with rapidly evolving neck swelling and subsequent airway compromise—a true surgical emergency.

INFECTION

With an incidence of 0.5%–3%, surgical site infections after thyroidectomy are rare [4,5]. Usually, for thyroid surgery, peri-operative antibiotics are not needed unless the field is contaminated by entry into the aerodigestive tract or a break in sterility during the procedure [6]. Obesity, extent of the surgery, diabetes, steroid use, smoking, and alcohol intake are predisposing factors for surgical site infection [5,7,8]. Peri-operative antibiotics can be considered in these patients, but no clear evidence exists for its efficacy in preventing infection following thyroid surgery [9]. While oral antibiotics and local wound care are sufficient for superficial wound infections, deep wound infection often requires admission, intravenous antibiotics, incision and drainage of the wound, culture of the wound, and identification of the potential source for the infection. Deep neck space infections following thyroidectomy are often associated with an undiagnosed aerodigestive tract injury and should be appropriately addressed, since underestimating such infections is perilous as these infections can often progress quickly, descend to the mediastinum, and can result in mortality [10].

HEMATOMA

Given the well-vascularized nature of the thyroid gland, meticulous hemostasis is paramount during its surgery. Post-thyroidectomy hemorrhage is a rare, but potentially life-threatening complication with an incidence of 0.1%–2.1% [11]. It needs emergent intervention.

With the new vessel sealing devices, it has been found that if post-operative hemorrhage does occur, it generally happens in the initial post-operative hours [12].

Risk factors for post-operative hemorrhage include male gender, malignancy, retrosternal extension, large goiters, Graves' disease, extent of the surgery, and anti-coagulant use [11,13–15]. This is particularly important given the new trend of outpatient surgery for thyroidectomy, so caution should be exercised on discharge of patients with multiple risk factors for post-operative bleeding.

Post-operative bleeding may occur due to a residual thyroid tissue, an unsealed vessel, an improperly tied knot, or a patient with a coagulation defect. Signs for a hematoma are evolving swelling in the neck, increasing pain, and developing respiratory distress. Drain usage in thyroidectomy has not been shown to reduce the rate of hematomas, has not been shown to be an effective "warning sign" following thyroidectomy, and indeed may actually contribute to hematoma occurrence [3]. Additionally, drains are associated with surgical site infection, longer hospital stay, and more post-operative pain [3]. Therefore, routine drain usage in thyroidectomy is not recommended [16].

Early diagnosis of hematoma development is essential. Larger, deeper hematomas, with bleeding deep to the strap muscles, may cause venous and lymphatic congestion with subsequent laryngopharyngeal edema, airway compromise, tracheal compression, and airway obstruction. Immediate evacuation and decompression of the hematoma is key and paramount to alleviating the impending airway compromise. Consequent intubation for airway control should be undertaken with subsequent return to the operating room for formal hematoma evacuation, washout, and identification of the bleeding source. The main preventive approach for post-operative hematoma is meticulous surgery and good hemostasis.

HYPERTROPHIC OR KELOID SCAR

Detailed history of previous surgeries, post-operative scar formation, and examination for hypertrophic scar or keloid suspicion are important. An adequate, symmetrical incision in a natural skin crease can avoid hypertrophic scarring [17]. Post-operative application of over-the-counter scar care products and avoidance of sun are helpful. Despite the precautions taken, patients prone to healing defects will develop hypertrophic scarring or keloids. Scar revision, intralesional steroid injection, or laser therapy might be helpful for treatment [18].

AERODIGESTIVE INJURY

Cervical esophagus perforation is a very rare complication after thyroidectomy. It usually occurs due to adherent thyroid malignancy affecting adjacent structures such as the trachea or the esophagus. For this reason, pre-operative work-up, imaging, and endoscopy should be performed rigorously and combined with a good surgical strategy. When an esophageal injury occurs, the edges of the perforation are debrided and closed in two layers (mucosa and the muscular layer) with absorbable sutures with or without a strap muscle buttress to the repair. The surgical site is copiously irrigated, a drain is placed, and IV antibiotics and total parenteral nutrition are initiated for 7–10 days [19,20]. An esophagram with

a water-soluble contrast material, is performed; if there is no leak, the patient can begin a soft diet. If a leak is detected, then further investigation and treatment options must be sought to avoid fistula or stricture formation.

Small tracheal injuries can be primarily repaired. Large defects may require segmental tracheal resection and subsequent repair, or alternatively a tracheostomy tube can be placed in the defect and removed at a later date.

AIRWAY CONCERNS

DIFFICULT INTUBATION
While planning the intubation, assessment of risk factors for difficult intubation is essential. Large goiters, invasive thyroid cancer, anaplastic thyroid cancer, increased neck circumference, older age, reduced mouth opening, history of difficult intubation, and substernal goiter can be predictors of difficult intubation [21,22].

In patients with large goiters, tracheal deviation may occur. Furthermore, in aggressive thyroid cancers vocal cord paralysis can be encountered at the pre-operative stage. Both of these conditions need safe airway management with proper intubation or tracheostomy [23]. Checking the larynx, vocal cords, and airway with a pre-operative laryngoscopic examination and imaging studies, such as chest x-ray or computed tomography, might anticipate a difficult intubation process. If necessary, anesthesiology should be consulted pre-operatively so that as a team the surgeon and the anesthesiologist can decide the best management for the patient. If managed properly, patients with a difficult intubation risk can be extubated safely. For a secure airway, awake fiberoptic intubation or direct laryngoscopy-aided intubation and intubation after induction with inhalational agents are recommended [24].

INJURY TO THE EXTERNAL BRANCH OF THE SUPERIOR LARYNGEAL NERVE
The external branch of the superior laryngeal nerve (EBSLN) innervates the cricothyroid muscle, which lengthens and tenses the vocal cords, providing timbre to the voice. Therefore, injury to this nerve can result in a lower pitched, husky voice that is easily fatigued with a substantial reduction in phonatory frequency range, modest increase in phonatory instability (jitter), increased laryngeal resistance with no objective evidence of glottic insufficiency, and mild deterioration in voice quality most evident during high pitched voice productions, which is particularly pronounced in women and the singing voice [25,26]. Injury to this nerve can be particularly devastating to professional voice users. This is most famously illustrated by Amelita Galli-Curci, the great operatic soprano, who underwent thyroid surgery in 1935 and found that her vocal range had been greatly impacted, and indeed the surgery ultimately ended her singing career.

The rate of injury to EBSLN following thyroid surgery has also been variable, depending upon the method of identification, ranging from 0%–6% when assessed via laryngoscopy and as high as 58% when assessed by laryngeal electroneuromyography [27].

Injury to the EBSLN commonly occurs during ligation of the superior pole vessels during release of the superior thyroid pole. Several surgical techniques have been proposed to avoid injury to the EBSLN during thyroid surgery and can essentially be divided into three main techniques:

1. Individual identification and ligation of the superior pole vessels as close as possible to the thyroid capsule without specific identification of the EBSLN [28].

2. Others advocate for the importance of intra-operative visual identification of the EBSLN during thyroid surgery [29]. The drawback of this technique is that up to 20% of EBSLN run a subfascial course, and hence cannot be visualized intra-operatively [30,31].

3. Employing electrical neural stimulation with visualization of contraction of the cricothyroid muscle with or without intra-operative nerve monitoring (IONM) with endotracheal electrodes [27]. Many researchers have further corroborated that IOMN improves identification and visualization and may improve subjective symptoms following thyroid surgery but have not shown definitive reduction in nerve injury rates [32–35]. However, given the widespread use of IONM during thyroid surgery, there is a growing consensus that its use for EBSLN monitoring is recommended and aids in identification of this nerve [35].

Presently, there is no surgical repair technique available to repair intra-operatively identified EBSLN injuries; the main stay of management is speech therapy, vocal training, and counseling.

RECURRENT LARYNGEAL NERVE INJURY

The recurrent laryngeal nerve (RLN) via its motor and sensory fibers supplies all of the intrinsic muscles of the larynx other than the cricothyroid while receiving sensory and secretomotor fibers from the glottis, sub-glottis, and trachea. A systematic review of 25,000 patients reveals an average incidence of temporary RLNP is 9.8% and permanent RLNP is 2.3% [36] (Figure 16.1).

Pre-operative assessment should help identify any risk factors for RLN injury including thyroid carcinoma, need for lymph node dissection, retrosternal extension, reoperation, and potentially abnormal anatomy [37,38]. At the time of pre-operative assessment, it is also prudent to perform flexible fiberoptic laryngoscopy to determine and document baseline vocal cord function. The thyroid surgeon should be aware of the risk factors for poor regrowth of the RLN following injury including age, diabetes, smoking, and systemic disease [39].

Since the pioneering work of Lahey and Hoover who advocated for identification of the RLN at the time of surgery and demonstrated extremely low rates of RLN injury, intra-operative RLN visualization

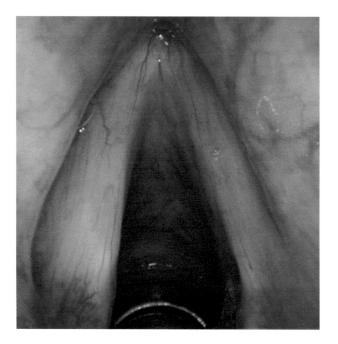

Figure 16.1 The laryngoscopic view of a vocal cord paralysis with atrophy of the paralyzed vocal cord on the right.

is the preferred method to minimize injury [40]. The thyroid surgeon must also be familiar with the occurrence of a non-recurrent laryngeal nerve (NRLN) and other anatomical and pathological variations [41].

The most consistent location of the RLN and NRLN is its most distal portion where it is covered by the tubercle of Zuckerkandl or a portion of the ligament of Berry (or both) before it turns below the inferior cricothyroid articulation, and the inferior cornu of the thyroid cartilage is an easily palpable landmark to approximate the RLN entry point into the larynx [42]. The nodule of Zuckerkandl and Berry's ligament are also where the plane of surgical dissection is most adherent and most closely approximates the RLN and therefore places the nerve at risk of severance, traction, clamping, or partial resection.

Another important adjunct to the visual identification of the RLN is IONM. IONM aids in identifying the nerve, mapping the nerve, assessing nerve function, and identifying the injured nerve segment. Additionally, IONM allows staging of total thyroidectomy after loss of signal in the first lobe avoiding contralateral lobe resection and subsequently avoiding the risk of bilateral vocal cord paralysis [43,44].

Notably, continuous IONM, a more recent advanced form of IONM, has the potential advantage of real-time nerve monitoring. It can detect adverse electromyography (EMG) changes that signify an impending RLN injury, thereby allowing a surgeon to prompt a corrective action, e.g., aborting or reversing associated maneuvers, thus likely avoiding permanent injury [45–47].

If transection of the nerve injury is identified at the time of surgery, attempts should be made to repair the defect. The techniques of RLN repair include primary end-to-end anastomosis, ansa cervicalis to RLN anastomosis, and a primary interposition graft [38]. End-to-end nerve approximation is preferred and can be achieved with three or four perineural stitches of 6.0 or 7.0 suture placed using microsurgical instruments. However, when there is a gap of >5 mm, or the anastomosis is under significant tension, a graft can be taken from the ansa cervicalis, transverse cervical nerve, or supraclavicular nerve [48]. These techniques also apply when sacrifice of the nerve is necessary for oncologic reasons and there is pre-operative vocal cord paralysis, as patients will experience a normal or improved voice post-operatively, secondary to the return of thyroarytenoid muscle tone and bulk, regardless of the length of time of vocal cord palsy [48]. IONM may also be helpful in these scenarios allowing the surgeon to identify the distal stump of the RLN. Non-surgical management for RLN injury includes voice therapy, vocal cord injection augmentation, medialization laryngoplasty (type 1 thyroplasty), arytenoid adduction, and cricothyroid subluxation [38].

Bilateral vocal cord palsy is a life threatening complication associated with thyroidectomy. Previous reports place its incidence at 0.6%, but the advent of IONM and staging procedures have likely decreased this incidence. A recent review by Sarkis et al. of 7,406 patients found the incidence to be much lower at 0.09% [49]. Their work and work by the International Neural Monitoring Study Group corroborate the importance of IONM to avoid this most dreaded complication [44,49]. The typical symptoms include inspiratory stridor, but phonation may be normal due to medial position of the vocal cords. Acutely, the majority of patients will require intubation and subsequent tracheostomy to stabilize the airway prior to definitive treatment [49].

HYPOPARATHYROIDISM

Prevention of hypoparathyroidism following thyroid surgery starts with pre-operative assessment of serum vitamin D, serum calcium, and parathyroid hormone (PTH) levels in patients at higher risk of hypoparathyroidism. A recent meta-analysis of pre-operative risk factors for hypoparathyroidism included female sex, Graves' disease and length of its duration, pre-operative beta-blockade, larger thyroid glands, retrosternal goiter, the need for a bilateral central neck dissection, reoperative thyroid surgery, and higher thyroid cancer stage [50–53]. Biochemical abnormalities identified should be corrected pre-operatively as this can decrease the impact and severity of hypocalcemia post-operatively particularly in vitamin D deficiency [54].

The incidence range of post-surgical hypocalcemia is generally wide with reports from 8.3%–38% for temporary cases lasting no greater than 6 months and 0.9%–1.7% for patients experiencing a more permanent complication across multiple series [52,55,56]. It has also been found by multiple studies to be the most common complication following thyroid surgery, namely for 63% of the complications [55]. Rosato et al. in their series of 14,934 patients also found the incidence of permanent hypocalcemia after surgical interventions for thyroid cancer was significantly higher (3.3%) [55].

Meticulous capsular dissection along the thyroid gland with subsequent preservation of the parathyroid glands and inadvertent disruption of their blood supply is recommended to avert hypoparathyroidism. The issue of routine identification of the parathyroid glands versus less gland identification has been controversial with some advocating for identification of at least two glands [57], while others advocate for less parathyroid gland identification citing a proportional rate of resulting hypocalcemia [58]. Puzziello et al. found a proportional association between gland identification and temporary hypocalcemia but an inversely proportional relationship with permanent hypocalcemia [56].

These findings support capsular dissection without extensive dissection and search for the parathyroid glands, but careful preservation of glands encountered during thyroid surgery by mobilization away from the plane of dissection while keeping the blood supply of the gland intact. A clearly ischemic and probable non-viable parathyroid gland identified during surgery should be confirmed pathologically through frozen section and then should be autotransplanted into the sternocleidomastoid. However, the surgeon should be aware that this practice may result initially in a temporary hypocalcemia but has no association with permanent hypocalcemia [50,57].

Traditionally hypocalcemia was post-operatively identified via serial serum calcium levels checked at regular intervals to determine the need for calcium supplementation. However, serum intact PTH (iPTH) levels have generally superseded this in locations where this is available. The timing of iPTH checks post-operatively to predict consequent hypocalcemia accurately is controversial. Most studies have found that most accuracy at 4 hours post op with a level greater than 10 pg/mL for iPTH and a drop no greater than 50% of the iPTH compared to pre-op levels is a reasonable indicator for adequate surgery [59–61]. Normal post-operative iPTH levels accurately predict normocalcemia after total thyroidectomy, and patients with PTH in the normal range can be safely discharged on an outpatient basis or on the first post-operative day. Regardless of serum calcium levels or iPTH levels, use of oral calcium supplements, either as needed or routinely, will avoid mild symptoms that may develop without treatment, and some advocate this for all their thyroidectomy patients [62].

If hypocalcemia is identified on serial calcium checks or predicted on iPTH levels, calcium replacement is recommended. In the acute setting with serum calcium levels less than 7 mg/dL, IV calcium gluconate is administered to alleviate symptoms which can include paresthesia, muscle cramps and spasms, twitching, tetany, seizures, and cardiopulmonary dysfunction. If serum calcium is at least 8 mg/dL, then it is treated with oral calcium carbonate and vitamin D. The starting dose of calcium is usually 500–1000 mg three times a day with upward titration if symptoms persist. Vitamin D plays a crucial role in calcium absorption and bone metabolism and should therefore be administrated, in the most active form, 1,25-dihydroxy D3 (calcitriol), 0.25 µg PO once daily, when the thyroid surgeon has identified a patient with hypocalcemia. In patients warranting IV calcium therapy, calcium gluconate is preferred to calcium chloride, as there is less risk of tissue necrosis if extravasation occurs [54]. Ionized calcium, phosphorous, PTH, and Vitamin D should be checked at regular intervals if the patient is not improving or getting worse. The goal is to maintain a low normal serum calcium with normal phosphorous levels and low urinary excretion of calcium. For patients with permanent hypoparathyroidism, maintaining calcium and phosphorous levels is more difficult and requires routine monitoring, adjustments to supplementation as needed, and long-term management by an endocrinologist with expertise in this area.

A promising new treatment option is recombinant PTH (rhPTH), an injectable synthetic human PTH, which has been shown to normalize and maintain serum calcium levels, allow discontinuation of vitamin D, and a decrease in calcium supplementation, as well as fewer clinical symptoms of hypocalcemia during treatment [63]. Unfortunately, the main concern relating to its more widespread use versus conventional treatments in patients with hypoparathyroidism is its cost [64].

HYPOTHYROIDISM
Hypothyroidism is an expected sequel following total thyroidectomy. Notably, it also occurs in 7%–35% of patients following thyroid lobectomy and is more likely to occur in patients with pre-existing high thyroid stimulating hormone (TSH), lower free T4, Hashimoto's disease, and small size of the remaining thyroid lobe [65]. The starting dose for Levothyroxine is 1.6–1.8 mcg/kg/day and is titrated based on thyroid function testing at 6–8 weeks after surgery [65,66]. Additional suppression of TSH beyond normal levels is also appropriate for management of higher risk well-differentiated thyroid cancer [66].

THYROID STORM
Patients undergoing thyroid surgery for hyperthyroidism are at risk of thyroid storm, a life threatening complication affecting multiple systems including the cardiopulmonary, thermoregulatory, metabolism, neurologic, and gastrointestinal systems [67]. Thyroid storm is associated with hyperthyroidism secondary to Graves' disease and less often with toxic nodule or multinodular goiter [67]. This complication is believed to precipitate due to the stress of surgery, anesthesia, or thyroid manipulation during surgery [68]. Recognition and appropriate management of thyrotoxicosis is vital to prevent associated high morbidity and mortality.

Pre-operatively, the surgeon should discuss the risk of thyroid storm and emphasize the importance of compliance with medication up to the day of surgery. Additionally, the American Thyroid Association guidelines recommend that the patient should be euthyroid pre-operatively and if this is not possible, beta blockers should be used to decrease the risk of a potentially lethal thyrotoxic crisis [69]. The surgeon and anesthesiologist should have experience in this situation [69].

In the operating room, a shift in vital signs alerts anesthesia to the possibility of thyroid storm. Systemic decompensation, tachycardia, dysrhythmia (usually atrial fibrillation), high fever, and respiratory changes are the most common symptoms [67,69]. A multimodality treatment approach to these patients should be used, including b-adrenergic blockade, antithyroid drug (ATD) therapy, inorganic iodide, corticosteroid therapy, cooling with acetaminophen and cooling blankets, and volume resuscitation initiated to mitigate the associated symptoms [69]. Subsequently, intensive care unit admission with nutritional support, and respiratory care and monitoring as concurrently, antithyroid medication Propylthiouracil or Methimazole is started to stop synthesis of new hormone and to prevent peripheral conversion of T4 [67]. Of note, the symptoms of malignant hyperthermia and thyroid storm are difficult to differentiate, therefore familiarity with the condition by the anesthesiologist is critical.

Post-operatively, patients with thyroid storm need close monitoring and continuation of supportive care and consultation with an endocrinologist until thyroid hormone levels normalize and the patient is no longer symptomatic.

SALIENT POINTS

1. Foundation of optimum post-operative outcomes is laid in the pre-operative assessment and discussions with patient, caregiver, anesthesiologist, and other involved physicians.

2. Excellent knowledge of the normal anatomy, variants of normal anatomy, and pathological anatomy along with meticulous surgical technique are essential for positive outcomes.

3. Early recognition of complications with prompt management lead to better outcomes.

AUTHORS' EXPERIENCE/PEARLS OF WISDOM

1. Pre-operative assessment of extent of disease, vocal cord paralysis, and preparing a surgical map can help avoid unexpected surgical outcomes.

2. IONM is a very useful adjunct and following the standards and guidelines published by the International Neural Monitoring Study Group (INMSG) allow for proper implementation of IONM with best outcomes.

3. Intra-operative meticulousness and vigilance along with excellent post-operative surveillance are key.

CONCLUDING REMARKS

Complications following thyroid surgery have a low incidence but have the prospect for high morbidity and potentially mortality. The avoidance of complications is governed by early detection, adequate management, and the astute surgeons' knowledge and preparation pre-operatively and at the time of surgery. Post-operative active surveillance for complications, especially in high risk patients, is vital. Additionally, an informed patient or caregiver educated to identify early signs of an evolving complication can at times be the difference between a minor setback versus a major complication.

REFERENCES

1. Ramouz A, Rasihashemi SZ, Daghigh F, Faraji E, Rouhani S. Predisposing factors for seroma formation in patients undergoing thyroidectomy: Cross-sectional study. *Ann Med Surg (Lond)*. 2017;23:8–12.

2. Samraj K, Gurusamy KS. Wound drains following thyroid surgery. Cochrane Wounds Group, ed. *Cochrane Database Syst Rev*. 2007;53(4):CD006099.

3. Portinari M, Carcoforo P. The application of drains in thyroid surgery. *Gland Surg*. 2017;6(5):563–73.

4. Bergenfelz A et al. Complications to thyroid surgery: Results as reported in a database from a multicenter audit comprising 3,660 patients. *Langenbecks Arch Surg*. 2008;393(5):667–73.

5. Dionigi G, Rovera F, Boni L, Dionigi R. Surveillance of surgical site infections after thyroidectomy in a one-day surgery setting. *Int J Surg*. 2008;6(Suppl 1):S13–5.

6. Mangram AJ, Horan TC, Pearson ML, Silver LC, Jarvis WR. *Guideline for Prevention of Surgical Site Infection*, 1999. Centers for Disease Control and Prevention (CDC) Hospital Infection Control Practices Advisory Committee. *Am J Infect Control*. 1999;27(2):97–132.quiz133–4–discussion96.

7. Avenia N et al. Antibiotic prophylaxis in thyroid surgery: A preliminary multicentric Italian experience. *Ann Surg Innov Res*. 2009;3(1):10.

8. Elfenbein DM, Schneider DF, Chen H, Sippel RS. Surgical site infection after thyroidectomy: A rare but significant complication. *J Surg Res*. 2014;190(1):170–6.

9. De Palma M, Grillo M, Borgia G, Pezzullo L, Lombardi CP, Gentile I. Antibiotic prophylaxis and risk of infections in thyroid surgery: Results from a national study (UEC-Italian Endocrine Surgery Units Association). *Updates Surg*. 2013;65(3):213–6.

10. Al-Qurayshi Z, Walsh J, Owen S, Kandil E. Surgical site infection in head and neck surgery: A National perspective. *Otolaryngol Head Neck Surg*. 2019;13(48):194599819832858.

11. Lang BH-H, Yih PC-L, Lo C-Y. A review of risk factors and timing for postoperative hematoma after thyroidectomy: Is outpatient thyroidectomy really safe? *World J Surg*. 2012;36(10):2497–502.

12. Materazzi G et al. Prevention and management of bleeding in thyroid surgery. *Gland Surg*. 2017;6(5):510–5.

13. Al-Qahtani AS, Abouzeid Osman T. Could post-thyroidectomy bleeding be the clue to modify the concept of postoperative drainage? A prospective randomized controlled study. *Asian J Surg*. 2018;41(5):511–6.

14. Weiss A, Lee KC, Brumund KT, Chang DC, Bouvet M. Risk factors for hematoma after thyroidectomy: Results from the nationwide inpatient sample. *Surgery*. 2014; 156(2):399–404.

15. Farooq MS, Nouraei R, Kaddour H, Saharay M. Patterns, timing and consequences of post-thyroidectomy haemorrhage. *Ann R Coll Surg Engl*. 2017;99(1):60–2.

16. Tian J, Li L, Liu P, Wang X. Comparison of drain versus no-drain thyroidectomy: A meta-analysis. *Eur Arch Otorhinolaryngol*. 2017;274(1):567–77.

17. Ma X, Xia Q-J, Li G, Wang T-X, Li Q. Aesthetic principles access thyroidectomy produces the best cosmetic outcomes as assessed using the patient and observer scar assessment scale. *BMC Cancer*. 2017;17(1):654.

18. Forbat E, Ali FR, Al-Niaimi F. Treatment of keloid scars using light-, laser- and energy-based devices: A contemporary review of the literature. *Lasers Med Sci*. 2017;32(9):2145–54.

19. Wu JT, Mattox KL, Wall MJ. Esophageal perforations: New perspectives and treatment paradigms. *J Trauma*. 2007;63(5):1173–84.

20. Sdralis EIK, Petousis S, Rashid F, Lorenzi B, Charalabopoulos A. Epidemiology, diagnosis, and management of esophageal perforations: Systematic review. *Dis Esophagus.* 2017;30(8):1–6.

21. Bouaggad A, Nejmi SE, Bouderka MA, Abbassi O. Prediction of difficult tracheal intubation in thyroid surgery. *Anesth Analg.* 2004;99(2):603–6, tableofcontents.

22. De Cassai A, Papaccio F, Betteto G, Schiavolin C, Iacobone M, Carron M. Prediction of difficult tracheal intubations in thyroid surgery. Predictive value of neck circumference to thyromental distance ratio. Ballotta A, ed. *PLOS ONE.* 2019;14(2):e0212976.

23. Shaha AR. Difficult airway and intubation in thyroid surgery. *Ann Otol Rhinol Laryngol.* 2015;124(4):334–5.

24. Agarwal A et al. High incidence of tracheomalacia in longstanding goiters: Experience from an endemic goiter region. *World J Surg.* 2007;31(4):832–7.

25. Kark AE, Kissin MW, Auerbach R, Meikle M. Voice changes after thyroidectomy: Role of the external laryngeal nerve. *Br Med J (Clin Res Ed).* 1984;289(6456):1412–5.

26. Roy N, Smith ME, Dromey C, Redd J, Neff S, Grennan D. Exploring the phonatory effects of external superior laryngeal nerve paralysis: An in vivo model. *Laryngoscope.* 2009;119(4):816–26.

27. Potenza AS, Araujo Filho VJF, Cernea CR. Injury of the external branch of the superior laryngeal nerve in thyroid surgery. *Gland Surg.* 2017;6(5):552–62.

28. Bellantone R et al. Is the identification of the external branch of the superior laryngeal nerve mandatory in thyroid operation? Results of a prospective randomized study. *Surgery.* 2001;130(6):1055–9.

29. Hurtado-Lopez LM, Pacheco-Alvarez MI, Montes-Castillo MDLL, Zaldivar-Ramirez FR. Importance of the intraoperative identification of the external branch of the superior laryngeal nerve during thyroidectomy: Electromyographic evaluation. *Thyroid.* 2005;15(5):449–54.

30. Lennquist S, Cahlin C, Smeds S. The superior laryngeal nerve in thyroid surgery. *Surgery.* 1987;102(6):999–1008.

31. Friedman M, Wilson MN, Ibrahim H. Superior laryngeal nerve identification and preservation in thyroidectomy. *Oper Tech Otolaryngol-Head Neck Surg.* 2009;20(2):145–51.

32. Lifante J-C, McGill J, Murry T, Aviv JE, Inabnet WB. A prospective, randomized trial of nerve monitoring of the external branch of the superior laryngeal nerve during thyroidectomy under local/regional anesthesia and IV sedation. *Surgery.* 2009;146(6):1167–73.

33. Masuoka H et al. Prospective randomized study on injury of the external branch of the superior laryngeal nerve during thyroidectomy comparing intraoperative nerve monitoring and a conventional technique. *Head Neck.* 2015;37(10):1456–60.

34. Uludag M, Aygun N, Kartal K, Besler E, Isgor A. Is intraoperative neural monitoring necessary for exploration of the superior laryngeal nerve? *Surgery.* 2017;161(4):1129–38.

35. Barczynski M et al. External branch of the superior laryngeal nerve monitoring during thyroid and parathyroid surgery: International Neural Monitoring Study Group standards guideline statement. *Laryngoscope.* 2013;123(Suppl 4):S1–S14.

36. Jeannon J-P, Orabi AA, Bruch GA, Abdalsalam HA, Simo R. Diagnosis of recurrent laryngeal nerve palsy after thyroidectomy: A systematic review. *Int J Clin Pract.* 2009;63(4):624–9.

37. Dralle H et al. Risk factors of paralysis and functional outcome after recurrent laryngeal nerve monitoring in thyroid surgery. *Surgery.* 2004;136(6):1310–22.

38. Lynch J, Parameswaran R. Management of unilateral recurrent laryngeal nerve injury after thyroid surgery: A review. *Head Neck.* 2017;39(7):1470–8.

39. Affleck BD, Swartz K, Brennan J. Surgical considerations and controversies in thyroid and parathyroid surgery. *Otolaryngol Clin North Am.* 2003;36(1):159–87, x.

40. Lahey FH, Hoover WB. Injuries to the recurrent laryngeal nerve in thyroid operations: Their management and avoidance. *Ann Surg.* 1938;108(4):545–62.

41. Randolph G. *Surgery of the Thyroid and Parathyroid Glands.* Elsevier Saunders Health Sciences, Philadelphia, PA, 2012.

42. Pelizzo MR, Toniato A, Gemo G. Zuckerkandl's tuberculum: An arrow pointing to the recurrent laryngeal nerve (constant anatomical landmark). *J Am Coll Surg.* 1998;187(3):333–6.

43. Goretzki PE, Schwarz K, Brinkmann J, Wirowski D, Lammers BJ. The impact of intraoperative neuromonitoring (IONM) on surgical strategy in bilateral thyroid diseases: Is it worth the effort? *World J Surg.* 2010;34(6):1274–84.

44. Schneider R et al. International neural monitoring study group guideline 2018 part I: Staging bilateral thyroid surgery with monitoring loss of signal. *Laryngoscope.* 2018;128(Suppl 3):S1–S17.

45. Schneider R et al. Continuous intraoperative vagus nerve stimulation for identification of imminent recurrent laryngeal nerve injury. *Head Neck.* 2013;35(11):1591–8.

46. Schneider R et al. Continuous intraoperative neural monitoring of the recurrent nerves in thyroid surgery: A quantum leap in technology. *Gland Surg.* 2016;5(6):607–16.

47. Schneider R, Machens A, Randolph GW, Kamani D, Lorenz K, Dralle H. Opportunities and challenges of intermittent and continuous intraoperative neural monitoring in thyroid surgery. *Gland Surg.* 2017;6(5):537–45.

48. Sanuki T, Yumoto E, Minoda R, Kodama N. The role of immediate recurrent laryngeal nerve reconstruction for thyroid cancer surgery. *J Oncol.* 2010;2010(3):846235–37.

49. Sarkis LM, Zaidi N, Norlén O, Delbridge LW, Sywak MS, Sidhu SB. Bilateral recurrent laryngeal nerve injury in a specialized thyroid surgery unit: Would routine intraoperative neuromonitoring alter outcomes? *ANZ J Surg.* 2017;87(5):364–7.

50. Edafe O, Antakia R, Laskar N, Uttley L, Balasubramanian SP. Systematic review and meta-analysis of predictors of post-thyroidectomy hypocalcaemia. *Br J Surg.* 2014;101(4):307–20.

51. Su A, Wang B, Gong Y, Gong R, Li Z, Zhu J. Risk factors of hypoparathyroidism following total thyroidectomy with central lymph node dissection. *Medicine (Baltimore).* 2017;96(39):e8162.

52. Edafe O, Balasubramanian SP. Incidence, prevalence and risk factors for post-surgical hypocalcaemia and hypoparathyroidism. *Gland Surg.* 2017;6(Suppl 1):S59–68.

53. Bai B, Chen Z, Chen W. Risk factors and outcomes of incidental parathyroidectomy in thyroidectomy: A systematic review and meta-analysis. Kidane B, ed. *PLOS ONE.* 2018;13(11):e0207088.

54. Walker Harris V, Jan De Beur S. Postoperative hypoparathyroidism: Medical and surgical therapeutic options. *Thyroid.* 2009;19(9):967–73.

55. Rosato L et al. Complications of thyroid surgery: Analysis of a multicentric study on 14,934 patients operated on in Italy over 5 years. *World J Surg.* 2004;28(3):271–6.

56. Puzziello A et al. Hypocalcemia following thyroid surgery: Incidence and risk factors. A longitudinal multicenter study comprising 2,631 patients. *Endocrine.* 2014;47(2):537–42.

57. Thomusch O, Machens A, Sekulla C, Ukkat J, Brauckhoff M, Dralle H. The impact of surgical technique on postoperative hypoparathyroidism in bilateral thyroid surgery: A multivariate analysis of 5846 consecutive patients. *Surgery.* 2003;133(2):180–5.

58. Praženica P, O'Keeffe L, Holý R. Dissection and identification of parathyroid glands during thyroidectomy: Association with hypocalcemia. *Head Neck.* 2015;37(3):393–9.

59. Barczynski M, Cichoń S, Konturek A. Which criterion of intraoperative iPTH assay is the most accurate in prediction of true serum calcium levels after thyroid surgery? *Langenbecks Arch Surg.* 2007;392(6):693–8.

60. Raffaelli M et al. Post-thyroidectomy hypocalcemia is related to parathyroid dysfunction even in patients with normal parathyroid hormone concentrations early after surgery. *Surgery.* 2016;159(1):78–84.

61. Filho EBY, Machry RV, Mesquita R, Scheffel RS, Maia AL. The timing of parathyroid hormone measurement defines the cut-off values to accurately predict postoperative hypocalcemia: A prospective study. *Endocrine.* 2018;61(2):224–31.

62. AES Guidelines 06/01 Group. Australian Endocrine Surgeons Guidelines AES06/01. Postoperative parathyroid hormone measurement and early discharge after total thyroidectomy: Analysis of Australian data and management recommendations. *ANZ J Surg.* 2007;77(4):199–202.

63. Mannstadt M et al. Efficacy and safety of recombinant human parathyroid hormone (1–84) in hypoparathyroidism (REPLACE): A double-blind, placebo-controlled, randomised, phase 3 study. *Lancet Diabetes Endocrinol.* 2013;1(4):275–83.

64. Chomsky-Higgins KH et al. Recombinant parathyroid hormone versus usual care: Do the outcomes justify the cost? *World J Surgery.* 2018;42(2):431–6.

65. McHenry CR, Slusarczyk SJ. Hypothyroidisim following hemithyroidectomy: Incidence, risk factors, and management. *Surgery.* 2000;128(6):994–8.

66. Haugen BR et al. 2015 American Thyroid Association Management Guidelines for Adult Patients with Thyroid Nodules and Differentiated Thyroid Cancer: The American Thyroid Association Guidelines Task Force on Thyroid Nodules and Differentiated Thyroid Cancer. *Thyroid.* 2016;26(1):1–133.

67. Nayak B, Burman K. Thyrotoxicosis and thyroid storm. *Endocrinol Metab Clin North Am.* 2006;35(4):663–86, vii.

68. Jassim Al A et al. A retrospective cohort study: Do patients with graves' disease need to be euthyroid prior to surgery? *J Otolaryngol Head Neck Surg.* 2018;47(1):37.

69. Ross DS et al. 2016 American Thyroid Association Guidelines for Diagnosis and Management of Hyperthyroidism and Other Causes of Thyrotoxicosis. *Thyroid.* 2016;26(10):1343–421.

Chapter 17

LOCALLY ADVANCED THYROID CANCER

Amit Agarwal and Roma Pradhan

CONTENTS

Introduction	127
Invasion of the Strap Muscles	127
Invasion of the Aerodigestive Tract (Larynx, Trachea, Hypopharynx, and/or Esophagus)	127
Surgical Management	129
Pharyngeal/Esophageal Involvement	132
Vascular Invasion	132
Conclusion	132
References	133

INTRODUCTION

Locally advanced thyroid cancer (LATC) occurs when there is either extrathyroidal extension from the primary tumor in the thyroid or extracapsular extension from involved lymph nodes into the surrounding structures. The incidence of invasive disease depends on the pathology of the thyroid cancer.

The structures that are in close association with the thyroid gland have more chance of invasion, like the strap muscles, recurrent laryngeal nerve, trachea, great vessels, vagus nerve, esophagus, and larynx.

The surgical treatment of thyroid lesions that invade adjacent structures is controversial but removing as much abnormal tissue as possible and maintaining the functional integrity of the neck structures are basic principles.

The type of thyroid cancer is an important criteria that decides our management strategy.

For aggressive thyroid cancer like anaplastic and medullary when present with airway compromise, palliative management is the treatment of choice because of poor prognosis. This is in contrast with the differentiated thyroid cancer where resection surgery with curative intent is the treatment option because of good survival in these patients.

According to the new American Joint Committee on Cancer (AJCC) Staging Manual, 8th Edition, a few changes are important as they relate to locally advanced thyroid cancer.

Minor extrathyroidal extension detected only on histological examination was removed from the definition of T3 disease and therefore has no impact on either T category or overall stages.

Older patients with tumors >4 cm confined to the thyroid (T3a) are classified as stage II regardless of the lymph node status.

T3b is a new category for tumors of any size demonstrating gross extrathyroidal extension into the strap muscles (sternohyoid, sternothyroid, thyrohyoid, or omohyoid muscles).

Older patients demonstrating gross extrathyroidal extension are classified as stage II if only the strap muscles are grossly invaded (T3b), stage III if there is gross invasion of the sub-cutaneous tissue, larynx, trachea, esophagus, or recurrent laryngeal nerve (T4a), and stage IVA if there is gross invasion of the prevertebral fascia or tumor encasing major vessels (T4b).

INVASION OF THE STRAP MUSCLES

The strap muscles (sternohyoid, sternothyroid, and omohyoid) are the most common structures involved in locally advanced thyroid cancer due to their proximity to the thyroid gland. The point that concerns the treating doctor is whether the invasion of strap muscles is an important prognostic factor or not. This was recently answered by a study from Amit M et al. [1]. Gross strap muscle invasion may not be an important survival prognostic factor for staging purposes. Although both gross strap muscle invasion and perithyroidal soft tissue extension may be predictive for locoregional recurrence, the distinction between them may not be as important for post-operative risk stratification.

The management of the invasion of the strap muscle includes resection of the involved muscle to obtain negative margins.

INVASION OF THE AERODIGESTIVE TRACT (LARYNX, TRACHEA, HYPOPHARYNX, AND/OR ESOPHAGUS)

Invasion of the aerodigestive tract (ADT) including the larynx, trachea, hypopharynx, and esophagus can be found in 1%–8% of all patients with thyroid cancer [2–4].

Due to anatomical proximity, respiratory tract invasion can be found in 50% and an esophagus invasion in 25% of locally advanced thyroid cancers [2].

The invasion of the aerodigestive tract in thyroid cancer occurs from the outer layer (superficial) of these organs to the deeper layer and then in lumen, which is different from the primary tumor of these organs. In about 3/4th of the patients, at the time of diagnosis, invasion does not affect the complete wall (non-transmural invasion), but in 1/4th of patients, transmural invasion with intraluminal tumor manifestation is usually found.

When the cartilage is penetrated, the tumor very often grows horizontally first and then vertically between the mucosa and the deeper layers before intraluminal manifestation occurs [2]. As a consequence, in intraluminal ADT invasion, the area of tumor invasion is very often much larger than expected from intraluminal assessment.

RESPIRATORY TRACT

Respiratory tract invasion can range from outer cartilaginous invasion to frank intraluminal ingrowth. It can involve the upper airway at multiple levels. Even in the presence of distant metastases, resection is recommended often because of the mortality rate that is associated with local disease and the need for primary tumor resection for the effectiveness of other adjuvant therapy.

LARYNX

PRESENTATION

1. Patient may present with voice change, dysphagia, dyspnea, or hemoptysis.
2. Vocal cord dysfunction on routine pre-operative examination.
3. FNA proven patient on cross sectional imaging demonstrating invasion.
4. Patient may present with recurrent disease.

All patients with suspicion of invasion must undergo tracheoscopy or esophagoscopy to know the extent of the disease and to allow for a better surgical road map.

IMAGING

Imaging is the most important investigation for thyroid cancer. High frequency ultrasound is the standard method to investigate for thyroid nodules and to detect lymph nodes in lateral compartment. However, its use in detecting extra thyroidal extension (ETE) and invasion of larynx, trachea, and esophagus is limited. Contrast enhanced computed tomography (CECT) has better sensitivity in detecting ETE and for detecting level VI and VII central compartment lymph nodes.

In some instances MRI may also be used to detect ETE.

Laryngeal Invasion

Laryngeal involvement can occur in various ways, directly or indirectly affecting the function or structure of the larynx:

1. It can affect the function of the larynx indirectly by involvement of the RLN either by primary tumor or by metastatic lymph node.
2. Laryngeal invasion can occur by direct extension of thyroid carcinoma through the cricoid/thyroid cartilage (Figure 17.1) or by posterior extension around the thyroid cartilage (Figure 17.2) into the piriform sinus or the cricotracheal invasion.
3. Metastasis to cartilage, which is rare.

Operative treatment of locally invasive thyroid cancer involving the larynx ranges from shave excision to extended laryngeal resections:

- Shave Excision.
- Partial laryngeal resection.
- Vertical hemilaryngectomy (lateral invasion of hemilarynx) (Figure 17.3): The defect can be covered with nearby soft tissue, regional myocutaneous flaps, or free flaps. If only the unilateral thyroid ala is removed without the underlying soft tissue, then no additional procedure is required.
- Total laryngopharyngectomy or total laryngectomy:

In LATC, when complete resection is performed, local recurrence is less common [5]. With a less radical procedure, even after adding post-operative I-131 therapy or radiotherapy, relapse is frequent. Persistent growth of an intraluminal mass, followed by vocal fold paralysis, airway obstruction, and death by asphyxiation or bleeding occurs.

INVASION OF THE TRACHEA

Tracheal invasion is more common than laryngeal invasion and is observed in about 6% of patients with differentiated thyroid cancer

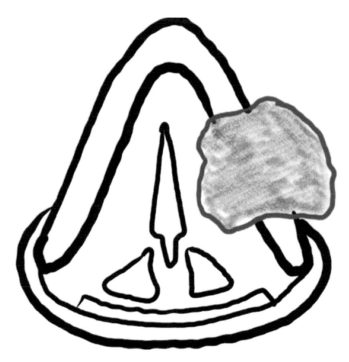

Figure 17.1   Laryngeal invasion by direct extension of thyroid carcinoma through the cricoid/thyroid cartilage.

(DTC), and surgery is accepted as the treatment of choice. However, it is mandatory to have a good pre-operative evaluation before any major surgical intervention in these cases.

Tracheal invasion may complicate with hemoptysis (Figure 17.4) or dyspnea, and patients often die of hemorrhage or airway obstruction [6]. Tracheal infiltration is associated with impaired tumor-free survival and increased disease-specific mortality [7,8].

EVALUATION

Initial evaluation with a thorough history and examination is important.

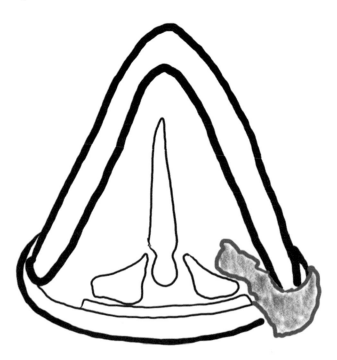

Figure 17.2   Laryngeal invasion by posterior extension around the thyroid cartilage into the piriform sinus or the cricotracheal invasion.

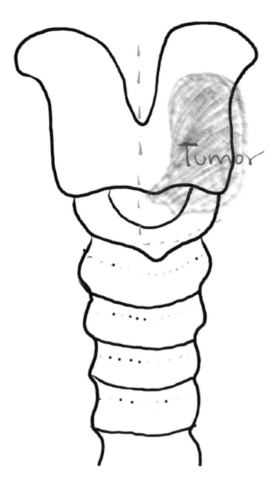

Figure 17.3   Vertical hemilaryngectomy (lateral invasion of hemilarynx).

A thorough physical examination will allow the clinician to suspect airway invasion. Usually, a palpable neck mass or nodule that has recently enlarged will be present. The mass is often hard and displace or fixed to the surrounding tissue (Figure 17.5).

Ultrasound scanning is typically not useful for the evaluation of intraluminal invasion. CT scanning is able to detect the presence and delineate the extent of cartilaginous and intraluminal invasion. It can also identify structures that are not involved by the carcinoma. CT scanning is a reliable tool to evaluate the thyroid gland and the tumor, identify tissue planes and vascular structures, provide images of the trachea at different levels, and determine the extent of any stenosis.

All intra-laryngotracheal luminal invasions should be confirmed by bronchoscopy and neck computed tomography imaging. Endoscopic diagnosis of luminal invasion is made by confirming localized redness that indicates neovascularity and telangiectasias [9].

Management to attain best outcome for patients:

1. Preoperative evaluation of the disease extent rather than surgical surprise.

2. Removal of all gross tumor.

3. Preservation of vital structures while maintaining a balance between satisfactory quality of life (QOL) and oncological resection.

4. Every effort should be made to preserve the recurrent laryngeal nerves.

As tracheal invasion is more common than laryngeal invasion, and a lot of discussion is available in the literature regarding its management, Shin has classified a staging system of tracheal invasion (Figure 17.6) [10]:

Stage 1: Invades through the thyroid capsule and abuts but does not invade the external perichondrium of trachea.

Stage 2: Invades in the cartilage or destroys it.

Stage 3: Extends into the lamina propria of the mucosa but does not breech the mucosa.

Stage 4: Full thickness invasion of the trachea with intraluminal growth.

SURGICAL MANAGEMENT

Management of differentiated thyroid cancer invading the trachea depends on:

•   Depth of invasion into the wall

•   Horizontal and vertical extent

Incomplete wall resections (without opening of the lumen) of the trachea (shaving) gives excellent results in terms of tumor-free resection margins and outcome [11]. Deeper invasions, however, require complete wall resections. Nishida et al. [12] and McCaffery [13] advocated for shave excision for stage I. The advocates of shave excision favor it because it avoids morbidity associated with tracheal resection and also its complications like tracheal stenosis. Nishida et al. [12] compared patients who underwent shave excision and those without any tracheal involvement and they found no difference in local recurrence or overall survival between the two groups. Five year survival was also similar in patients who underwent radical resection compared to shave excision of macroscopic disease and radioactive iodine for microscopic residual disease [14]. However, it is unclear if shave resection with post-operative radioiodine ablation and/or external radiation therapy is clearly associated with a higher recurrence rate and worse prognosis as compared to aggressive resection with airway reconstruction. This is due to the fact that studies comparing these surgical approaches have had small study cohorts, the extent of disease was different among patients with DTC, different surgical techniques were used, and retrospective, non-randomized or unmatched cohorts were compared.

In contrast to these previously discussed studies, the study by Gaissert et al. [15] proved that disease-free survival was significantly higher after early resection, with 10- and 20-year disease-free survival rates of 67% and 50%, respectively, whereas after delayed resection (i.e., patients who underwent shave resection initially) disease-free survival at 10 years was only 7%, and none of the patients were alive without disease after 20 years. Different studies by different authors studied on shave and full thickness resection are shown in Tables 17.1–17.3.

The important point to note and discuss in patients in which we plan to do shave resection is the histology of the thyroid cancer. Aggressive variants of PTC or tumors with undifferentiated components, such as Hurthle cell carcinomas, may not be radioactive iodine avid, hence formal resection instead of shave resection needs to be done [16].

When the thyroid cancer invades into the cartilage or destroys it (Shin stage 2), then the shave procedure is not sufficient and the patient requires formal tracheal resection as mentioned by Nishida et al. [13].

Shave resection of all gross tumor involving the trachea and larynx is possible when DTC is not infiltrating the tracheal perichondrium. Several studies have demonstrated that this approach has a lower morbidity and similar survival rates when compared to full-thickness resection. In patients who have laryngotracheal wall invasion, shave resection may be associated with a higher recurrence rate than extended resection. Some small retrospective studies comparing shave resection to extended resection (en bloc) in patients with tracheal wall invasion have documented improved survival rates in patients who had an extended resection.

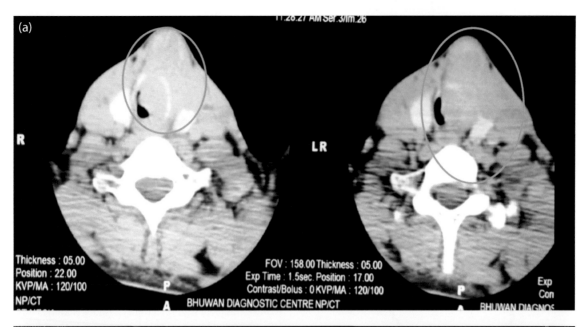

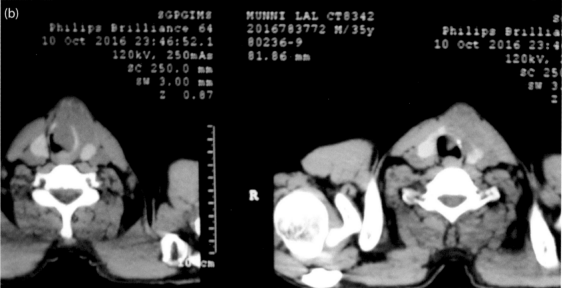

Figure 17.4   (a and b) CECT of a patient who presented with breathlessness and hemoptysis, showing intra-luminal invasion by thyroid carcinoma.

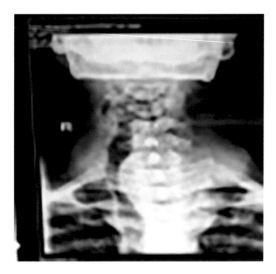

Figure 17.5   X-ray of chest and neck: soft tissue shadow displacing or narrowing the trachea.

The complete wall resection on the trachea has been classified by Dralle et al. [2] according to the extent of involvement.

In patients with limited involvement of the trachea (anterolateral wall, Dralle type 2) with maximal extent 2 cm vertically and less than 1/4th of circumference, window resection of the trachea is possible with either primary closure or muscle patch (strap muscle or SCM muscle). An anteriorly placed tumor can be managed with window resection and the defect converted to tracheostomy which can be downsized and decannulated post-operatively.

In tumors involving >2 cm vertically or >1/4th of circumference (Dralle type 4), circular wall resection (sleeve) is required with primary anastomosis. A primary anastomosis can be performed with maximum resection of 5–6 cm of trachea or 7–8 tracheal rings (Figures 17.7 through 17.9).

To ensure a tension free repair in such circumstances, various procedures can be performed:

- Supralaryngeal release to gain extra 2 cm
- Division of suprahyoid muscle
- Hilar mobilization of trachea through sternotomy

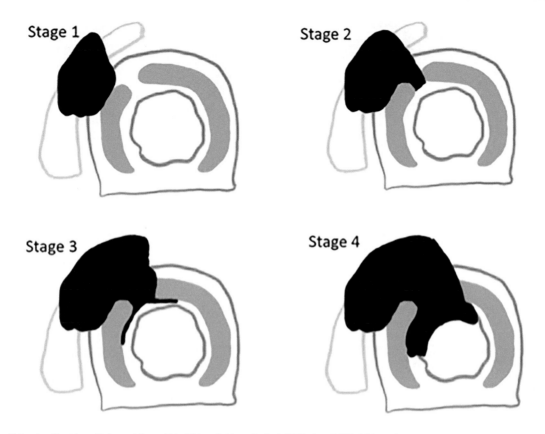

Figure 17.6 Shin classification. (Adapted from Shin DH etal. *Hum Pathol.* 1993 Aug;24(8):866–70.)

Table 17.1 Comparative studies of shave and full thickness resection

Authors	Locally invasive DTC/Total ca thyroid pts	Procedure: Shave/ full-thickness	RAI/RT	FUP period	Survival	Authors conclusion	Comments
Cody HS (1981) [19]	12	Shave = 9 Full-thickness = 3	3/2	8.7 years	10 yr: 64%	Shave as good as full resection	Small cohort
Czaja JM et al. (1997) [20]	109	Shave = 75 Full-thickness = 34	Yes/yes	40 yrs	Shave = 48% Full-thickness = 58%	Equal survival with both. No gross tumor should be left behind in shave procedures	Good number of patients and very long
Kasperbauer (2004) [21]	49	Shave = 33 Full-thickness = 16	Yes/yes	10.3 yrs	5-year survival Shave = 79% Full-thickness = 75%	Equal results with both procedures	
Musholt [22]	33	Shave = 17 Full-thickness = 17	Yes/yes	Shave = 19 mo Full = 25 mo		Procedures resulting in primary end-to-end anastomosis of the upper airways were associated with lower peri-operative morbidity and improved recurrence-free survival when compared with "window" resections with muscle flap reconstruction. In cases of superficial tracheal tumor infiltration, laminar ablations were sufficient for local tumor control.	

Table 17.2 Studies of full-thickness resection

Authors	Locally invasive DTC/Total ca thyroid pts	Procedure: Shave/full-thickness	RAI/RT	FUP period	Survival	Authors conclusion	Comments
Nakao et al. (2004) [23]	40		–/–		10 yr: 67.7%	Combined resection is a good treatment choice for survival and good QOL when performed for local control in patients with differentiated thyroid cancer	
Sywak 2003 [24]	7		Yes/yes	19 mo	Recurrence = 2	Tracheal resection for locally invasive thyroid cancer is associated with a return to full dietary intake within 4 weeks of surgery in most cases. Function and QOL after this type of surgery are acceptable	
Yang (2000) [25]	8		Yes/–	91 mo	Alive = 7 Disease free = 5	Tracheal resection for locally invasive thyroid cancer is associated with a return to full dietary intake within 4 weeks of surgery in most cases. Function and QOL after this type of surgery are acceptable	All patients had mucosal involvement

Table 17.3 Studies with shave excision only

Authors	Locally invasive DTC/Total ca thyroid pts	Procedure: Shave/full-thickness	RAI/RT	FUP period	Survival	Authors conclusion	Comments
Park (1993) [17]	16	Shave in all	Yes/yes	70.7 mo	Recurrence = 12 Mortality = 7	We feel that a more extensive resection procedure than cartilage shaving should be considered, even in patients with superficial tracheal invasion, to increase the disease-free survival rate.	

Points to be kept in mind while mobilizing the trachea:

Tracheal blood supply enters laterally from the inferior thyroid artery to join two longitudinal vascular anastomoses. One should never mobilize the trachea circumferentially in order to avoid damage to these vessels.

PHARYNGEAL/ESOPHAGEAL INVOLVEMENT

The pharynx and esophagus can be invaded by the primary tumor or by metastatic lymph nodes.

Pharyngeal invasion usually occurs after laryngeal invasion, and esophageal invasion usually occurs after tracheal invasion. Invasion tends to penetrate the muscular layer with relative sparing of the mucosa and submucosa. Typically, a well-differentiated thyroid carcinoma will invade only the outer muscular layer.

Dysphagia is the common complaint and may be because of compression from the mass or direct involvement of the esophagus. A thorough pre-operative evaluation is necessary if esophageal involvement is suspected. Besides cross-sectional imaging, endoscopic ultrasound may be useful in these cases. During surgery, a Ryles tube or feeding tube placement can be helpful in identification of the esophageal lumen.

For esophageal involvement of only the muscular layer, no repair or simple suture repair is all that is required if an intact submucosal layer can be maintained. Full-thickness invasion may require partial resection and immediate repair. However, it should be kept in mind that the repair should be tension free, watertight, and multilayer. Moderately sized intraluminal defects after resection can be reconstructed with myocutaneous flaps. Larger defects may require a jejunal free flap. For inoperable patients, the esophagus can be stented for palliation [16,18].

Extensive pharyngeal tumors may require radical surgery like total laryngopharyngectomy.

VASCULAR INVASION

Major artery and venous involvement are rare. Venous invasion is more common than arterial. CECT scan can be used to detect vascular involvement. Angiography is used to evaluate the full extent of vascular invasion.

CONCLUSION

Reasonable survival and quality of life can be given even to patients with locally advanced thyroid cancer. Hence, every attempt should be made to achieve R0 resection but without causing extreme morbidity. Full-thickness resection in cases of airway invasion is desirable to control symptoms like hemoptysis or breathlessness, as well as to improve survival. Therefore, such patients should be referred to expert endocrine surgeons for a radical operation. Various factors like histology, vascular invasion, distant metastases, available expertise, age of the patient, and operative fitness has to be taken into account before making the decision of radical excision in patients of locally advanced thyroid cancer.

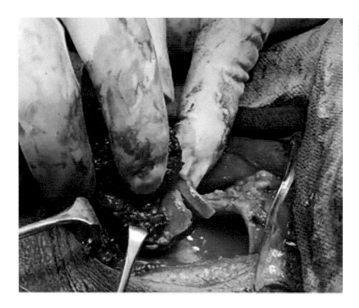

Figure 17.7 Intra-operative photograph of a patient undergoing excision of a crico-tracheal segment.

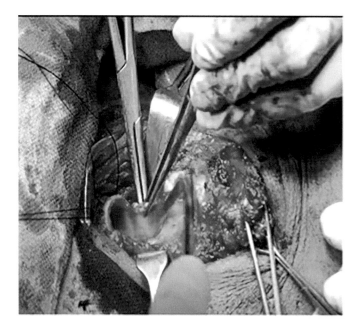

Figure 17.8 Crico-tracheal anastomosis in progress.

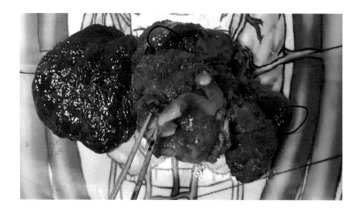

Figure 17.9 Specimen showing the thyroid mass infiltrating the cricoid and tracheal rings.

REFERENCES

1. Amit M et al. Extrathyroidal extension: Does strap muscle invasion alone influence recurrence and survival in patients with differentiated thyroid cancer? *Ann Surg Oncol.* 2018 Oct;25(11):3380–8.

2. Dralle H, Brauckhoff M, Machens A, Gimm O. Surgical management of advanced thyroid cancer invading the aerodigestive tract. In: Clark OH, Duh QY, Kebebew E (eds) *Textbook on Endocrine Surgery*, 2nd edn. Elsevier Saunders, Philadelphia, 2005, pp. 318–33.

3. Brauckhoff M, Dralle H. Extrathyroidal thyroid cancer: Results of tracheal shaving and tracheal resection. *Chirurg.* 2011;82:134–40.

4. Brauckhoff M, Dralle H. Cervicovisceral resection in invasive thyroid tumors. *Chirurg.* 2009;80:88–98.

5. Ballantyne AJ. Resections of the upper aerodigestive tract for locally invasive thyroid cancer. *Am J Surg.* 1994;168: 636–9.

6. Su SY et al. Well-differentiated thyroid cancer with aerodigestive tract invasion: Long-term control and functional outcomes. *Head Neck.* 2016;38:72–8.

7. Shindo ML et al. Management of invasive well-differentiated thyroid cancer: An American Head and Neck Society consensus statement. AHNS consensus statement. *Head Neck.* 2014;36:1379–90.

8. Lin S et al. Treatments for complications of tracheal sleeve resection for papillary thyroid carcinoma with tracheal invasion. *Eur J Surg Oncol.* 2014;40:176–81.

9. Koike E, Yamashita H, Noguchi S, Yamashita H, Ohshima A, Watanabe S, Uchino S, Takatsu K, Nishii R. Bronchoscopic diagnosis of thyroid cancer with laryngotracheal invasion. *Arch Surg.* 2001;136:1185–9.

10. Shin DH, Mark EJ, Suen HC, Grillo HC. Pathologic staging of papillary carcinoma of the thyroid with airway invasion based on the anatomic manner of extension to the trachea: A clinicopathologic study based on 22 patients who underwent thyroidectomy and airway resection. *Hum Pathol.* 1993 Aug;24(8):866–70.

11. Brauckhoff M et al. Impact of extent of resection for thyroid cancer invading the aerodigestive tract on surgical morbidity, local recurrence, and cancer-specific survival. *Surgery.* 2010;148:1257–66.

12. McCaffrey JC. Aerodigestive tract invasion by well-differentiated thyroid carcinoma: Diagnosis, management, prognosis, and biology. *Laryngoscope.* 2006;116:1–11.

13. Nishida T, Nakao K, Hamaji M. Differentiated thyroid carcinoma with airway invasion: Indication for tracheal resection based on the extent of cancer invasion. *J Thorac Cardiovasc Surg.* 1997;114:84–92.

14. Segal K, Shpitzer T, Hazan A, Bachar G, Marshak G, Popovtzer A. Invasive well-differentiated thyroid carcinoma: Effect of treatment modalities on outcome. *Otolaryngol Head Neck Surg.* 2006;134:819–22.

15. Gaissert HA, Honings J, Grillo HC, Donahue DM, Wain JC, Wright CD, Mathisen DJ. Segmental laryngotracheal and tracheal resection for invasive thyroid carcinoma. *Ann Thorac Surg.* 2007 Jun;83(6):1952–9.

16. Price DL, Wong RJ, Randolph GW. Invasive thyroid cancer: Management of the trachea and esophagus. *Otolaryngol Clin North Am*. 2008;41(6):1155–68, ix-x.

17. Park CS, Suh KW, Min JS. Cartilage-shaving procedure for the control of tracheal cartilage invasion by thyroid carcinoma. *Head Neck*. 1993 Jul-Aug;15(4):289–91.

18. Ginsberg GG. Palliation of malignant esophageal dysphagia: Would you like plastic or metal? *Am J Gastroenterol*. 2007;102(12):2678–9.

19. Cody HS 3rd, Shah JP. Locally invasive, well-differentiated thyroid cancer. 22 years' experience at Memorial Sloan-Kettering Cancer Center. *Am J Surg*. 1981 Oct;142(4):480–3.

20. Czaja JM, McCaffrey TV. The surgical management of laryngotracheal invasion by well-differentiated papillary thyroid carcinoma. *Arch Otolaryngol Head Neck Surg*. 1997 May;123(5):484–90.

21. Kasperbauer JL. Locally advanced thyroid carcinoma. *Ann Otol Rhinol Laryngol*. 2004 Sep;113(9):749–53.

22. Musholt TJ, Musholt PB, Behrend M, Raab R, Scheumann GF, Klempnauer J. Invasive differentiated thyroid carcinoma: Tracheal resection and reconstruction procedures in the hands of the endocrine surgeon. *Surgery*. 1999 Dec;126(6):1078–87; discussion 1087–8.

23. Nakao K, Kurozumi K, Nakahara M, Kido T. Resection and reconstruction of the airway in patients with advanced thyroid cancer. *World J Surg*. 2004 Dec;28(12):1204–6.

24. Sywak M, Pasieka JL, McFadden S, Gelfand G, Terrell J, Dort J. Functional results and quality of life after tracheal resection for locally invasive thyroid cancer. *Am J Surg*. 2003 May;185(5):462–7.

25. Yang CC, Lee CH, Wang LS, Huang BS, Hsu WH, Huang MH. Resectional treatment for thyroid cancer with tracheal invasion: A long-term follow-up study. *Arch Surg*. 2000 Jun;135(6):704–7.

Chapter 18

SURGICAL MANAGEMENT OF MEDULLARY THYROID CANCERS

Anuja Deshmukh and Anand Thomas

CONTENTS

Introduction 135
Work-Up 135
TNM Classification AJCC, 8th Edition, for MTC 138
Recurrence/Metastasis/Residual MTC 142
Adjuvant External Beam Radiotherapy (EBRT) 142
Prophylactic Cancer Surgery 142
Salient Points 143
Authors' Experience/Pearls of Wisdom 144
Concluding Remarks 144
Acknowledgments 144
References 144

INTRODUCTION

Medullary thyroid cancer (MTC) is a rare malignant neuroendocrine tumor comprising 5%–10% of all thyroid cancers. It arises from the parafollicular or C-cells of the thyroid gland, which secretes calcitonin.

Hazard et al. recognized the presence of amyloid as a unique feature of medullary thyroid cancer [1].

A. It presents in the sporadic form (75%) or the hereditary form (25%). The hereditary form is autosomal dominant and part of the MEN 2A and MEN 2B syndrome.

B. Sporadic MTC is more aggressive than hereditary and commonly presents with metastatic cervical lymph nodes (70%). They are mainly solitary (68%) and less likely bilateral or multifocal (32%).

C. The RET (REarranged during Transfection), proto-oncogene on chromosome 10q11.2, is the germline mutation in the hereditary form. All patients with medullary thyroid cancer should be screened for germline RET mutation (Figure 18.1).

    i.   It can identify the index case of a germline mutation in <10% of cases of sporadic MTC without any family history. This may benefit the whole family to detect MTC in the carrier stage.

    ii.   De novo RET mutation is seen in 75% of MEN 2B patients.

    iii.   It detects the familial cases before an abnormal biochemical test.

    iv.   Abnormal serum calcitonin test does not mean harboring the MTC gene, as various conditions like chronic renal failure, pancreatitis, small cell lung carcinoma, and pernicious carcinoma can result in the same.

    v.   It is done once in a lifetime to detect asymptomatic carriers instead of doing serial biochemical tests.

    vi.   It helps in prognostication depending on age-related progression pattern and in deciding about the optimal timing for prophylactic surgery.

    vii.   It helps to work up the patient for associated endocrinopathy, such as hyperparathyroidism and pheochromocytoma. Also, it predicts the approach to surgical management and the risk of recurrence [2].

D. Somatic mutations involving RET have been identified in 40%–50% of sporadic MTCs. Mutation with M918 T have a more advanced stage, higher rates of recurrences and persistent disease, and poor long-term survival [2].

E. Because of its origin from the parafollicular C-cells that do not express the sodium/iodide symporter, medullary tumors do not concentrate radioiodine. Therefore, there is no role of radioiodine therapy or TSH suppression. It is more aggressive than differentiated thyroid cancer. There is a very high rate of recurrence and mortality. Surgery is the mainstay of treatment.

F. The parafollicular cells are situated predominantly at the junction of the upper and middle one-third of the thyroid gland. Hence a total thyroidectomy is mandatory in medullary thyroid cancer.

G. The various histological types described are classic (48.9%), amyloid-rich (38.3%), insular, trabecular, and epithelial variants. Some may histologically divide into a small cell variant, a giant cell variant, a papillary variant, oncocytic, squamoid, and clear cell variant type [3] (Figures 18.2 and 18.3). Immunohistochemistry (IHC) analysis shows the presence of markers for calcitonin, chromogranin, carcinoembryonic antigen CEA, and the absence of thyroglobulin (Figure 18.4).

H. Serum calcitonin and serum (CEA) are useful biomarkers for assessment of disease burden and prognostication during the preoperative and postoperative period. Serum carcinoembryonic antigen (CEA) has long half-life and lower specificity than calcitonin [2].

I. Use of serum calcitonin test for screening for MTC is controversial. Measurement of basal serum calcitonin levels is adequate. Provocative calcitonin stimulation tests are not required [2].

WORK-UP

Pre-operative evaluation is crucial in medullary thyroid cancer management.

A. *Clinical evaluation*: Sporadic MTC presents in the fourth to sixth decades of life, whereas hereditary MTC presents early in life depending on the germline mutation.

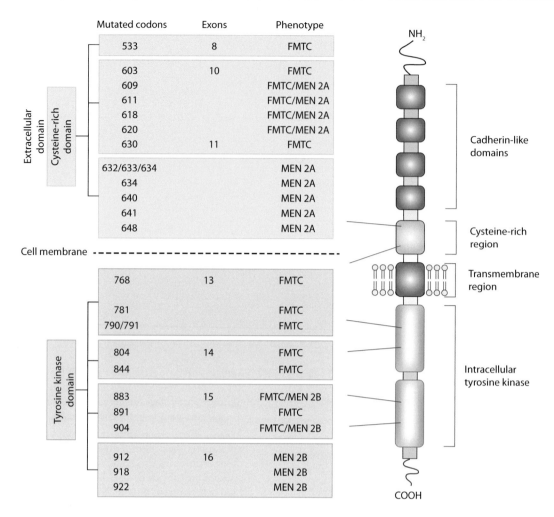

Mutated codons	Exons	Phenotype
533	8	FMTC
603	10	FMTC
609		FMTC/MEN 2A
611		FMTC/MEN 2A
618		FMTC/MEN 2A
620		FMTC/MEN 2A
630	11	FMTC
632/633/634		MEN 2A
634		MEN 2A
640		MEN 2A
641		MEN 2A
648		MEN 2A
768	13	FMTC
781		FMTC
790/791		FMTC
804	14	FMTC
844		FMTC
883	15	FMTC/MEN 2B
891		FMTC
904		FMTC/MEN 2B
912	16	MEN 2B
918		MEN 2B
922		MEN 2B

Figure 18.1   Schematic representation of RET proto-oncogene.

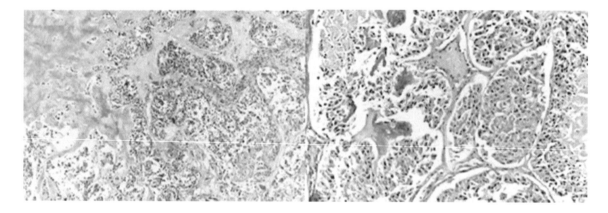

Figure 18.2   Histological features of classical MTC: 1A low power (×40) and 1B high power (×400). The tumor cells are present in nests and clusters and have a plasmacytoid morphology with eccentrically placed nuclei and abundant amount of cytoplasm with intranuclear inclusions. Also shows collection of eosinophilic amorphous material (top left-hand corner) consistent with Amyloid.

History of thyroid, parathyroid, or adrenal disorder in the family; history of sudden death in the family following any general anesthesia procedure (undetected secretary pheochromocytoma); presence of marfanoid body habitus; thickened everted eyelids mucosal neuromas (Figure 18.5); intestinal ganglioneuromatosis (phenotypic appearance of MEN 2B); presence of pruritic lesion involving interscapular area (Lichen planus amyloidosis); history of headache, palpitation, anxiety, tremor and diaphoresis (pheochromocytoma); and Hirschsprung's disease may suggest hereditary MTC.

The typical clinical presentation is a thyroid swelling with neck node metastases (75%–90%) (Figure 18.6). Generally, the pattern of lymph node spread is from central compartment nodes to the ipsilateral neck node and then to the contralateral neck node and then to the superior mediastinal nodes.

Some patients present with diarrhea secondary to substances secreted by the MTC tumors, viz calcitonin, calcitonin gene-related peptide, and other substances. They may present with ectopic Cushing syndrome with facial flushing due to corticotropin (ACTH) secretions.

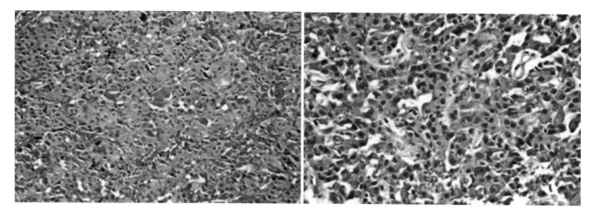

Figure 18.3   Histological features of oncocytic variant of MTC: 1C (×100) and 1D (×200). Tumor cells in follicular arrangement with centrally placed nuclei, intranuclear inclusions, and abundant granular cytoplasm, resembling Hurthle cell variant of PTC.

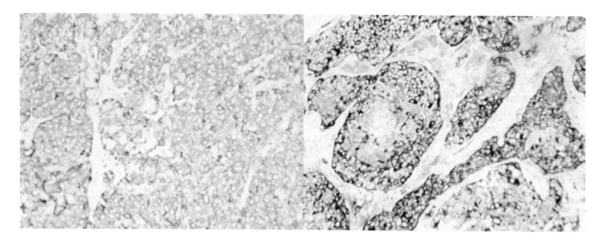

Figure 18.4   Immunohistochemical features of MTC. A panel showing that MTC cells are diffusely positive for synaptophysin, chromogranin, and calcitonin (hallmark of MTC).

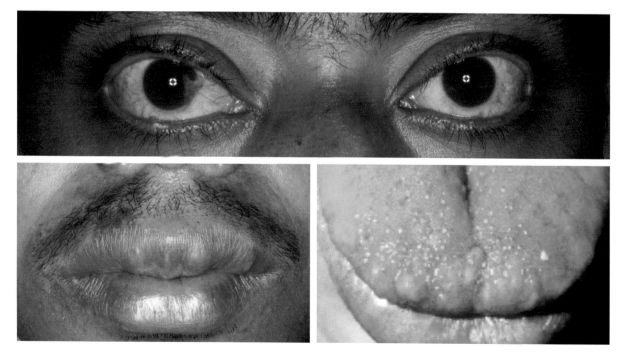

Figure 18.5   Phenotypic characteristics of MEN 2B syndrome.

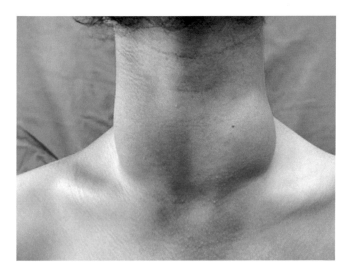

Figure 18.6 Medullary thyroid swelling with left thyroid nodule with C634G positivity.

Locally invasive MTC (10%–15%) may present with dysphagia, stridor, hoarseness, or dyspnea. Hematogenous spread (5%–10%) may be to the liver, bones, lung, brain, and soft tissues.

Any previous surgery of the thyroid or neck should be noted along with the histopathological report. The vocal cord mobility is assessed pre-operatively irrespective of the voice status.

A thyroid function test is done to assess the functional status of the gland.

B. Investigations

    a. Fine needle aspiration cytology (FNAC): It is performed under ultrasonography guidance from the suspicious thyroid nodule for tissue diagnosis. False-negative report for MTC is <20%. An inconclusive report should have the FNAC washout fluid for calcitonin measurement and IHC staining.

    b. Serum calcitonin: It is done pre-operatively and post-operatively for MTC confirmation, to decide the extent of surgery and prognostication. Low serum calcitonin has a limited lymph node burden and higher calcitonin levels suggest a considerable disease burden.

    Total thyroidectomy with central compartment neck dissection with ipsilateral neck dissection is done for serum calcitonin level between 40–200 pg/mL. Contralateral neck dissection is added for more than 200 pg/mL and superior mediastinal clearance is added to this for more than 500 pg/mL of serum calcitonin level. Less than 1000 pg/mL serum calcitonin patient may achieve 50% biochemical cure rates while more than 10,000 pg/mL serum calcitonin may not achieve biochemical cure. Calcitonin is a late marker for terminal differentiation and is lost in aggressive tumors [4].

    A poorly differentiated MTC, a defect in the cellular level and mutation involving calcitonin gene-related peptide (CGRP) gene may present with normal serum calcitonin and carcinogenic embryonic antigen CEA levels despite having advanced disease [5,6].

    c. Serum carcinogenic embryonic antigen (CEA): Low level of serum CEA indicates a low incidence of nodal metastasis to the central, ipsilateral, or contralateral compartment. As the serum CEA level reaches >100 ng/mL, the patient has a high chance of lymph node metastasis to central and bilateral compartment

along with distant metastasis and low chances of biochemical cure. Unlike calcitonin, CEA is a marker for early differentiation and is retained even in aggressive tumors [4].

    d. Serum calcium and serum parathyroid hormone levels are done to rule out hyperparathyroidism.

    e. RET proto-oncogene analysis: This is done for all to evaluate the germline mutation (Figure 18.7).

    f. Plasma free metanephrines and normetanephrine should be done for every medullary thyroid cancer before surgery.

    g. Imaging

      – Ultrasonography (USG) of the neck has to be done for evaluation of the thyroid and cervical lymph nodes.

      – Distant metastatic workup is done whenever there are cervical lymph node metastasis or serum calcitonin level above 500 pg/mL. Computed tomography (CT scan) of the neck and chest is done to evaluate the extent of neck disease, lung metastasis, and mediastinal nodes. Three-phase multi-detector contrast-enhanced (CE) CT scan or CE MRI is done for liver metastasis. Axial magnetic resonance imaging (MRI scan) with contrast and bone scintigraphy is done to rule out bony metastasis. FDG-PETCT scan is done to evaluate distant metastatic disease. With high serum calcitonin levels, the sensitivity of the PET scan increases [7].

    h. In case of locally advanced MTC, fiberoptic bronchoscopy and flexible esophagoscopy are done to assess the involvement of aerodigestive tract with transesophageal ultrasound to assess esophageal involvement.

TNM CLASSIFICATION AJCC, 8TH EDITION, FOR MTC

It lacks certain prognostic factors (Table 18.1) like age, biochemical parameters (serum calcitonin and CEA levels), number of lymph node metastasis, involved compartment by lymph nodes, completeness of resection, and genetic mutation analysis [3].

UNRESECTABILITY CRITERIA

- Extensive disease involvement of internal carotid artery
- Prevertebral fascia involvement
- Involvement of mediastinal structures
- Extensive distant metastasis with extensive locally advanced MTC

PALLIATIVE SURGERY

Locally advanced MTC is treated with less aggressive surgery with minimal morbidity for palliation. The decision is based on structures involved, extent of disease, life expectancy, medical comorbidity, and quality of life. Palliative surgery may be offered to cutaneous, hepatic, lung, brain, and bony metastasis. A multidisciplinary team plays an important role in decision-making.

SURGICAL TREATMENT

In the past, a total thyroidectomy without neck dissection was done for MTC. However, current recommendations are a total thyroidectomy with a systematic lymph node clearance (central, lateral, and mediastinum). This compartment oriented dissection avoids removal of only involved nodes (Berry picking). Sensitivity of intra-operative palpation to detect lymph node metastasis is very low (64%) [8]. This avoids the repeated recurrences in the same compartment, increased morbidity, and poor survival.

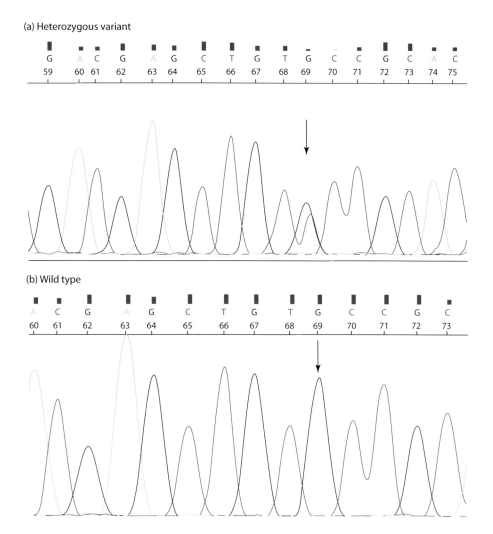

Figure 18.7 Germline mutation C634G (ATA-H, high risk) in RET proto-oncogene.

Miyauchi et al. have advocated unilateral thyroidectomy with ipsilateral central compartment clearance with neck dissection in nonhereditary, unifocal, small MTC with low serum calcitonin in patients without germline RET mutation [9].

However, this is rarely done as they usually present as advanced disease with abnormal serum calcitonin levels. The surgical technique for total thyroidectomy is the same as for the differentiated thyroid cancer. However, the clearance is more aggressive than DTC as there is no RAI back up. Size of the primary tumor does not decide the extent of surgery for thyroid or for neck nodes. Bilateral thyroid tumors have high chances of bilateral lateral compartment nodal metastasis. In the presence of upper pole thyroid tumor, the patient may present with lateral compartment nodal metastasis with skip central compartment.

SURGICAL STEPS

Surgical steps are the same for MTC or DTC for performing total thyroidectomy. However, the disease clearance is more aggressive than DTC. Intra-operative nerve monitoring and magnification may be used as adjunct for surgery.

Based on location and size of the primary MTC, USG findings, cross-sectional studies, serum calcitonin and serum CEA levels, and intra-operative frozen section, the extent of the initial neck node compartment dissection is determined.

Patients with lymph node metastasis and higher serum calcitonin levels are systematically not curable. However, a compartment oriented surgery may decrease the risk of local recurrences and further morbidity such as infiltration of local structures.

Following are the special considerations from the MTC point of view:

- The neck extension is given so as to aid dissection of the superior mediastinum. Even though generally MTC warrants extensive bilateral neck dissection, Kocher's incision is still preferred without any vertical extension.

- Cutting strap muscles leads to adherence of neck skin to the tracheal cartilage directly giving "cobra deformity" which is cosmetically not acceptable. Therefore, mere large thyroid gland and MTC histology do not warrant a strap muscles sacrifice. Only in case of extrathyroidal extension, the strap muscles are partially sacrificed.

- The parathyroid and recurrent laryngeal nerve makes the thyroidectomy an interesting and skillful surgery. Parathyroid glands receive the blood supply from the inferior thyroid artery. Occasionally the superior parathyroid gland may be supplied by the superior thyroid artery. The dissection over the thyroid and fascia on the lateral aspect and then proceeding superiorly helps to preserve this branch instead of taking superior pole vessels directly. Due to extensive central compartment dissection, it is essential to safe guard the blood supply of the bilateral superior parathyroid gland. The technique of identification of the parathyroid gland is the same as in DTC. Indocyanine green (ICG) dye injection along

Table 18.1 AJCC 8th edition staging for medullary thyroid cancer

T category	T criteria
Definition of primary tumor (T)	
TX	Primary tumor cannot be assessed
T0	No evidence of primary tumor
T1	Tumor 2 cm or less in greatest dimension, limited to the thyroid
T1a	Tumor 1 cm or less, limited to the thyroid
T1b	Tumor more than 1 cm, but less than or equal to 2 cm, in greatest dimension, limited to the thyroid
T2	Tumor more than 2 cm, but less than or equal to 4 cm in greatest dimension, limited to the thyroid
T3	Tumor more than 4 cm in greatest dimension or with extrathyroidal extension
T3a	Tumor more than 4 cm in greatest dimension limited to the thyroid
T3b	Tumor of any size with gross extrathyroidal extension invading only to strap muscles (sternohyoid, sternothyroid, thyrohyoid, or omohyoid muscles)
T4	Advanced disease
T4a	Moderately advanced disease: Tumor of any size with gross extrathyroidal extension into the nearby tissues of the neck, including subcutaneous soft tissues, larynx, trachea, esophagus, or recurrent laryngeal nerve.
T4b	Very advanced disease: Tumor of any size with extension toward the spine or into nearby large blood vessels, gross extrathyroidal extension invading the prevertebral fascia or encasing the carotid artery or mediastinal vessels.
N category	**N criteria**
Definition of regional lymph nodes (N)	
NX	Regional lymph nodes cannot be assessed
N0	No evidence of locoregional lymph node metastasis
N0a	One or more cytologically or histologically confirmed benign lymph nodes
N0b	No radiological or clinical evidence of locoregional lymph node metastasis
N1	Regional lymph node metastasis
N1a	Metastasis to level VI or VII (pretracheal, paratracheal, and prelaryngeal/Delphian or upper mediastinal) lymph nodes. This can be unilateral or bilateral disease.
N1b	Metastasis to unilateral, bilateral, or contralateral lateral neck lymph nodes levels I, II, III, IV, or V) or retropharyngeal lymph nodes
M category	**M criteria**
Definition of distant metastasis (M)	
M0	No distant metastasis
M1	Distant metastasis

AJCC stage	Stage grouping		
Prognostic stage groups			
I	T1	N0	M0
II	T2/T3	N0	M0
III	T1/T2/T3	N1a	M0
IV A	T4a	Any N	M0
IV A	T1/T2/T3	N1b	M0
IV B	T4b	Any N	M0
IV C	Any T	Any N	M1

with near infrared camera may be used for parathyroid glands identification [10].

- A thorough knowledge of the anatomical variation in this area is essential for performing total thyroidectomy. Thermal damage to the cricothyroid muscle should be avoided which leads to cricothyroiditis, fibrosis, and change in voice pitch. Exposure of the RLN in its entire course should be avoided if possible. In case of infiltration of RLN by disease or nodes, a plane of dissection is attempted. If not possible, then the nerve is sacrificed after securing the functional contralateral RLN. Intra-operative nerve monitoring may help to trace the nerve and assess the functional aspect of the RLN and EBSLN.

- Central compartment neck node dissection is done with serum calcitonin level >40 pg/mL. It constitutes prelaryngeal, pretracheal, and bilateral paratracheal lymph nodes. The central compartment is cleared from hyoid to suprasternal notch and between internal carotid arteries either side laterally. The prelaryngeal and pretracheal dissection is done to clear the lymph nodes. Upper mediastinal clearance is done if serum calcitonin is >500 pg/mL. It is cleared from the suprasternal level to innominate artery on the right side

Table 18.2   Clinico-radiological and biochemical combined criteria for extent of nodal clearance

Clinical/imaging criteria	Serum calcitonin criteria	Extent of surgery for central, lateral, and superior mediastinal compartment
No central compartment nodes	Serum calcitonin <20 pg/mL	Central: Ipsilateral
No central compartment nodes or Ipsilateral central compartment nodal metastasis or Ipsilateral lateral cervical nodal metastasis	Serum calcitonin 20–50 pg/mL	Central: Ipsilateral Lateral: Ipsilateral SND (II–V)
Central compartment nodal metastasis or Ipsilateral lateral cervical nodal metastasis	Serum calcitonin 50–200 pg/mL	Central: Bilateral Lateral: Ipsilateral SND (II–V)
Contralateral nodal metastasis	Serum calcitonin >200 pg/mL	Central: Bilateral Lateral: Bilateral SND (II–V)
Superior mediastinal nodal metastasis	Serum calcitonin level >500 pg/mL	Upper mediastinal clearance Central: Bilateral Lateral: Bilateral SND (II–V)

and corresponding axial plane on the left side. Meticulous dissection and securing the vessels with ligation or clip is important.

- Bilateral paratracheal dissection is important as it is crucial for functionality of the RLN and parathyroid viability. The tissue between hyoid and cricoid cartilage rarely harbors lymph nodes. The dissection is started from the carotid artery laterally and inferiorly. The inferior thyroid artery is preserved and the inferior parathyroid gland along with its blood supply is flipped laterally. The fibrofatty tissue along with all lymph nodes are dissected out. The course of the right RLN is more oblique and ventral. The left side RLN is vertical and close to the tracheoesophageal groove.

- Any devascularized parathyroid is removed and stored in ice cold isotonic sodium chloride solution and frozen confirmation is achieved. All the parathyroid glands, except in high incidence of hyperparathyroidism MEN 2A cases, are autotransplanted in sternocleidomastoid muscle and tagged by nonabsorbable suture for future identification. In MEN 2A cases with high incidence of hyperparathyroidism, the devascularized parathyroids are autotransplanted in non-dominant forearm brachioradialis muscle (heterotopic muscle bed) after mincing into 1 mm × 3 mm fragments. A portion of the graft can be removed if graft dependent hyperparathyroidism develops [2].

- There is no role of prophylactic parathyroidectomy as hyperparathyroidism is age dependent and requires a second hit with low penetrance depending on the germline mutation. The normal well vascularized parathyroid glands are left in situ.

- The term "compartmental oriented cervical lymphadenectomy" was coined by Dralle et al. They divided the neck compartment into cervicocentral right C1a and left C1b compartments, cervicolateral right C2 and left C3, and mediastinal right C4a and left C4b compartments [11].

- The lateral neck dissection is usually done from level II to level V for clearance of all micrometastasis in the neck. Some surgeons advocate performing less than level II to level V neck dissection [12]. Table 18.2 shows the extent of neck dissection based on clinic radio-biochemical criterion [13,14].

- In view of bulky lymph nodal burden and aggressive thyroid pathology, dissection is done with meticulous hemostasis. The important three non-lymphatic structures (sternocleidomastoid muscle, internal jugular vein, and

spinal accessory nerve) are saved if not involved. If infiltrated due to disease, then these structures are sacrificed. Bilateral internal jugular veins should not be sacrificed as this leads to severe facial edema and cerebral edema. If it is indicated bilaterally, then the jugular vein has been resected as a two-stage procedure. Also, sacrificing the vagus nerve, if necessary, should be attempted only after securing the contralateral vagus nerve and the RLN. The chyle duct should be preserved and any damage to small chyle duct collaterals should be secured and confirmed by the valsalva maneuver. Figure 18.8 shows the intra-operative thyroid bed after excision, and Figure 18.9 shows the specimen of the same patient.

- Hemostasis is achieved and strap muscles are approximated in midline. No drains are kept in the central compartment. Avoid taking out the drain in the midline or below the clavicle. The suction drain is placed on either side in the line

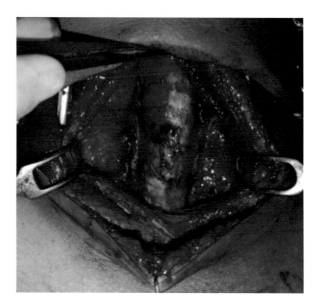

Figure 18.8   Intra-operative thyroid bed after total thyroidectomy with bilateral central compartment clearance and bilateral selective neck dissection (II–V).

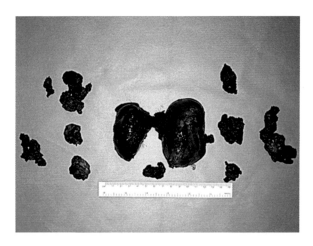

Figure 18.9 Surgical specimen following total thyroidectomy, bilateral central compartment clearance, and bilateral selective neck dissection (II–V) with C634G positivity.

of the incision. The wound is closed in layers and subcuticular sutures are taken.

- All patients undergo post-operative laryngeal examination to assess the vocal cord mobility and are started on Thyroxine supplement. Hypocalcemic patients are treated with oral and intravenous calcium supplements or oral calcium supplements along with calcitriol depending on the severity of clinical symptoms and biochemically corrected calcium levels.
- *Coexisting pheochromocytoma with MTC*: The pheochromocytoma should always be addressed first and MTC surgery later.
- *Coexisting hyperparathyroidism with MTC*: Single staged surgery is done. The involved gland is excised and, if required, subtotal or total parathyroidectomy is done for three or four gland disease.
- *Isolated pheochromacytoma following initial thyroidectomy*: Work-up is done for the pheochromocytoma and laproscopic subtotal adrenalectomy or retroperitoneoscopic subtotal adrenalectomy with cortical area sparing surgery is done. Pheochromocytoma should be excluded in patients with MEN 2 who wish to become pregnant, and if detected during pregnancy, it should be resected prior to the third trimester if possible.

RECURRENCE/METASTASIS/RESIDUAL MTC

During the post-operative period, serum calcitonin is done at 3 months. If it is normal, then it is done every 6 months for 1 year and then yearly [2].

In patients with serum calcitonin >150 pg/mL or where serum calcitonin is doubled, a whole-body evaluation is warranted. Patients with calcitonin doubling time less than 6 months have poor 5-year and 10-year survival rates. Patients with calcitonin doubling time of more than 24 months have the best 5-year and 10-year survival rates. Calcitonin doubling time is a better predictor of survival than the CEA doubling time [15]. In patients with post-operative elevated calcitonin levels, one forth of patients may have false negative imaging in spite of having fine military pattern liver metastasis, which may be visible only on laparoscopic examination [16].

If resectable disease is detected, revision surgery is done to achieve biochemical cure. Even during revision surgery, compartment

oriented lymph node dissection is done instead of Berry picking. Only in extensively operated fields is selective resection of the disease done.

Indications for revision surgery are:

1. Incomplete surgery in RET germline mutation positive patient
2. Post-operatively elevated calcitonin >150 pg/mL or with calcitonin double the baseline post-operative value with resectable disease
3. Residual MTC on imaging
4. Pre-operative serum calcitonin high, however, histopathology suggestive of incomplete and inadequate clearance
5. Initial surgery showing C-cell hyperplasia with incomplete surgery
6. Multicentric tumor with positive tumor margin, less than five lymph nodes dissection, and extrathyroid extension at the initial surgery with incomplete surgery [2]
7. Compartmental microdissection to bring down the serum calcitonin level—initial concept described by Norton et al. (1980) [17], Tisell et al. (1986) [18], Dralle et al. (1994), etc. [11]

ADJUVANT EXTERNAL BEAM RADIOTHERAPY (EBRT)

Dose: 60–66 Gy/6 weeks/4–6 MV photons for adjuvant treatment and 70 Gy for gross residual disease.

Adjuvant EBRT should be considered in patients at high risk for local recurrence (microscopic or macroscopic residual MTC, extrathyroidal extension, or extensive lymph node metastases) and those at risk of airway obstruction [2].

PROPHYLACTIC CANCER SURGERY

This is the pre-emptive operative removal of an organ prior to malignant transformation or while the cancer is "in situ" from an asymptomatic individual.

To perform any prophylactic cancer surgery, certain criteria need to be fulfilled. You et al. have given the following ideal criteria for prophylactic surgery in cancer. The criteria are fulfilled by MEN 2A and MEN 2B [19].

1. Gene mutation complete or near complete penetrance: MTC penetrance is 100%
2. Highly reliable test: RET proto oncogene is highly reliable test to detect germline mutation
3. Organ at risk is expendable or replacement therapy is available: Thyroxin supplement is available following prophylactic total thyroidectomy
4. Minimal surgical morbidity and mortality: Thyroid surgery is with minimal morbidity
5. Reliable test for cure: Serum calcitonin is used during follow-up with its doubling time

Factors affecting the timing of prophylactic thyroid surgery for mutation positive MTC are [20]:

1. DNA analysis and genotype and phenotype correlation
2. Age of onset of MTC: Germline mutation carrier 918 present with early (<1 yr) onset MTC than rest

3. Aggressiveness of MTC: Germline mutation 918 is more aggressive, followed by 634, and then the rest

4. Lymph node propensity and distant metastatic spread: Germline mutation 918 present with early lymph node and distant metastasis

5. Not reliable to use calcitonin levels during early life as the levels are high <3 years

6. In older patients, depending on clinical data and serum calcitonin levels. This should be used cautiously as loss to follow up for periodic visits is common and may present with clinically evident disease.

7. Issues with early age thyroid surgery
   - Higher rates of complication
   - Small, translucent parathyroid glands and difficult to distinguish parathyroids from surrounding tissues
   - Warrants experienced surgeons
   - Magnification
   - Low compliance for follow up and evaluation
   - Detrimental effect of insufficient thyroid hormone replacement due to poor compliance leading to impaired brain development and retarded growth
   - Surgery for <2 years age is more challenging [2]

SURGERY EXTENT

Prophylactic total thyroidectomy is done to clear all C-cell precursors. Central compartment clearance is done when serum calcitonin is >40 pg/mL (serum calcitonin is very high <3 years, therefore not useful). In 918 germline mutation (MEN 2B) patients, with age >1 year, if parathyroid glands are identified, then central compartment clearance is done. There is no role for any prophylactic parathyroidectomy [2]. Table 18.3 shows the guidelines for screening and timing of prophylactic thyroid surgery in MEN syndrome.

OUTCOME

Risk of having stage III/IV MTC at the time of diagnosis increased 12% per year of age at thyroidectomy [21]. Rate of recurrence is 0% versus 34–42% when compared prophylactic versus therapeutic respectively [22,23]. There is a strong correlation between age at surgery and the rate of disease recurrence following surgery.

SURVIVAL

Ten-year survival rate ranges from 21%–100%. Ten-year survival rate for stages I, II, III, and IV MTC are 100%, 93%, 71%, and 21% respectively [24].

Survival depends on the pre-operative serum calcitonin levels and their normalization after surgery. It also depends on the age, tumor size, stage, lymph node status, distant metastasis, and adequacy of surgery. However, stage adjustment may show a similar progression between sporadic and hereditary MTC.

SALIENT POINTS

- Medullary thyroid cancer is an aggressive disease that falls between DTC and anaplastic cancer.
- RET proto oncogene testing, serum calcitonin, serum CEA, imaging, and ruling out secretary pheochromocytoma comprise the essential pre-operative work-up before surgery.
- An undiagnosed pheochromocytoma in a patient undergoing any procedure under general anesthesia may result in substantial morbidity and even death.
- Medullary thyroid cancer is rare cancer arising from parafollicular C-cells. Therefore, they do not concentrate RAI, and there is no role of TSH suppression.

Table 18.3 Guidelines for screening and prophylactic surgery in MEN syndrome

Hereditary	Types	Associated endocrinopathy/ abnormality with MTC	Incidence	Screening for MTC	Timing of prophylactic surgery for MTC	Screening for PHEO/HPTH
Autosomal Dominant	MEN 2A 1) 634 (High risk; ATA-H)	(A) Classic MEN 2A with (634) Pheochromocytoma (PHEO) Hyperparathyroidism (HPTH)	50% 20%–30%	High risk; ATA-H (634): 3 yrs	ATA-H Before 5 yrs or earlier based on elevated serum calcitonin levels	11 yrs PHEO for ATA- H and ATA- HST
MTC: Bilateral, multicentre		(B) MEN 2A with Cutaneous lichen planus CLA (634)	Rare 36% MEN2A;634			
C cells are precursor for MTC	2) Rest (excluding 918,883,634) (Moderate risk; ATA-MOD)	(C) MEN 2A with Hirschsprung disease HD (609/611/618/620)	Rare 7% MEN2A PHEO 20%–30% HPTH 10%	Moderate risk; ATA- MOD (Rest): 5 yrs	ATA- MOD May be delayed beyond 5 yrs depending on serum calcitonin levels	11 yrs HPTH for ATA- H
		(D) Familial MTC	None			
	MEN 2B 3) 918 (Highest risk; ATA -HST)	Pheochromocytoma Multiple mucosal neuroma Marfanoid body habitus Mucosal Neuroma Intestinal ganglioneuromatosis	50% >95% 80%	Highest risk; ATA- HST (918): Soon after the birth	ATA- HST As soon as possible and within 1st year of life perhaps even in 1st month	16 yrs PHEO/HPTH for ATA-MOD
	4) 883 (High risk; ATA- H)			ATA-H (883): 3 yrs	ATA- H: Before 5 yrs or earlier based on elevated serum calcitonin levels	

- Distant metastatic work-up is done for serum calcitonin level more than 500 pg/mL.
- Do not perform hemithyroidectomy or subtotal thyroidectomy in MTC.
- Surgery is the mainstay of treatment in MTC.
- Subcapsular plane of dissection, thorough knowledge of anatomy and its variation, and meticulous dissection are essential steps for the MTC surgery.
- Systematic compartment wise neck dissection is done under the pre-operative serum calcitonin level guidance rather than Berry picking.
- Use pressure to control bleeding instead of the use of electrocautery near the entry point of the RLN.
- Prophylactic thyroidectomy is a way forward toward personalized medicine for carriers.
- Regular follow up with a multidisciplinary approach to MTC patients and their family is required.

AUTHORS' EXPERIENCE/PEARLS OF WISDOM

- Initial adequate surgery is a key to achieve the biochemical cure with less morbidity.
- Do not ligate inferior thyroid artery and vein and superior thyroid artery as a mass ligation, but meticulous dissection and individual vessels are ligated or clipped.
- Do not dissect the RLN in its entire course but only in few skip segments. This preserves the functionality of the RLN.
- Do not leave any thyroid tissue at the superior pole, inferior pole, Berry's ligament, and pyramidal lobe.
- Do not cut any structure transversely in the inferior aspect until the RLN is identified.
- Before sacrificing the RLN, securing the other side RLN is essential. Also, before sacrificing any important structure, R0 resection should be achieved elsewhere.
- Preservation of structures anatomically and functionally, meticulous dissection in the correct plane of dissection, and handling the structures carefully reduces long term morbidity of the surgery.

CONCLUDING REMARKS

The low incidence of medullary thyroid cancer has made detailed research and establishment of management guidelines strenuous. All diagnosed cases of medullary thyroid cancer patients should undergo a physical examination, laboratory analysis for serum CEA and serum calcitonin, appropriate imaging, laboratory tests to rule out pheochromocytoma, and genetic testing for germline mutation of RET proto-oncogene. Surgical intervention is the mainstay of treatment for medullary thyroid cancer. The decision on locoregional lymphadenectomy is best driven by imaging features, central and lateral compartment nodal status, and serum calcitonin levels. Compartment oriented nodal clearance is practiced in per primum and also in recurrent cases. Prophylactic thyroidectomy is a way forward toward personalized medicine for RET proto-oncogene mutation positive carriers.

ACKNOWLEDGMENTS

The authors would like to acknowledge Dr. Neha Mittal, Assistant Professor in Pathology Department for microphotographs; Mr. Nilesh N Ganthade, Officer in charge of Medical Graphics, Tata Memorial Centre, Mumbai for graphics; Dr Rajiv Sarin, Professor in Radiation Oncology Department for germline mutation photograph; and Dr. Gouri Pantvaidya for surgical photographs.

REFERENCES

1. Hazard JB, Hawk WA, Crile G Jr. Medullary (solid) carcinoma of the thyroid; a clinicopathologic entity. *J Clin Endocrinol Metab.* 1959;19:152–61.

2. Wells SA Jr et al. Revised American Thyroid Association guidelines for the management of medullary thyroid carcinoma. American Thyroid Association Guidelines Task Force on Medullary Thyroid Carcinoma. *Thyroid.* 2015;25(6):567.

3. Amin MB et al. (eds.) *AJCC Cancer Staging Manual*, 8th edn. Springer International Publishing, American Joint Commission on Cancer; 2017.

4. Mendelsohn G, Wells SA Jr, Baylin SB. Relationship of tissue carcinoembryonic antigen and calcitonin to tumor virulence in medullary thyroid carcinoma. An immunohistochemical study in early, localized, and virulent disseminated stages of disease. *Cancer.* 1984;54:657–62.

5. Nakazawa T, Cameselle-Teijeiro J, Vinagre J, Soares P, Rousseau E, Eloy C, Sobrinho-Simões M. C-cell-derived calcitonin-free neuroendocrine carcinoma of the thyroid: The diagnostic importance of CGRP immunoreactivity. *Int J Surg Pathol.* 2014;22(6):530–5.

6. Sand M, Gelos M, Sand D, Bechara FG, Bonhag G, Welsing E, Mann B. Serum calcitonin negative medullary thyroid carcinoma. *World J Surg Oncol.* 2006 Dec;4:97.

7. Kushchayev SV, Kushchayeva YS, Tella SH, Glushko T, Pacak K, Teytelboym OM. Medullary thyroid carcinoma: An update on imaging. *J Thyroid Res.* 2019 Jul;2019:1893047.

8. Moley JF, DeBenedetti MK. Patterns of nodal metastases in palpable medullary thyroid carcinoma: Recommendations for extent of node dissection. *Ann Surg.* 1999;229:880–7; discussion 887–8.

9. Miyauchi A, Matsuzuka F, Hirai K, Yokozawa T, Kobayashi K, Ito Y, Nakano K, Kuma K, Futami H, Yamaguchi K. Prospective trial of unilateral surgery for nonhereditary medullary thyroid carcinoma in patients without germline RET mutations. *World J Surg.* 2002 Aug;26(8):1023–8.

10. Vidal Fortuny J, Sadowski SM, Belfontali V, Guigard S, Poncet A, Ris F, Karenovics W, Triponez F. Randomized clinical trial of intraoperative parathyroid gland angiography with indocyanine green fluorescence predicting parathyroid function after thyroid surgery. *Br J Surg.* 2018 Mar;105(4):350–7.

11. Dralle H, Damm I, Scheumann GF, Kotzerke J, Kupsch E, Geerlings H, Pichlmayr R. Compartment-oriented

microdissection of regional lymph nodes in medullary thyroid carcinoma. *Surg Today.* 1994;24(2):112–21.

12. Pena I et al. Management of the lateral neck compartment in patients with sporadic medullary thyroid cancer. *Head Neck.* 2018 Jan;40(1):79–85.

13. Machens A, Dralle H. Biomarker-based risk stratification for previously untreated medullary thyroid cancer. *J Clin Endocrinol Metab.* 2010 Jun;95(6):2655–63.

14. Machens A, Hauptmann S, Dralle H. Prediction of lateral lymph node metastases in medullary thyroid cancer. *Br J Surg.* 2008;95(5):586–91.

15. Barbet J, Campion L, Kraeber-Bodéré F, Chatal JF; GTE Study Group. Prognostic impact of serum calcitonin and carcinoembryonic antigen doubling-times in patients with medullary thyroid carcinoma. *J Clin Endocrinol Metab.* 2005;90:6077–84.

16. Tung WS, Vesely TM, Moley JF. Laparoscopic detection of hepatic metastases in patients with residual or recurrent medullary thyroid cancer. *Surgery.* 1995;118:1024–9; discussion 1029–30.

17. Norton JA, Doppman JL, Brennan MF. Localization and resection of clinically inapparent medullary carcinoma of the thyroid. *Surgery.* 1980 Jun;87(6):616–22.

18. Tisell LE, Hansson G, Jansson S, Salander H. Reoperation in the treatment of asymptomatic metastasizing medullary thyroid carcinoma. *Surgery.* 1986;99:60–6.

19. You YN, Lakhani VT, Wells SA Jr. The role of prophylactic surgery in cancer prevention. *World J Surg.* 2007 Mar;31(3):450–64.

20. Waguespack SG, Rich TA, Perrier ND, Jimenez C, Cote GJ. Management of medullary thyroid carcinoma and MEN2 syndromes in childhood. *Nat Rev Endocrinol.* 2011 Aug; 7(10):596–607.

21. Yip L, Cote GJ, Shapiro SE, Ayers GD, Herzog CE, Sellin RV, Sherman SI, Gagel RF, Lee JE, Evans DB. Multiple endocrine neoplasia type 2: Evaluation of the genotype-phenotype relationship. *Arch Surg.* 2003 Apr; 138(4):409–16.

22. Shepet K, Alhefdhi A, Lai N, Mazeh H, Sippel R, Chen H. Hereditary medullary thyroid cancer: Age-appropriate thyroidectomy improves disease-free survival. *Ann Surg Oncol.* 2013 May;20(5):1451–5.

23. Schreinemakers JM, Vriens MR, Valk GD, de Groot JW, Plukker JT, Bax K, Hamming JF, van der Luijt RB, Aronson DC, Borel Rinkes IH. Factors predicting outcome of total thyroidectomy in young patients with multiple endocrine neoplasia type 2: A nationwide long-term follow-up study. *World J Surg.* 2010 Apr;34(4):852–60.

24. Modigliani E et al. Prognostic factors for survival and for biochemical cure in medullary thyroid carcinoma: Results in 899 patients. The GETC Study Group. Groupe d'etude des tumeurs a calcitonine. *Clin Endocrinol (Oxf).* 1998; 48:265–73.

Chapter 19

SURGICAL MANAGEMENT OF ANAPLASTIC THYROID CANCERS

Deepa Nair and K.S. Rathan Shetty

CONTENTS

Introduction   147
Clinical Presentation   147
Treatment   148
Role of Neoadjuvant Treatment   149
References   149

INTRODUCTION

Anaplastic thyroid cancers (ATC) are extremely aggressive undifferentiated tumors arising from the thyroid follicular epithelium. They are characterized by rapid progression of the disease, poor outcomes, and with a disease-specific mortality close to 100% [1–3]. The diagnosis of ATC is agonizing news to the patient, and early diagnosis of the disease remains paramount to initiate treatment. The age-adjusted annual incidence of anaplastic cancer ranges from one to two per million persons [4,5] and accounts for 0.9%–9.8% of all thyroid cancers in the world [6]. ATC, like all thyroid cancers, have a female predominance and affect older individuals, most commonly in the 6th–7th decade of life, and fewer than 10% occur in individuals younger than 50 years [7]. It has been hypothesized that ATC develops from pre-existing differentiated thyroid tumors due to dedifferentiation, which is supported by the finding that approximately 20% have a history of differentiated thyroid cancer and 20%–30% have coexisting differentiated thyroid cancer [8,9].

CLINICAL PRESENTATION

The most common clinical symptom is a rapidly enlarging neck mass with other concomitant symptoms like pain, dyspnea, dysphagia, hoarseness, and cough. These symptoms arise due to involvement of aerodigestive structures like the trachea, larynx, esophagus, recurrent laryngeal nerves, and great vessels [2,8,10]. Another hallmark of ATC is the frequency of distant metastasis at presentation, which can be seen in up to 50% of cases, leading to symptoms like chest pain, bone pain, dyspnea, cough, weight loss, and fatigue. Hyperthyroidism may also be a feature due to a rapidly enlarging mass leading to destruction of normal thyroid tissue causing release of thyroid hormones into the bloodstream or thyroiditis [2,8,10].

Lungs are the most common site of distant metastases, where they can occur in up to 90% of the cases, followed by bony metastases in 5%–15% of cases; other not so frequent sites are brain, abdomen, and pancreas [6,10–12]. Death is usually due to obstruction or invasion of the aerodigestive tract along with distant metastasis [13].

CLINICAL FINDINGS

On clinical examination, the most common clinical finding is a hard thyroid mass involving one or both lobes of the thyroid and may be frequently associated with an enlarged neck node [14]. The tumor may be tender on palpation with features such as redness of external skin, local rise in temperature, and skin necrosis which may be due to rapid tumor growth. The tumor is usually hard on palpation and may be fixed to surrounding structures like the trachea, larynx, esophagus, great vessels, and also may have retrosternal/mediastinal extension. Involvement of extrathyroidal structures may lead to vocal cord palsy, stridor, dysphagia, and neck venous engorgement [15]. Another pathognomonic feature of ATC is rapid disease progression due to which the clinical symptoms and signs may evolve during the course of clinical assessment; hence, early diagnosis is the key to achieve meaningful treatment outcomes [2,6,16].

DIAGNOSIS

ATC can be confirmed by cytological examination like FNAC or core biopsy from the neck mass [17,18]. In a case series of 113 fine-needle aspirates in patients with anaplastic thyroid cancer, 107 (94.7%) were diagnostic of malignancy, and 96 of 107 were diagnosed with anaplastic thyroid cancer. The remaining 11 were diagnosed with differentiated thyroid cancer and malignant tumor not otherwise specified [17]. Ultrasonography guided fine-needle aspiration of solid, non-necrotic tumor is advisable to assist cytological diagnosis [19]. Core biopsy or infrequently open biopsy may be required if FNAC shows necrotic or inflamed tissue without a specific diagnosis. If core biopsy or open biopsy is to be done, then the site of biopsy should be along the line of the likely surgical incision in case of resectable disease. Cytology or biopsy specimen should be subjected to immunohistochemistry to aid in diagnosis. A highly dedifferentiated ATC may lose TTF1, Tg positivity which is of help in differentiating from poorly differentiated thyroid carcinoma in which it is retained. Various cytomorphological patterns of ATC are spindle cell, pleomorphic giant cell, and squamoid and may have a mixture of two or more patterns of varying proportions [6]. On cytopathology, there may be a coexisting differentiated thyroid cancer, usually papillary carcinoma of the thyroid or infrequently follicular carcinoma of the thyroid. ATC has been reported in up to 10% of Hurthle cell carcinomas [20].

EVALUATION

Clinical evaluation should include laryngoscopy and upper GI endoscopy to assess the involvement of the aerodigestive tract. Appropriate imaging to assess extent and staging should involve ultrasonography of the neck along with a PET scan as recommended by ATA [21]. A PET scan would show intense uptake of 18 FDG in the primary as well as metastatic nodes as ATC are found to be highly GLUT1 positive [22]. Patients with anaplastic thyroid cancer may have coexisting differentiated thyroid cancer. The appearance of distant metastases may not necessarily be from ATC and should not preclude curative intent. PET scan may help in differentiating between these two as ATC are hypermetabolic and have more avid uptake on PET scanning when compared to differentiated thyroid cancer [22–24].

If PET scan is not available, then CECT/MRI of the neck, brain, chest, abdomen, pelvis, and a bone scan can be done to assess the extent of the thyroid tumor and to identify tumor invasion of the great vessels, upper aerodigestive tract, and distant metastatic sites [25]. Brain MRI is recommended as part of an initial work-up in the presence of neurological symptoms. Laboratory investigations are done as part of the general work-up [26]. In patients with surgically resectable primary tumor, FNAC or biopsy of distant metastatic sites may be required to differentiate between well differentiated cancer and ATC when considering surgery. Thyroglobulin level will be markedly elevated in distant metastasis due to well differentiated thyroid cancers unlike in anaplastic carcinoma of the thyroid [27].

Laboratory investigations should include thyroid hormonal profile, complete blood count, serum biochemistry including BUN, electrolytes, calcium, and phosphorous, which may be deranged in distant metastases. Serum thyroglobulin may have a role to assess the possibility of metastatic well-differentiated thyroid cancer which is markedly elevated if metastatic lesions are from the well-differentiated component of the tumor rather than ATC; however, it cannot be relied upon as it may also be raised in inflammatory thyroid disease and goiter.

STAGING

Only about 10% of patients have ATC confined to the thyroid gland. About 40% of ATC have extrathyroidal extension and/or neck metastases, and up to 50% may have distant metastases at presentation [28,29].

As per AJCC, 8th Edition, all anaplastic cancers are now classified according to the same T definitions as differentiated thyroid cancer. All anaplastic cancers are considered stage IV cancers, intrathyroidal disease is stage IVa, gross extrathyroidal extension or cervical lymph node metastases are stage IVb, and distant metastases are stage IVc [21].

TREATMENT

Management of ATC involves multidisciplinary teams made up of surgeons, radiation oncologists, medical oncologists, and ancillary specialists. The best definitive treatment involves surgical extirpation followed by post-operative external beam radiotherapy (EBRT) and chemotherapy [30–32]. EBRT and chemotherapy is generally preferred in unresectable disease [6,11,21,33].

Accurate assessment of performance status, staging, and resectability is important when contemplating surgery. Treatment decisions and its initiation should be undertaken as early as possible as the tumor may become unresectable within months if not weeks. Surgical treatment may not be feasible in a majority of cases due to the advanced nature of the disease at presentation; however, if the disease is confined to the neck and is resectable, then surgery should be considered if gross tumor resection is possible with minimal morbidity. Combined modality treatment, i.e., surgery followed by adjuvant radiotherapy with chemotherapy, has shown the best survival among patients with resectable tumors [30–32].

Pre-operative staging determines surgical intervention. For patients with stage IVa or stage IVb disease, in whom gross total resection is feasible, surgery should be expedited as complete resection is associated with prolonged disease-free and overall survival [29–32].

Total thyroidectomy with central and lateral neck lymph node dissection is the preferred treatment in ATC. In intrathyroidal tumors without coexisting well-differentiated thyroid cancer, thyroid lobectomy with wide margins of adjacent soft tissue on the side of the tumor has been tried as it has been shown that total thyroidectomy with complete tumor resection does not prolong survival compared to ipsilateral thyroid lobectomy and is associated with a higher complication rate [16,21]. However, total thyroidectomy is generally preferred in ATC to ensure complete tumor resection. Total thyroidectomy with therapeutic central and lateral neck node dissection is recommended for stage IVb disease [6,21,34].

Neoadjuvant pre-operative radiotherapy (XRT) can be considered to downstage locally unresectable disease so as to subsequently enable complete gross resection; however, the surgical dissection may become challenging in a radiated field along with increased risk of complications. The intent of surgery should be gross total resection as debulking surgery may not necessarily prolong survival and the extent of resection should be weighed against the morbidity of the procedure, especially in an aggressive disease such as ATC characterized by dismal survival. Limited resection of the trachea or larynx can be performed if the morbidity is minimal; however, laryngectomy, esophagectomy, or sternotomy is generally avoided as it is associated with higher complications and morbidity rates with poor quality of life. De Crevoisier et al. in a prospective study report that in a multivariate analysis, gross tumor resection (i.e., R0 or R1) is associated with longer survival [35].

Surgery should be attempted only when R0 or R1 resection is possible and is almost always followed by adjuvant radiotherapy with or without chemotherapy [35–38].

When ATC is detected incidentally as a microscopic focus within a differentiated thyroid cancer after thyroidectomy, there is no adequate evidence to guide a surgical strategy; however, a completion thyroidectomy is preferred by most followed by radioiodine ablation [29]. ATA guidelines recommend close observation with frequent anatomic imaging [21].

When ATC is detected after a hemithyroidectomy, completion thyroidectomy is preferred by most surgeons, and this surgical strategy is also determined by the stage of the coexisting differentiated thyroid tumor component if present. Thyroid lobectomy with wide margins for intrathyroidal tumors has been shown to have similar survival compared to total thyroidectomy in such a scenario and it should always be followed by adjuvant radiation to the neck. Completion thyroidectomy is preferred if the stage of coexisting differentiated thyroid tumor component dictates total thyroidectomy and is followed by radioiodine ablation along with adjuvant radiotherapy. Several large retrospective studies studies have shown that surgery combined with radiotherapy provides the longest survival. A meta-analysis of 17 retrospective studies by Kwon et al. has shown that radiotherapy improves survival in ATC patients. However, it is not certain as to which cumulative doses, and whether radiotherapy versus combined radiochemotherapy before or after surgery is beneficial [39]. In aggressive surgeries involving limited tracheal resection, laryngectomy is warranted only if R0 resection can be achieved without grossly compromising the quality of life [13,40,41]. Surgery is avoided for tumors involving the upper mediastinum, esophagus, and great vessels as it is associated with higher morbidity rates and poorer survival.

Palliative surgery of the resectable primary tumor may be considered in stage IVc disease in order to avoid subsequent aerodigestive tract obstruction and it may enhance quality of life. Complications of surgery are usually higher compared to differentiated thyroid cancers and include hemorrhage, dysphagia, salivary fistulae, hypoparathyroidism, chylous fistulae, vocal cord paralysis, and surgical site infection [38]. A case series by Brignardello et al.

reported complications like recurrent laryngeal nerve injury in 2 of 55 patients (3.6%), hypoparathyrodism in 11 of 55 patients (20%), 2 of 55 patients required a tracheostoma (3.6%), and hemorrhage was found in 1 of 55 patients (1.8%) [38].

In a study by Sugitani et al. [8] 233 patients with stage IVb were evaluated retrospectively. Outcomes of patients who underwent super-radical resection (n = 23) were compared to patients who underwent curative surgery (n = 49), palliative surgery (n = 72), or no surgery (n = 80). The one-year cause-specific survival rate for patients who underwent super-radical surgery was similar to patients who underwent restricted curative surgery, and significantly better than patients who underwent palliative surgery or no surgery (level IV) [42].

Securing a patent airway may be challenging in patients with large tumors. Routine tracheostomy is generally avoided as it worsens the quality of life and has not been shown to prolong survival. Tracheostomy is considered during acute airway compromise and for those patients presenting with impending stridor not responsive to medical management with corticosteroids. Palliative tracheostomy is generally avoided as the tumor may cause bleeding, obstruction of stoma, or may subsequently erode into the trachea with significant worsening of quality of life. Tracheostomy is challenging in a case of ATC as the presence of hard thyroid mass, a surgical landmark, may not be visible during the procedure and critical neck structures like carotid artery, internal jugular vein, along with trachea may be encased and displaced by the tumor. Cricothyroidotomy with jet ventilation may be a useful procedure to buy time before formal tracheostomy in certain cases. Fiber optic guided endotracheal intubation is preferred if feasible before embarking on a formal tracheostomy, however, this may not be possible in a rapidly emergent condition. A larger incision is preferred while performing tracheostomy to better identify the structures as dissection through the tumor mass is usually accompanied by a copious amount of bleeding. An appropriately sized cuffed tracheostomy tube should be inserted to secure the airway. The ultimate decision regarding tracheostomy should be made according to the patient's and family's wishes [13,43].

ROLE OF NEOADJUVANT TREATMENT

Neoadjuvant chemotherapy has been tried in stage IVa and IVb tumors that were initially deemed unresectable often with an intent to assess disease biology. There are no large trials to assess the efficacy of neoadjuvant chemotherapy, and whenever feasible surgery should be the first line of treatment. Higashiyama et al. reported a response rate of 33% with weekly paclitaxel in nine patients with stage IVb disease. Four patients became amenable to curative intent surgery and adjuvant therapy and were alive and disease free at 32 months [43] A Japanese series of 40 patients with anaplastic thyroid carcinoma who were treated with neoadjuvant weekly paclitaxel for 4–8 weeks revealed that 33 patients (82.5%) achieved stable disease or partial response (PR). Of these 33 patients, 25 underwent surgery followed by additional paclitaxel for 4–8 weeks in the adjuvant setting, and 16 patients proceed to consolidation radiation therapy. The group that completed multimodality treatment achieved long-term survival.

There are several case reports and case series regarding the use of tyrosine kinase inhibitors in neoadjuvant setting usually in unresectable or borderline resectable cases. No meaningful conclusions can be made as responses to TKIs are variable as ATC is characterized by multistep dedifferentiation. Mutational screening of known oncogenes has been tried with subsequent targeted therapies using multikinase inhibitors and checkpoint inhibitors; however, the results of mutational screening may take weeks, by which time the tumor may have progressed.

SURVEILLANCE

Patients who have undergone a complete resection should undergo aggressive surveillance with cross-sectional imaging every 1–3 months for the first year, and every 4–6 months thereafter. FDG PET is a useful tool to monitor recurrence or to assess the success of treatment. Thyroglobulin measurements and radioactive iodine scanning are not useful in ATC [21].

To conclude, surgical extirpation of the tumor followed by adjuvant radiotherapy with or without chemotherapy is the optimal treatment modality in operable anaplastic thyroid cancer. Integration of targeted therapy in the multimodality management of anaplastic thyroid cancer needs to be further investigated to design an optimal treatment strategy to deal with aggressive tumors.

REFERENCES

1. Nilsson O et al. Anaplastic giant cell carcinoma of the thyroid gland: Treatment and survival over a 25-year period. *World J Surg.* 1998 Jul 1;22(7):725–30.

2. Kebebew E, Greenspan FS, Clark OH, Woeber KA, McMillan A. Anaplastic thyroid carcinoma: Treatment outcome and prognostic factors. *Cancer.* 2005 Feb 28;103(7):1330–5.

3. Harada T, Ito K, Shimaoka K, Hosoda Y, Yakumaru K. Fatal thyroid carcinoma: Anaplastic transformation of adenocarcinoma. *Cancer.* 1977 Jun;39(6):2588–96.

4. Burke JP et al. Long-term trends in thyroid carcinoma: A population-based study in Olmsted county, Minnesota, 1935–1999. *Mayo Clin Proc.* 2005 Jun;80(6):753–8.

5. Davies L, Welch HG. Increasing incidence of thyroid cancer in the United States, 1973–2002. *JAMA.* 2006 May;295(18):2164–7.

6. Smallridge RC, Bible KC. Anaplastic thyroid carcinoma. In: Luster M, Duntas LH, Wartofsky L (eds) *The Thyroid and Its Diseases* [Internet], Springer International Publishing, Cham, 2019 [cited 2019 Jun 8]. pp. 693–700. Available from: http://link.springer.com/10.1007/978-3-319-72102-6_45

7. Nagaiah G, Hossain A, Mooney CJ, Parmentier J, Remick SC. Anaplastic thyroid cancer: A review of epidemiology, pathogenesis, and treatment. *J Oncol.* 2011;2011:1–13.

8. Venkatesh YSS, Ordonez NG, Schultz PN, Hickey RC, Goepfert H, Samaan NA. Anaplastic carcinoma of the thyroid: A clinicopathologic study of 121 cases. *Cancer.* 1990 Jul 15;66(2):321–30.

9. McIver B et al. Anaplastic thyroid carcinoma: A 50-year experience at a single institution. *Surgery.* 2001 Dec;130(6):1028–34.

10. Tan RK, Finley RK, Driscoll D, Bakamjian V, Hicks WL, Shedd DP. Anaplastic carcinoma of the thyroid: A 24-year experience. *Head Neck.* 1995 Jan;17(1):41–8.

11. Veness MJ, Porter GS, Morgan GJ. Anaplastic thyroid carcinoma: Dismal outcome despite current treatment approach. *ANZ J Surg.* 2004 Jul;74(7):559–62.

12. Derbel O et al. Results of combined treatment of anaplastic thyroid carcinoma (ATC). *BMC Cancer* [Internet]. 2011 Dec [cited 2019 Sep 30];11(1). Available from: http://bmccancer.biomedcentral.com/articles/10.1186/1471-2407-11-469

13. Shaha AR et al. Airway issues in anaplastic thyroid carcinoma. *Eur Arch Oto-Rhino-Laryngol.* 2013 Sep;270(10):2579–83.

14. Neff RL, Farrar WB, Kloos RT, Burman KD. Anaplastic thyroid cancer. *Endocrinol Metab Clin N Am.* 2008 Jun;37(2):525–38.

15. Wendler J et al. Clinical presentation, treatment and outcome of anaplastic thyroid carcinoma: Results of a multicenter study in Germany. *Eur J Endocrinol.* 2016 Dec;175(6):521–9.

16. Haddad RI et al. Anaplastic thyroid carcinoma, version 2.2015. *J Natl Compr Canc Netw.* 2015 Sep;13(9):1140–50.

17. Us-Krasovec M, Golouh R, Auersperg M, Besic N, Ruparcic-Oblak L. Anaplastic thyroid carcinoma in fine needle aspirates. *Acta Cytol.* 1996 Oct;40(5):953–8.

18. Chang TC, Liaw KY, Kuo SH, Chang CC, Chen FW. Anaplastic thyroid carcinoma: Review of 24 cases, with emphasis on cytodiagnosis and leukocytosis. *Taiwan Yi Xue Hui Za Zhi.* 1989 Jun;88(6):551–6.

19. Suh HJ, Moon HJ, Kwak JY, Choi JS, Kim E-K. Anaplastic thyroid cancer: Ultrasonographic findings and the role of ultrasonography-guided fine needle aspiration biopsy. *Yonsei Med J.* 2013 Nov;54(6):1400–6.

20. Moore JH, Bacharach B, Choi HY. Anaplastic transformation of metastatic follicular carcinoma of the thyroid. *J Surg Oncol.* 1985 Aug;29(4):216–21.

21. Smallridge RC et al. American Thyroid Association guidelines for management of patients with anaplastic thyroid cancer. *Thyroid.* 2012 Nov;22(11):1104–39.

22. Poisson T et al. 18F-fluorodeoxyglucose positron emission tomography and computed tomography in anaplastic thyroid cancer. *Eur J Nucl Med Mol Imaging.* 2010 Dec;37(12):2277–85.

23. Bogsrud TV et al. 18F-FDG PET in the management of patients with anaplastic thyroid carcinoma. *Thyroid.* 2008 Jul;18(7):713–9.

24. Nguyen BD, Ram PC. PET/CT staging and posttherapeutic monitoring of anaplastic thyroid carcinoma. *Clin Nucl Med.* 2007 Feb;32(2):145–9.

25. Takashima S et al. CT evaluation of anaplastic thyroid carcinoma. *AJR Am J Roentgenol.* 1990 May;154(5):1079–85.

26. Miyakoshi A, Dalley RW, Anzai Y. Magnetic resonance imaging of thyroid cancer. *Top Magn Reson Imaging.* 2007 Aug;18(4):293–302.

27. Ragazzi M, Ciarrocchi A, Sancisi V, Gandolfi G, Bisagni A, Piana S. Update on anaplastic thyroid carcinoma: Morphological, molecular, and genetic features of the most aggressive thyroid cancer. *Int J Endocrinol.* 2014;2014:1–13.

28. Akaishi J et al. Prognostic factors and treatment outcomes of 100 cases of anaplastic thyroid carcinoma. *Thyroid.* 2011 Nov;21(11):1183–9.

29. Sugitani I, Miyauchi A, Sugino K, Okamoto T, Yoshida A, Suzuki S. Prognostic factors and treatment outcomes for anaplastic thyroid carcinoma: ATC Research Consortium of Japan Cohort study of 677 patients. *World J Surg.* 2012 Jun;36(6):1247–54.

30. Xia Q, Wang W, Xu J, Chen X, Zhong Z, Sun C. Evidence from an updated meta-analysis of the prognostic impacts of postoperative radiotherapy and chemotherapy in patients with anaplastic thyroid carcinoma. *Onco Targets Ther.* 2018;11:2251–7.

31. Chen J, Tward JD, Shrieve DC, Hitchcock YJ. Surgery and radiotherapy improves survival in patients with anaplastic thyroid carcinoma: Analysis of the surveillance, epidemiology, and end results 1983-2002. *Am J Clin Oncol.* 2008 Oct;31(5):460–4.

32. Swaak-Kragten AT, de Wilt JHW, Schmitz PIM, Bontenbal M, Levendag PC. Multimodality treatment for anaplastic thyroid carcinoma–treatment outcome in 75 patients. *Radiother Oncol.* 2009 Jul;92(1):100–4.

33. Kim TY et al. Prognostic factors for Korean patients with anaplastic thyroid carcinoma. *Head Neck.* 2007 Aug;29(8):765–72.

34. for the German Societies of General and Visceral Surgery; Endocrinology; Nuclear Medicine; Pathology; Radiooncology; Oncological Hematology; and the German Thyroid Cancer Patient Support Organization Ohne Schilddrüse leben e.V., Dralle H et al. German Association of Endocrine Surgeons practice guideline for the surgical management of malignant thyroid tumors. *Langenbeck's Arch Surg.* 2013 Mar;398(3):347–75.

35. De Crevoisier R et al. Combined treatment of anaplastic thyroid carcinoma with surgery, chemotherapy, and hyperfractionated accelerated external radiotherapy. *Int J Radiat Oncol Biol Phys.* 2004 Nov;60(4):1137–43.

36. Haigh PI et al. Completely resected anaplastic thyroid carcinoma combined with adjuvant chemotherapy and irradiation is associated with prolonged survival. *Cancer.* 2001 Jun 15;91(12):2335–42.

37. Goffredo P, Thomas SM, Adam MA, Sosa JA, Roman SA. Impact of timeliness of resection and thyroidectomy margin status on survival for patients with anaplastic thyroid cancer: An analysis of 335 cases. *Ann Surg Oncol.* 2015 Dec;22(13):4166–74.

38. Brignardello E et al. Early surgery and survival of patients with anaplastic thyroid carcinoma: Analysis of a case series referred to a single institution between 1999 and 2012. *Thyroid.* 2014 Nov;24(11):1600–6.

39. Kwon J, Kim BH, Jung H-W, Besic N, Sugitani I, Wu H-G. The prognostic impacts of postoperative radiotherapy in the patients with resected anaplastic thyroid carcinoma: A systematic review and meta-analysis. *Eur J Cancer.* 2016 May;59:34–45.

40. Gaissert HA et al. Segmental laryngotracheal and tracheal resection for invasive thyroid carcinoma. *Ann Thorac Surg.* 2007 Jun;83(6):1952–9.

41. Grillo HC, Suen HC, Mathisen DJ, Wain JC. Resectional management of thyroid carcinoma invading the airway. *Ann Thorac Surg.* 1992 Jul;54(1):3–10.

42. Sugitani I et al. Super-radical surgery for anaplastic thyroid carcinoma: A large cohort study using the anaplastic thyroid carcinoma research consortium of Japan database: Super-radical surgery for anaplastic thyroid carcinoma. *Head Neck.* 2014 Mar;36(3):328–33.

43. Xu J, Liao Z, Li J-J, Wu X-F, Zhuang S-M. The role of tracheostomy in anaplastic thyroid carcinoma. *World J Oncol.* 2015;6(1):262–4.

Chapter 20

POST-TREATMENT SURVEILLANCE OF THYROID CANCER

Abhishek Vaidya

CONTENTS

Introduction 151
Surveillance Tools for DTC 151
Initial Risk Stratification 153
Dynamic Risk Stratification 155
Surveillance Strategies 157
Summary 158
Acknowledgments 158
References 158

INTRODUCTION

There has been a recent increase in the incidence of thyroid cancer worldwide [1–3]. However, a significant proportion of this has been due to overdiagnosis of subclinical disease, and the disease-specific mortality remains unchanged [3]. Differentiated thyroid cancers (DTCs) carry a low global mortality rate of about 0.5/100,000 [4], with most disease specific mortality occurring in a few patients with advanced disease [2]. Overall, most thyroid cancers have a good prognosis with a low risk of mortality. But there remains a significant risk of residual disease and recurrence, only a minority of which is clinically significant [5]. The combination of increased diagnosis and treatment on one hand and low mortality on the other hand results in a large group of treated thyroid cancer patients who need post-treatment surveillance [5]. Surveillance strategies for DTCs have a significant economic impact, with a study in the United States showing that the cost to detect a recurrence in low-risk patient is 6–7 times more than the cost for intermediate-risk and high-risk patients [6]. The aim of the surveillance strategy, therefore, should be to accurately identify recurrences in high-risk patients and spare additional investigations in those patients at low risk of recurrence. High specificity tools allow identification of those unlikely to have a recurrence; such that safer, cheaper, and less aggressive surveillance strategies could be directed towards this group, whereas those with a high risk for recurrence are monitored more aggressively since early recurrence diagnosis allows optimal treatment [7]. This chapter focuses on the surveillance and follow-up strategies in DTC, in the context of existing guidelines, including the 2015 guidelines of the American Thyroid Association. We look at the surveillance tools available, the initial and dynamic risk stratification system, and follow-up schedules and strategies.

SURVEILLANCE TOOLS FOR DTC

SERUM THYROGLOBULIN

Thyroglobulin (Tg) is a circulating protein exclusively synthesized by thyroid tissue. Its serum levels are a highly sensitive and specific marker for the presence of thyroid tissue in the body. Tg can be produced both by normal thyroid and neoplastic thyroid cells.

The level of serum Tg is an aggregate of three variables: the mass of thyroid tissue (benign or neoplastic) in the body, the degree of thyroid-stimulating hormone (TSH) stimulation, and the thyrocyte's innate ability to produce Tg [8].

Since Tg is dependent on TSH levels, Tg measurements should always be interpreted relative to TSH levels in the patient. Higher TSH levels increase serum Tg levels and thus increase its sensitivity as a tumor marker for DTC. Serum Tg levels measured in presence of normal TSH level are called "unstimulated Tg levels" or "suppressed Tg levels," while Tg measured in presence of elevated TSH is called "stimulated Tg level." In a patient who has received initial therapy, the TSH level can be increased by two methods: (1) The withdrawal of exogenous Levothyroxine (T4), such that endogenous TSH levels increase. This is known as thyroid hormone withdrawal TSH stimulation and may require about 2–4 weeks of T4 withdrawal. (2) The administration of exogenous recombinant TSH (rTSH). This is known as rTSH stimulation of Tg and takes 2–3 days only. After two doses of rTSH (0.9 mg intramuscularly daily), Tg values have been shown to be as accurate as those obtained after endogenous TSH elevation after T4 withdrawal [9]. Tg levels typically increase 10 times after TSH stimulation in DTCs, whereas this rise may be less than three times in poorly differentiated thyroid cancers [8]. RAI ablation also increases Tg sensitivity as a tumor marker by removing normal residual remnant thyroid tissue after surgery. Thus, the Tg threshold used to define response to treatment depends on residual remnant thyroid tissue, whether the patient has undergone total thyroidectomy + RAI ablation or total thyroidectomy alone or lobectomy alone (Tables 20.3 and 20.4).

A single Tg level measurement (stimulated or unstimulated) may not give an accurate and complete picture in the context of ongoing management. Hence it is recommended that serial Tg measurements should be used to determine disease progress, the response to treatment, and the need for any additional imaging or therapy. Several assays are available for Tg measurement, and there is a lack of standardization across assays. Hence Tg should always be measured by the same method, preferably from the same laboratory. Classic Tg assays have a sensitivity of about 1 ng/mL, while newer ultra-sensitive assays have a sensitivity of about 0.1–0.2 ng/mL. The sensitivity of classic assays can be improved by TSH stimulation. Negative predictive value of TSH-stimulated Tg level approaches 100% [10]. The likelihood of disease recurrence is extremely low in the presence of TSH-stimulated Tg levels <1 ng/mL (with the possible exception

BOX 20.1   ROLES OF SERIAL TG MEASUREMENT
DURING DTC FOLLOW-UP [14]

- In low-risk patients, very low/undetectable Tg may obviate the need for imaging and stringent surveillance
- Tg levels can validate or question the significance of suspicious imaging findings
- Rising Tg trend identifies patients who need further imaging or therapy
- In suspected neck nodal recurrence, if FNAC is not convincing, needle washout of Tg may be helpful in diagnosing disease
- In patients with proven loco-regional or metastatic disease, changes in serial Tg levels help monitor therapy response and guide regarding the need for additional therapy
- Whether Tg level is proportionate or disproportionate to imaging evidence of disease load may indicate the extent of tumor differentiation, and its likelihood of responding to RAI
- Rapid Tg-doubling time (<1 year) is associated with worse prognosis

BOX 20.2   EUROPEAN THYROID ASSOCIATION NECK
LYMPH NODE CLASSIFICATION [17]

Normal Node
- Normal size, ovoid shape, hilum preserved, no hilar vascularity. No suspicious signs (e.g., microcalcifications, cystic appearance)

Indeterminate Node
- Absence of a hilum
- At least one of the following characteristics:
  - Round shape (PPV 63%)
  - Increased short axis, ≥8 mm in size in level II and ≥5 mm in size in levels III and IV
  - Increased central vascularity

Suspicious Node
- At least one of these features:
  - Microcalcifications (PPV 88%–100%)
  - Partially cystic appearance (PPV 77%–100%)
  - Peripheral or diffuse vascularity (PPV 77%–80%)
  - Parenchymal hyperechoic-looking thyroid tissue (PPV 66%–96%)

Abbreviation: PPV, Positive Predictive Value.

of initial high-risk disease). Risk of residual disease increases as post-operative thyroglobulin approaches 5–10 ng/mL [7]. Ultrasensitive Tg assays may obviate the need for TSH stimulation [11]. The cut-off using basal ultrasensitive Tg is reported as 0.2–0.3 ng/mL [12]. As stated, serial measurements of Tg are more informative than a single measurement, and the doubling time of Tg over serial measurements has prognostic significance. A Tg-doubling time of less than 12 months has been shown to be associated with increased risk of recurrence and decreased cause-specific survival [13].

Box 20.1 illustrates the roles that serial Tg measurements may play during surveillance.

ANTI-THYROGLOBULIN ANTIBODIES (ANTI-TG AB)

Anti-thyroglobulin antibodies may interfere with serum Tg measurements. These are found in about 20% of patients, represent an important limitation to the interpretation of individual Tg values, and may produce both false negative or less commonly false positive results. Hence, anti-Tg Ab should always be measured in conjunction with Tg measurements. In patients with anti-Tg Ab, serial measurements of these antibodies (preferably using the same assay) may be a surrogate marker of disease recurrence [15]. Declining or steady titers of anti-Tg Ab are associated with disease remission/NED [10].

ULTRASONOGRAPHY OF THE NECK (USG NECK)

Most of PTC recurrences occur in the neck. As such, USG neck provides a highly sensitive tool for detection of DTC persistence or recurrence. The sensitivity of a good USG neck in identifying neck recurrences is as high as 94% compared to about 50% of RAI scan [16].

ATA guidelines recommend using a 10-MHz frequency USG neck for detection of neck nodes [7]. The European guidelines recommend examination of the thyroid bed and levels II-VI in both necks using a 12-MHz neck USG [17]. These guidelines also specify characteristics to help identify suspicions from benign and indeterminate findings (Box 20.2). This is important as up to 18% of benign nodes may exhibit suspicious features on USG.

About 2/3 of neck nodes labeled indeterminate spontaneously resolve over time [18], thus waiting and watching may be done for small indeterminate nodes [10]. It is common to find small (<5 mm) thyroid bed nodules, but less than 10% of these may progress over a 5-year follow-up [19]. Further false positive results of thyroid bed nodules may be seen in about a quarter due to scar tissue or granuloma which may mimic recurrent disease [10].

A USG guided fine needle aspiration cytology (FNAC) should be done for central compartment nodes more than 8 mm in short-axis, lateral compartment nodes more than 10 mm in short-axis, and those showing persistent suspicious findings [7]. Thyroglobulin assays in the FNAC needle washout fluid is highly accurate and has an adjunctive value for detection of recurrence [20].

WHOLE BODY RAI SCANS (WBS)

RAI scan is based on the thyroid tissue's preferential concentration of radioactive iodine (I-131), which allows detection of normal or neoplastic remnant thyroid tissue for potential ablation; it also identifies, localizes, and monitors RAI avid DTC metastases [14] (Figures 20.1 and 20.2).

Prior to the current usage of Tg and USG for surveillance, RAI scans were the mainstay of thyroid cancer surveillance. RAI scan is usually done in a TSH-stimulated state, which requires T4 withdrawal of 3–4 weeks. This causes hypothyroidism, which may be clinically very symptomatic in many patients; furthermore, it has the risk of accelerated progression of metastases since these are also TSH sensitive and may be a cause of concern, especially at critical sites like the spinal cord or weight bearing bones. Further, the specificity of RAI scans in picking recurrent disease is not perfect [14]. Hence, the response to treatment and completeness is now defined by a normal neck USG and very low or undetectable Tg levels [10].

In patients who have achieved an excellent response to treatment, a normal post-treatment RAI scan (no RAI uptake outside the thyroid bed) obviates the need for further diagnostic whole-body RAI scans [21]. In current practice, WBS are done for those patients in whom the disease stage and risk estimate may warrant further RAI therapy/ablation. A diagnostic post-surgery RAI WBS may be useful if the extent of the thyroid remnant or residual disease cannot be accurately ascertained from surgical report or neck ultrasonography, and when the result may influence further treatment decisions [7]. It is important to note the different terminology used with regard to RAI scans and treatment. While *RAI ablation* refers to the use of RAI to ablate functional normal residual thyroid tissue post-surgery, *RAI therapy* refers to use of RAI to treat structural disease persistence/recurrence, and *adjuvant RAI therapy*

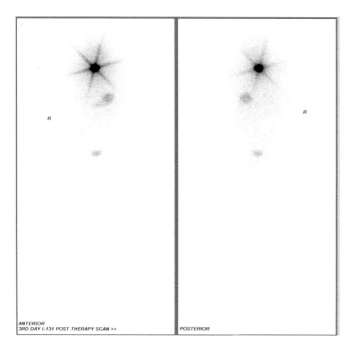

ANTERIOR
3RD DAY I-131 POST THERAPY SCAN >>

POSTERIOR

Figure 20.1   Post-treatment whole body RAI scan showing intense uptake in thyroid bed. (Figure courtesy of Dr. Shefali Gokhale.)

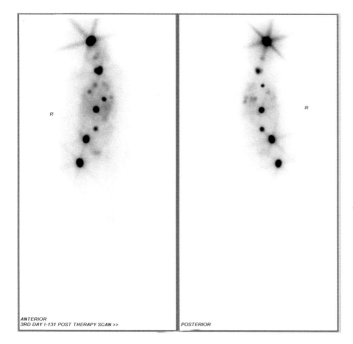

ANTERIOR
3RD DAY I-131 POST THERAPY SCAN >>

POSTERIOR

Figure 20.2   Post-treatment whole body RAI scan showing local disease with multiple metastases. (Figure courtesy of Dr. Shefali Gokhale.)

refers to RAI for treating possible microscopic foci of disease not seen on imaging [22].

COMPUTED TOMOGRAPHY (CT) SCANS

Cross-sectional imaging using CT scan of the neck and thorax can complement USG in localizing and mapping disease particularly in the central compartment before initial surgery. However, as a surveillance tool post-treatment, CT scan does not find routine recommendation. But CT scans can provide valuable information in a selected subset with lower neck, mediastinal, or distant disease.

For neck and chest, a contrast CT is preferred, while for lung metastases CT without contrast may be used [23]. MRI scan may provide complementary information for the neck, and especially for respiratory and gastrointestinal tract disease [23].

According to ATA guidelines, CT scan may be considered in patients with elevated Tg (especially >10 ng/mL or rising trend), and negative USG neck [7]. Thus, though CT neck is not a part of the routine surveillance plan for DTC, it is important when suspected recurrence is not picked up on USG neck.

POSITRON EMISSION TOMOGRAPHY (FDG-PET) SCANS

FDG-PET is based on the principle of coincidence detection, i.e., release of two high energy photons after a positron and electron collide. The basis of disease localization is the high uptake by malignant tissues of glucose labeled with a radioisotope (18-FDG) which is seen on scanning; whereas the CT component provides spatial resolution.

In DTC surveillance, PET-CT has a role when there is a suspicion of metastases based on high/rising Tg or clinical findings, but imaging modalities (RAI scan, USG, or CT) have been unable to localize the disease [14]. PET-CT may pick up suspected recurrent/metastatic disease in DTC, which has not been localized by USG, CT scan, or RAI in about 45%–100% patients, and this may alter management in about 50% [24]. PET-CT showed a sensitivity of 83% and specificity of 84% for detection of non-RAI avid recurrent DTC in a large meta-analysis [24]. The sensitivity of PET-CT improves with rising Tg levels, with a maximum sensitivity and specificity at Tg range of 12–32 ng/mL [14].

According to ATA guidelines, FDG-PET scan may be considered in patients with elevated Tg (especially >10 ng/mL or rising trend) and negative RAI scan [7]. They also recommend considering FDG-PET for: (a) part of initial staging in poorly differentiated thyroid cancers and invasive Hurthle cell carcinomas, (b) a prognostic tool in patients with metastatic disease to identify lesions and patients at highest risk of mortality, and (c) evaluation of post-treatment response after systemic or local therapy of metastatic or locally invasive disease [7].

INITIAL RISK STRATIFICATION

THYROID CANCER MORTALITY RISK

Several risk stratification systems have been developed to predict mortality in thyroid cancer. These recognize the importance of age, distant metastases, extra-thyroidal extension (ETE), tumor size, and histological grade/differentiation. More commonly the American Joint Committee on Cancer (AJCC) Tumor-Node-Metastasis (TNM) staging is used for assessing initial thyroid cancer mortality risk. The 8th edition of AJCC (2017) brought some changes to the previous edition for thyroid cancer staging, including the age of increased mortality risk was increased from 45 to 55 years; tumors with microscopic extrathyroid extension to perithyroidal soft tissues were no longer staged T3; and tumors with central and lateral compartment metastases were re-staged to stage II [25]. These changes are expected to cause down-staging in about a third of DTC patients. A salient point of TNM staging for DTCs is that age is an independent prognostic factor. Patients below the age of 55 years are staged I (without distant metastases) or II (with distant metastases) only. Young patients (<55 years) are not categorized in stages III and IV, reflecting the excellent prognosis of this group. The detailed TNM classification can be found elsewhere in this book; however, the stages are briefly described in Box 20.3.

It is noteworthy that TNM staging efficiently predicts mortality; however, within each TNM stage, patients have different risk of recurrence, as outlined in the following section.

THYROID CANCER RECURRENCE RISK

The goal of any surveillance strategy is to detect any recurrence, so that appropriate treatment can be instituted and the risk of disease related mortality decreased. As outlined previously, in thyroid cancer, the risks of recurrence and mortality do not always go hand in hand [5]. Though the global DTC related mortality is

low (<2% at 5 years), there is greater risk of disease residual and recurrence. Further, the TNM staging does not adequately predict the recurrence risk in thyroid cancers [7,26]. The American Thyroid Association (ATA) has devised a risk stratification system to predict the risk of disease persistence and recurrence. The 2009 ATA recommendations gave an initial three-tiered stratification system that classifies the recurrence risk into low, intermediate, and high risk categories [27]. Low risk patients are those who have intrathyroidal DTC, without ETE, vascular invasion, or metastases, and carry a risk of structural recurrence of <5%. Intermediate risk patients are defined as those who have microscopic ETE, neck node metastases, radioiodine (RAI) avid disease in the neck outside the thyroid bed, vascular invasion, or aggressive histology type, and carry a risk of structural recurrence of >5%–20%. High risk patients have gross ETE, incomplete surgical resection, distant metastases, or elevated post-operative thyroglobulin (Tg) values suggestive of distant disease and carry a risk of structural disease persistence/recurrence of more than 20% [7].

This system has been validated by analyzing datasets from four studies, and the estimates of patients achieving "No evidence of disease" (NED) after initial therapy are as follows: (1) low risk: 78%–91% NED, (2) intermediate risk: 52%–64% NED, (3) high risk: 14%–32% NED [26,28–30]. Similarly, the risk of structural incomplete response was 2%–3% in low-risk patients, 20%–34% in intermediate-risk patients, and 56%–72% for high-risk patients [26,28–30]. The 2009 stratification system has been validated and is a useful tool in initial risk stratification, but better understanding of recurrence risk associated with the extent of lymph node metastases, specific follicular thyroid cancer (FTC) histologies, and mutational status led the ATA to modify the initial risk stratification in its 2015 guidelines (Table 20.1) [7]. In this classification, the low-risk category also includes low-volume lymph nodal metastases (clinical N0 or ≤5 pathologic N1 micrometastases, all less than 0.2 cm in

Table 20.1   American thyroid association (ATA) initial risk stratification system for disease recurrence [7]

Risk category	Definition	Structural recurrence risk estimate
Low Risk	*Papillary Thyroid Cancers*[a]: (with all the below) • Intrathyroidal, no ETE • No neck or distant metastases • No tumor invasion • Clinical N0 or ≤5 pathologic N1 micrometastases, (<0.2 cm in greatest dimension) • No vascular invasion • No aggressive histology • Complete macroscopic tumor excision • If RAI given: no avid foci outside thyroid bed	<5%
	Papillary Microcarcinoma: Intrathyroidal, unifocal/multifocal, no ETE, B-RAF mutated (if known)	<5%
	Follicular Thyroid Cancers: • Intrathyroidal, well differentiated FTC • Capsular invasion only or minimal (<4 foci) vascular invasion	–
Intermediate Risk	• Microscopic tumor invasion into perithyroidal soft tissue • Papillary thyroid cancer with vascular invasion • Clinically N1 or >5 Pathological N1 lymph node metastases (all <3 cm in size) • Aggressive histology • Multifocal papillary thyroid carcinoma with B-RAF[V600E] mutation (if known) • If RAI post-treatment scan is done: avid foci in neck outside thyroid bed	5%–20%
High Risk	• Macroscopic invasion of tumor into perithyroidal soft tissues (gross ETE) • Incomplete tumor resection • Distant metastases • Post-operative Tg level suggestive of distant metastases • Pathologic N1 with any metastatic lymph node ≥3 cm in largest dimension • Follicular thyroid cancer with extensive vascular invasion (>4 foci of vascular invasion)	>20%

[a] For low risk category, all of these criteria should be present; ETE: Extrathyroidal extension; RAI: Radioactive Iodine; Aggressive histology includes tall cell, columnar cell, hobnail variant, diffuse sclerosing.

greatest dimension), intrathyroidal encapsulated follicular variant of papillary thyroid carcinoma (FVPTC), intrathyroidal FTC with minor capsular or vascular invasion (<4 foci of vascular invasion), and intrathyroidal papillary microcarcinomas (<1 cm in size) which are B-RAF wild-type or B-RAF mutated. The intermediate-risk category has been modified to include those patients with certain lymph nodal metastases (that are clinical N1 or >5 pathological N1, all <3 cm in greatest dimension), multifocal papillary microcarcinoma, extrathyroidal extension, or B-RAF mutated. The high-risk category now also includes large volume lymph nodal metastases (≥3 cm), and FTC with extensive vascular invasion (>4 foci). Thus, the size of the metastatic lymph nodes (≤2 mm, >2 mm or ≥3 cm), their number (<5 or >5), nodes with extra-capsular extension, and their location (central or lateral compartment) should also be taken into consideration when estimating recurrence risks [10]. Several other stratification systems have also been proposed, including one by a European Consensus Conference [31]. The ATA and European risk stratification systems are shown in Tables 20.1 and 20.2.

It is important to understand that though risk stratification systems give a category-wise classification, the actual risk of recurrence/persistence is a continuum, with different and often overlapping risk estimate for each specific clinico-pathological or imaging feature. Indeed, the risk of recurrence may vary from less than 1% in very low risk DTCs to more than 50% in some high-risk cases. Therefore, individualized management recommendations should be based not only on the risk category, but also on individual clinico-pathological or imaging risk determinants.

Application of the risk stratification system requires a comprehensive histopathological reporting. The reporting should necessarily include the histological type (e.g., PTC versus DTC), subtype or variant (e.g., tall cell, columnar cell), tumor size, any presence of ETE, details of capsular and vascular invasion (i.e., absent, <4 foci, ≥4 foci), lymph node involvement, lymph node size, and any presence of extranodal extension.

If a post-operative RAI scan is done, it will show areas of uptake within or outside the thyroid bed in the neck or at distant locations. The ATA recommends that post-operative RAI scans may be useful when the extent of thyroid remnant/residual is not clear from surgical report or neck sonography, and if the results may alter the decision to administer RAI or the dose of RAI used for treatment [7].

Table 20.2   European consensus conference risk stratification system [31]

Risk group	Definition	Implication for RAI ablation
Very low Risk	• Unifocal microcarcinoma (≤1 cm) • No ETE • Favorable histology • Complete surgical excision	No indication for RAI ablation
Low Risk	• Age <18 years • T1 >1 cm or T2N0M0 • Less than total thyroidectomy • No lymph nodal dissection • Unfavorable histology: 1. Papillary: tall cell, columnar, diffuse sclerosing 2. Follicular: widely invasive, poorly differentiated	Probable indication for RAI ablation
High Risk	• Incomplete surgical excision • Gross ETE (T3/T4) • Lymph nodal involvement • Distant metastases	Definite indication for RAI ablation

MOLECULAR MARKERS

Profiling of molecular markers of thyroid cancer is an attractive prospect since it may help in identifying tumor types that need more intensive treatment and surveillance. A large body of work has focused on molecular markers for predicting thyroid cancer outcomes. Incorporation of these markers in existing stratification systems is an attractive concept for tailoring patient management and surveillance [32].

B-RAF MUTATIONS

The most common mutation studied for prognostic implication in thyroid cancer is B-RAF. B-RAF^{V600E} is the most common driver mutation, being present in 40%–60% of all PTCs, especially in classical and tall cell variants [33]. In several series, this mutation was associated with adverse pathological factors like multifocality, ETE, lymph nodal metastases, distant metastases, and increased risk of recurrence and mortality [32]. However, the impact of B-RAF positivity in some studies was not independent of other tumor features, thus making the interpretation difficult. Furthermore, the clinical application of B-RAF^{V600E} as a prognostic marker is marred by its low specificity [32]. Thus, B-RAF is unlikely to be used in isolation, but only in conjunction with other prognostic variables in a multivariable context [34]. Though B-RAF features in the ATA risk stratification model (see Table 20.1) for its incremental prognostic value, the ATA does not routinely recommend B-RAF evaluation for initial post-operative risk stratification [7].

RAS MUTATIONS

These are found in about 40% of FTCs. Some studies have reported correlation between RAS mutations and metastases and poor survival in FTC and FVPTC [35]. However, RAS mutations are also seen in some follicular adenomas and encapsulated FVPTCs which are indolent, thus limiting their role owing to specificity issues [32].

TERT PROMOTER MUTATIONS

Recent studies have focused on TERT promoter mutations as a prognosticator for unfavorable outcomes in thyroid cancers. Though these mutations are found in 7%–22% of PTCs and 14%–17% of FTCs, these are commoner in dedifferentiated thyroid cancers, and portend a worse prognosis [7,36]. Furthermore, TERT mutations are common in PTCs with B-RAF mutation, and are associated with high risk of structural disease recurrence [37].

At present, B-RAF and TERT promoter mutations are included in risk stratification for recurrence; however, guidelines do not recommend their routine evaluation for initial risk stratification [7,32].

DYNAMIC RISK STRATIFICATION

The initial risk of recurrence needs to be modified in real-time during follow-up, in accordance with the patient's response to treatment and current findings. While initial stratification yields vital information about a patient's recurrence and mortality risk, it generates a static, time-point specific estimate based on data available initially. To exemplify, if a young patient with a low risk thyroid cancer develops neck nodes with high Tg levels after initial treatment, it would still be classified as low risk according to initial stratification. Therefore, there is a critical need of a risk stratification system that includes an individual patient's response to therapy and current clinical, laboratory, and imaging details. Such a real-time, dynamic risk assessment mechanism will help tailor ongoing management and follow-up. This concept forms the basis of the 2015 ATA Guidelines' Dynamic Risk Stratification system [7]; which is based on the work of Tuttle et al. [26]. It has been found that long-term outcomes can be more reliably predicted and surveillance strategies adapted using a system that adjusts to new data over time.

ATA's Dynamic Risk Stratification System incorporates information obtained mainly from surveillance tools like serum thyroglobulin (Tg), serum anti-thyroglobulin antibodies (anti-Tg Ab), and neck ultrasonography (USG), and may also include ancillary imaging modalities like RAI scan, cross sectional CT scan, and FDG-PET scan. This information is used to classify the response to therapy into four categories (Table 20.3) [7]:

A. *Excellent Response*: This implies that there is no clinical, biochemical, or structural (imaging) evidence of disease after initial treatment. If the initial treatment had been total thyroidectomy and RAI ablation, "excellent response" is defined as stimulated Tg <1 ng/mL, with absence of structural and functional evidence of disease, and absence of anti-Tg Ab [7,26,28]. Excellent response after initial therapy is seen in 86%–91% of ATA low-risk cases, 57%–63% intermediate-risk cases, and 14%–16% of high-risk cases [7,26,28]. Several studies have shown that in patients classified as excellent response, the 5- to 10-year risk of recurrence is as low as 1%–4%. The impact of this dynamic classification is most evident in those initial intermediate or high-risk patients who achieve excellent response, whose risk of recurrence drops from initial 30%–40% (ATA risk stratification) to 1%–2% (response to therapy re-classification).

B. *Biochemical Incomplete Response*: This implies that there is persistently abnormal unstimulated/stimulated Tg levels or increasing anti-Tg Ab levels in the absence of structural evidence of disease. The definition specifies unstimulated Tg >1 ng/mL or TSH-stimulated Tg >10 ng/mL. Biochemical incomplete response after initial therapy is seen in 11%–19% of ATA low-risk patients, 21%–22% intermediate-risk patients,

and 16%–18% of high-risk patients [7,26,30]. About half of these patients eventually achieve NED, about 20% develop structural recurrent disease, and about 30% continue to have thyroglobulinemia without structural disease at 5–10 years [7,26,30].

C. *Structurally Incomplete Response*: This implies that there is structural (imaging) or functional (RAI scan/FDG-PET) evidence of disease at loco-regional or distant sites. This definition is irrespective of Tg or anti-Tg Ab levels. This kind of response is seen in 2%–6% of ATA low-risk, 19%–28% intermediate-risk, and 67%–75% of high-risk patients [7,26,30]. Within this category, the risk of mortality is about 11% for loco-regional disease, while it is as high as 57% for distant metastatic disease [7,30,38].

D. *Indeterminate Response*: This implies that the clinical, biochemical, structural, and functional findings are neither classifiable as excellent response nor persistent disease. The category definition includes sub-centimeter thyroid bed nodules or neck nodes (non-specific structural), faint RAI uptake in the thyroid bed (non-specific functional), or unstimulated Tg <1 ng/mL or TSH-stimulated Tg 1–10 ng/mL (non-specific biochemical), in the absence of anti-Tg Ab [7]. This kind of response is present in 12%–29% of ATA low-risk, 8%–23% intermediate-risk, and 0%–4% of high-risk cases. In about 80%–90% of these, the non-specific findings may resolve or may remain stable over time. In the remainder 10%–20%, the disease will evolve to either structural or biochemical recurrence [7].

The definitions, management pathways, and TSH suppression goals for patients falling into different response to therapy groups is elucidated in Figure 20.3.

It is important to understand that the previously discussed dynamic risk stratification applies to patients who have received total

Table 20.3 Response to therapy reclassification: Based on ATA 2015 guidelines [7]

Response category	Definition	Outcomes	Management principles
Excellent Response	1. Imaging: Negative *and* 2. Non-stimulated Tg <0.2 *or* stimulated Tg <1	• Recurrence: 1%–4% • DSM: <1%	1. Decrease intensity and frequency of follow-up 2. Decrease degree of TSH suppression
Biochemical Incomplete Response	1. Imaging: Negative *and* 2. Suppressed Tg ≥1 *or* stimulated Tg ≥10 *or* rising anti-Tg Ab	• 30% spontaneously become NED • 20% achieve NED after additional therapy • 20% have structural disease • DSM: <1%	1. If Tg stable or declining: continue observation with ongoing TSH suppression 2. If Tg/anti-Tg Ab rising: additional investigations and additional therapy as required
Structural Incomplete Response	1. Structural or functional evidence of disease 2. Any Tg level Any anti-Tg Ab	• 50%–85% have persistent disease despite additional therapy • DSM 11% in those with loco-regional disease • DSM 50% in those with distant metastases	Based on factors like size, location, rate of growth, RAI avidity, 18-FDG avidity, either: 1. Additional therapy *or* 2. Ongoing Observation
Indeterminate Response	1. Imaging: Non-specific findings 2. RAI scan: faint uptake in thyroid bed 3. Suppressed Tg <1 *or* stimulated Tg <10 *or* anti-Tg Ab stable or declining in absence of structural/ functional disease	• 15%–20% show structural disease at follow-up • The remainder resolve or show stable non-specific changes • DSM: <1%	1. Continued observation with appropriate serial imaging and Tg level monitoring 2. If non-specific changes evolve to suspicious: additional imaging and biopsy

Note: Tg levels are in ng/mL.
Abbreviations: DSM, Disease Specific Mortality; NED, No Evidence of Disease.

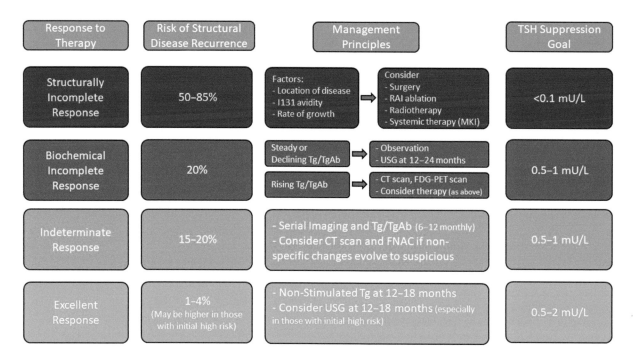

Figure 20.3   Dynamic Risk Stratification System: Definitions, management pathways, and TSH suppression goals.

thyroidectomy with RAI ablation as their initial treatment. However, for low-risk, intrathyroidal PTCs up to 4 cm in size, lobectomy is proposed. Similarly, the guidelines do not recommend RAI ablation for low risk PTCs. Hence, dynamic risk stratification was modified to make it applicable to those cases where either lobectomy or total thyroidectomy without RAI ablation was performed [39]. The category definitions for these subsets of patients are shown in Table 20.4.

SURVEILLANCE STRATEGIES

There is a lack of high-quality evidence-based guidelines for surveillance in DTCs [40]. As a result, there are marked differences in surveillance protocols, with the strategy being influenced by patient profile, individual preferences, and local resources available. The surveillance frequency and tools used currently have a high sensitivity, leading to early detection of recurrent/persistent disease. However, it is unclear whether this leads to better quality of life or survival [10,40]. A judicious use of these surveillance tools is therefore required to ensure optimum follow-up on one hand and unnecessary investigations on the other.

A brief initial timetable for surveillance tools in different risk groups is provided in Table 20.5. During initial follow-up, unstimulated Tg measurements (using a sensitive assay) should be done at 6–12 months, with this frequency being more for high-risk patients [7]. After surgery, an initial USG of the neck to assess the central and lateral compartments should be done at 6–12 months, and then repeated periodically, according to patient's Tg levels and risk status [7]. Whole Body RAI Scan has a role mainly in intermediate- and high-risk groups. In these, RAI scans may be done after thyroxine withdrawal or rTSH stimulation, at a frequency of 12 months.

The surveillance strategy varies according to the risk stratification and response to therapy, and is given for different groups, as follows.

Table 20.4   Response to therapy reclassification definitions in patients not receiving total thyroidectomy and RAI ablation [39]

Response category	Definition	
	Total thyroidectomy without RAI	Lobectomy
Excellent Response	• Negative imaging • Unstimulated Tg <0.2 or stimulated Tg <2 • Undetectable anti-Tg Ab	• Stable, unstimulated Tg <30 • Undetectable anti-Tg Ab • Negative imaging
Biochemical Incomplete Response	• Unstimulated Tg >5 or stimulated Tg >10 • Increasing anti-Tg Ab value • Negative imaging	• Unstimulated Tg >30 • Increasing Tg over time • Increasing anti-Tg Ab value • Negative imaging
Structural Incomplete Response	• Structural or functional evidence of disease • Any Tg or anti-Tg Ab value	• Structural or functional evidence of disease • Any Tg or anti-Tg Ab value
Indeterminate Response	• Imaging: Non-specific findings • RAI scan: faint uptake • Unstimulated Tg 0.2–5 or stimulated Tg 2–10 • Anti-Tg Ab stable or declining	• Imaging: Non-specific findings • Anti-Tg Ab stable or declining

Note: Tg levels are in ng/mL.

LOW-RISK/INTERMEDIATE-RISK PATIENTS

Excellent Response to Therapy after Total Thyroidectomy and RAI Ablation: If a low-/intermediate-risk patient has an excellent response to therapy as assessed by Tg and USG (see Table 20.3), the subsequent recurrence rate is very low. In these patients,

Table 20.5 Timetable for initial use of surveillance tools in DTC (after initial thyroidectomy +/− RAI scan)

Initial risk category	Timeframe (after initial treatment)			
	6 months	12 months	18 months	24 months
Low Risk	Tg	Tg USG neck	Tg	Tg USG neck
Intermediate Risk	Tg	Tg USG neck RAI scan	Tg USG neck	Tg USG neck RAI scan
High Risk	Tg USG neck RAI scan	Tg USG neck RAI scan Additional CT/ PET if indicated	Tg USG neck	Tg USG neck RAI scan Additional CT/PET if indicated

surveillance can be limited to unstimulated-Tg and anti-Tg Ab every 12–18 months. USG neck may be done at 18–24 months. A USG-guided FNAC should be done only for lesions with suspicious features and size >8–10 mm (in central and lateral compartments). If the USG is normal, further USG may be done at 3–5 years [10]. The goal for TSH suppression should be a level of 0.5–2 mU/L. (See Figure 20.3 and Box 20.4.)

Biochemical Incomplete Response to Therapy: As stated previously, this may be seen in about 10% of low-risk and 20% of intermediate-risk cases. In these patients, a trend of serial Tg levels is most important. In these, subsequent TSH-stimulated or sensitive Tg measurements along with anti-Tg Ab may be done at 6–12 months. A Tg-doubling time of less than 1 year portends a worse prognosis. USG neck should also be done every 12–24 months. The level of TSH aimed at is 0.1–0.5 mU/L. In those with an initial intermediate risk, aggressive histology, or rising trend of Tg/anti-Tg Ab, additional imaging may be done in the form of RAI scan, CT scan, or PET scan.

Total Thyroidectomy, No RAI Ablation: These patients may be followed-up with unstimulated sensitive Tg levels and anti-Tg Ab levels every 6–12 months. USG neck may be done every 6–12 months in those not achieving an excellent response.

HIGH-RISK PATIENTS

Excellent Response to Therapy: In these patients, if initial post-treatment evaluation shows excellent response to therapy, surveillance is done every 6–12 months; sensitive Tg and anti-Tg Ab levels, along with USG neck, are also done every 6–12 months.

Biochemical Incomplete Response to Therapy: If Tg/anti-Tg Ab levels are rising, further tests in form of RAI scan, CT scan, or PET scan are done.

The aimed TSH level in high-risk patients is <0.1 mU/L.

SUMMARY

The increasing incidence of thyroid cancers, along with the indolent nature of most of these, has caused the need for surveillance of a large set of such patients. With evolving understanding of the biology of thyroid cancer and better surveillance tools, current policy has shifted away from prolonged surveillance for all, to the current recommendation of less-intensive shorter surveillance for low-risk patients. Intensive surveillance strategy is reserved for those at a high risk of recurrence. It is advisable that the initial risk estimates be tempered depending on the response to therapy, such that a dynamic risk status guides ongoing surveillance and management. Serum Tg, anti-Tg Ab, and USG neck play frontline roles as surveillance tools. Most patients of DTC have an initial low risk and an excellent response to therapy. These may be followed up with annual Tg, anti-Tg Ab, and TSH levels for 5 years, with neck USG reserved for patients with abnormal findings. Selected subset of patients having a higher recurrence and mortality risk benefit from further imaging and therapy. In the future, incorporation of molecular proofing may further refine risk groups, and allow delivery of precision surveillance and medicine.

ACKNOWLEDGMENTS

The author would like to acknowledge Dr. Shefali Gokhale, Senior Consultant in Nuclear Medicine at Inlaks & Budhrani Hospital, Pune, India for Figures 20.2 and 20.3.

BOX 20.4 SURVEILLANCE STRATEGIES ACCORDING TO RISK AND RESPONSE TO TREATMENT

A. Initial Low/Intermediate Risk
  1. Excellent Response:
     a. TSH level 0.5–2 mU/L
     b. Unstimulated Tg and anti-Tg Ab: Every 12–18 monthly
     c. USG neck: 18–24 months; thereafter at 3–5 years
  2. Biochemical Incomplete/Indeterminate Response:
     a. TSH level 0.1–0.5 mU/L
     b. Stimulated Tg or sensitive Tg with anti-Tg Ab: every 6–12 monthly
     c. USG neck: 6–12 monthly
     d. RAI scan/FDG scan: if trend of Tg/anti-Tg Ab is rising
B. Initial High Risk
  1. Excellent Response:
     a. TSH level 0.1–0.5 mU/L
     b. Stimulated Tg or sensitive Tg with anti-Tg Ab: every 6–12 monthly
     c. USG neck: 6–12 monthly
  2. Biochemical Incomplete/Indeterminate Response:
     a. TSH level <0.1 mU/L
     b. Stimulated Tg or sensitive Tg with anti-Tg Ab: every 6–12 monthly
     c. USG neck: 6–12 monthly
     d. RAI scan/FDG scan: if trend of Tg/anti-Tg Ab is rising

REFERENCES

1. Ahn HS, Kim HJ, Welch HG. Korea's thyroid-cancer "epidemic"—screening and overdiagnosis. *N Engl J Med.* 2014;371(19):1765–7.

2. Davies L, Welch HG. Current thyroid cancer trends in the United States. *JAMA Otolaryngol — Head Neck Surg.* 2014;140(4):317–22.

3. Vaccarella S, Franceschi S, Bray F, Wild CP, Plummer M, Dal Maso L. Worldwide thyroid-cancer epidemic? the increasing impact of overdiagnosis. *N Engl J Med.* 2016;375(7):614–7.

4. La Vecchia C et al. Thyroid cancer mortality and incidence: A global overview. *Int J Cancer.* 2015;136(9):2187–95.

5. Wang LY, Ganly I. Post-treatment surveillance of thyroid cancer. *Eur J Surg Oncol.* 2018;44(3):357–66.

6. Wang LY et al. Cost-effectiveness analysis of papillary thyroid cancer surveillance. *Cancer.* 2015;121(23):4132–40.

7. Haugen BR et al. 2015 American Thyroid Association management guidelines for adult patients with thyroid nodules and differentiated thyroid cancer: The American Thyroid Association guidelines task force on thyroid nodules and differentiated thyroid cancer. *Thyroid.* 2016; 26(1):1–133.

8. Spencer CA, LoPresti JS, Fatemi S, Nicoloff JT. Detection of residual and recurrent differentiated thyroid carcinoma by serum thyroglobulin measurement. *Thyroid.* 1999; 9(5):435–41.

9. Haugen BR et al. A comparison of recombinant human thyrotropin and thyroid hormone withdrawal for the detection of thyroid remnant or cancer. *J Clin Endocrinol Metab.* 1999;84(11):3877–85.

10. Lamartina L, Grani G, Durante C, Borget I, Filetti S, Schlumberger M. Follow-up of differentiated thyroid cancer – what should (and what should not) be done. *Nat Rev Endocrinol.* 2018;14(9):538–51.

11. Schlumberger M et al. Comparison of seven serum thyroglobulin assays in the follow-up of papillary and follicular thyroid cancer patients. *J Clin Endocrinol Metab.* 2007;92(7):2487–95.

12. Malandrino P et al. Risk-adapted management of differentiated thyroid cancer assessed by a sensitive measurement of basal serum thyroglobulin. *J Clin Endocrinol Metab.* 2011;96(6):1703–9.

13. Miyauchi A et al. Prognostic impact of serum thyroglobulin doubling-time under thyrotropin suppression in patients with papillary thyroid carcinoma who underwent total thyroidectomy. *Thyroid.* 2011;21(7):707–16.

14. Santhanam P, Ladenson PW. Surveillance for differentiated thyroid cancer recurrence. *Endocrinol Metab Clin N Am.* 2019;48(1):239–52.

15. Rosario PW, Carvalho M, Mourao GF, Calsolari MR. Comparison of antithyroglobulin antibody concentrations before and after ablation with 131I as a predictor of structural disease in differentiated thyroid carcinoma patients with undetectable basal thyroglobulin and negative neck ultrasonography. *Thyroid.* 2016;26(4):525–31.

16. Frasoldati A, Pesenti M, Gallo M, Caroggio A, Salvo D, Valcavi R. Diagnosis of neck recurrences in patients with differentiated thyroid carcinoma. *Cancer.* 2003;97(1):90–6.

17. Leenhardt L et al. 2013 European thyroid association guidelines for cervical ultrasound scan and ultrasound-guided techniques in the postoperative management of patients with thyroid cancer. *Eur Thyroid J.* 2013;2(3):147–59.

18. Lamartina L et al. Risk stratification of neck lesions detected sonographically during the follow-up of differentiated thyroid cancer. *J Clin Endocrinol Metab.* 2016;101(8):3036–44.

19. Rondeau G, Fish S, Hann LE, Fagin JA, Tuttle RM. Ultrasonographically detected small thyroid bed nodules identified after total thyroidectomy for differentiated thyroid cancer seldom show clinically significant structural progression. *Thyroid.* 2011;21(8):845–53.

20. Grani G, Fumarola A. Thyroglobulin in lymph node fine-needle aspiration washout: A systematic review and meta-analysis of diagnostic accuracy. *J Clin Endocrinol Metab.* 2014;99(6):1970–82.

21. Pacini F, Capezzone M, Elisei R, Ceccarelli C, Taddei D, Pinchera A. Diagnostic 131-iodine whole-body scan may be avoided in thyroid cancer patients who have undetectable stimulated serum Tg levels after initial treatment. *J Clin Endocrinol Metab.* 2002;87(4):1499–501.

22. Lamartina L, Cooper DS. Radioiodine remnant ablation in low-risk differentiated thyroid cancer: The "con" point of view. *Endocrine.* 2015;50(1):67–71.

23. Lamartina L, Deandreis D, Durante C, Filetti S. Endocrine tumours: Imaging in the follow-up of differentiated thyroid cancer: Current evidence and future perspectives for a risk-adapted approach. *Eur J Endocrinol.* 2016;175(5): R185–202.

24. Leboulleux S, Schroeder PR, Schlumberger M, Ladenson PW. The role of PET in follow-up of patients treated for differentiated epithelial thyroid cancers. *Nat Clin Pract Endocrinol Metab.* 2007;3(2):112–21.

25. Tuttle RM, Haugen B, Perrier ND. Updated American Joint Committee on cancer/tumor-node-metastasis staging system for differentiated and anaplastic thyroid cancer (Eighth Edition): What changed and why? *Thyroid.* 2017;27(6):751–6.

26. Tuttle RM et al. Estimating risk of recurrence in differentiated thyroid cancer after total thyroidectomy and radioactive iodine remnant ablation: Using response to therapy variables to modify the initial risk estimates predicted by the new American Thyroid Association staging system. *Thyroid.* 2010;20(12):1341–9.

27. American Thyroid Association Guidelines Taskforce on Thyroid N, Differentiated Thyroid C, Cooper DS et al. Revised American Thyroid Association management guidelines for patients with thyroid nodules and differentiated thyroid cancer. *Thyroid.* 2009;19(11):1167–214.

28. Castagna MG et al. Delayed risk stratification, to include the response to initial treatment (surgery and radioiodine ablation), has better outcome predictivity in differentiated thyroid cancer patients. *Eur J Endocrinol.* 2011;165(3):441–6.

29. Pitoia F, Bueno F, Urciuoli C, Abelleira E, Cross G, Tuttle RM. Outcomes of patients with differentiated thyroid cancer risk-stratified according to the American thyroid association and Latin American thyroid society risk of recurrence classification systems. *Thyroid.* 2013;23(11):1401–7.

30. Vaisman F et al. Spontaneous remission in thyroid cancer patients after biochemical incomplete response to initial therapy. *Clin Endocrinol.* 2012;77(1):132–8.

31. Pacini F et al. European consensus for the management of patients with differentiated thyroid carcinoma of the follicular epithelium. *Eur J Endocrinol.* 2006;154(6):787–803.

32. D'Cruz AK et al. Molecular markers in well-differentiated thyroid cancer. *Eur Arch Oto-Rhino-Laryngol.* 2018;275(6):1375–84.

33. Vuong HG et al. A meta-analysis of prognostic roles of molecular markers in papillary thyroid carcinoma. *Endocr Connect.* 2017;6(3):R8–R17.

34. Tufano RP, Teixeira GV, Bishop J, Carson KA, Xing M. BRAF mutation in papillary thyroid cancer and its value in tailoring initial treatment: A systematic review and meta-analysis. *Medicine.* 2012;91(5):274–86.

35. Garcia-Rostan G et al. RAS mutations are associated with aggressive tumor phenotypes and poor prognosis in thyroid cancer. *J Clin Oncol.* 2003;21(17):3226–35.

36. Landa I et al. Frequent somatic TERT promoter mutations in thyroid cancer: Higher prevalence in advanced forms of the disease. *J Clin Endocrinol Metab.* 2013;98(9):E1562–6.

37. Xing M et al. BRAF V600E and TERT promoter mutations cooperatively identify the most aggressive papillary thyroid cancer with highest recurrence. *J Clin Oncol.* 2014;32(25):2718–26.

38. Vaisman F, Tala H, Grewal R, Tuttle RM. In differentiated thyroid cancer, an incomplete structural response to therapy is associated with significantly worse clinical outcomes than only an incomplete thyroglobulin response. *Thyroid.* 2011;21(12):1317–22.

39. Momesso DP et al. Dynamic risk stratification in patients with differentiated thyroid cancer treated without radioactive iodine. *J Clin Endocrinol Metab.* 2016;101(7):2692–700.

40. Gray JL, Singh G, Uttley L, Balasubramanian SP. Routine thyroglobulin, neck ultrasound and physical examination in the routine follow up of patients with differentiated thyroid cancer-Where is the evidence? *Endocrine.* 2018;62(1):26–33.

Chapter 21

APPLICATIONS OF RADIOISOTOPES IN THE DIAGNOSIS AND TREATMENT OF THYROID DISORDERS

Chandrasekhar Bal, Meghana Prabhu, Dhritiman Chakraborty, K. Sreenivasa Reddy, and Saurabh Arora

CONTENTS

Introduction 161
Molecular Basis of Imaging with RAI 161
Non-Radioactive Iodine Imaging 165
Salient Points 169
References 169

INTRODUCTION

Historical background: The suggestion by Enrico Fermi about the potential use of radioactive isotopes of iodine-127, the naturally occurring iodine isotope, in medicine began consequently to his group's production of new radioisotopes by neutron bombardment of natural elements in 1934 [1]. The first radioactive isotope of iodine, iodine-128, was produced by Robert Evans at the Massachusetts Institute of Technology [2]. Herz et al. suggested that RAI could be used for studying the physiology of the thyroid gland and for therapy [3]. Iodine-123 was discovered by I. Pearlman at the Crocker Medical Cyclotron at Berkeley in 1949 [4]. In the mid-1940s, the U.S. Atomic Energy Commission provided a plentiful supply of I-131, and the first human subject received RAI at MIT in 1946 [2].

MOLECULAR BASIS OF IMAGING WITH RAI

RAI follows the same physiological and biochemical pathways as non-radioactive iodine in the diet, where iodine is rapidly absorbed in the upper gastrointestinal tract. The recommended intake for an adult is 150 µg per day and 200 µg per day during pregnancy. Within the blood, iodine is preferentially carried by the red blood cells (RBCs) (60%), compared to 40% in plasma [5]. From the bloodstream, iodine freely diffuses into the interstitial space. Besides the thyroid, other organs involved in the clearance of iodide from the blood are the kidneys, salivary glands, gastric mucosa, sweat glands, and mammary glands. There is also placental transport of RAI (human thyroid begins to concentrate RAI after the first 12 weeks of gestation) [6]. The thyroid follicular cells trap iodine and incorporate it into thyroid hormones. The iodide trap/sodium iodide symporter (NIS) is located on the basolateral membrane of follicular cells through which two atoms of sodium are transported along with one of iodide. The ability of thyroid tissue and thyroid cancers to concentrate RAI depends upon the expression and functional integrity of NIS. Some differentiated thyroid cancer (DTC) and most anaplastic thyroid cancer (ATC) lose NIS and thus do not show uptake of RAI on diagnostic imaging and are hence insensitive to RAI therapy. Once trapped, the iodine becomes activated by oxidation and then organified through binding with the tyrosine

group of the thyroglobulin protein to form monoiodotyrosine and diiodotyrosine. These moieties undergo a coupling reaction to form the hormones triiodothyronine (T3) and thyroxine (T4), which are then stored in colloid form and released into the systemic circulation. RAI is incorporated into thyroid tissue, stored, and released from the thyroid in the same way as non-radioactive iodine, and this is a useful tool to study thyroid gland physiology [5]. The excretion of RAI is mainly by glomerular filtration; however, in hypothyroid patients, a lowered mean glomerular filtration rate (GFR) is observed [7] (Table 21.1).

THYROID UPTAKE STUDY

The percentage of radioactive iodine uptake by the thyroid gland is a simple and routine procedure.

INDICATIONS

1. Guidance in determining the activity of 131I to be administered. The uptake measurement should be performed as close in time as possible to the treatment.

2. Differentiation of sub-acute thyroiditis from Graves' disease is an essential requirement before administering radioiodine and other forms of thyrotoxicosis.

3. Confirmation of the diagnosis of hyperthyroidism due to Graves' disease.

PROCEDURE

Patients should preferably be fasting for approximately four hours (hr) before radioiodine ingestion to ensure good absorption. I-131 (10–20 uCi) is administered to the patient, and the same activity in the same volume is kept as standard. Both the neck counts and standard counts are measured at a given distance (around 25 cm) from the thyroid probe under identical geometry. The ratio of the neck counts to the standard counts (after background subtraction) multiplied by 100 provides the percentage of thyroid uptake. Room background for standard and thigh counts after voiding the urinary bladder provides the background counts for the standard and neck, respectively. The background subtracted neck counts can be measured at 2 hr and 24 hr post-administration of tracer dose of 131I. Percentage uptake at 24 hr is important for dosimetry. Uptake is calculated as follows:

Neck counts–thigh counts (background corrected)/administered activity ×100 (%).

Normal thyroid uptake values are at 2 hr: 1%–7% and at 24 hr: 7%–18% [8].

Table 21.1   Properties of radionuclides used for thyroid scintigraphy

SI no	Radionuclide	Physical half-life	Mode of decay	Principle photons	Energy (keV)
1	99m-Technetium	6 hours	Isomeric transition	Gamma	140
2	Thallium-201	73.1 hours	Electron capture	Mercury x-rays; Gamma	67–83 135, 167
3	131I-Iodine	8.02 days	Beta minus	Gamma	364, 637, 285
4	123I-Iodine	13.2 hours	Electron capture	Gamma	159
5	124I-Iodine	4.2 days	Beta plus (23%), Electron capture (74%)	Gamma	603, 723, 1691
6	18F-FDG	110 minutes	Beta plus (97%), electron capture (3%)	Gamma	633

THYROID SCAN
INDICATIONS

1. To relate the general structure of the thyroid gland (e.g., nodular or diffuse enlargement) to its function. The scan may be useful in distinguishing Graves' disease from toxic nodular goiter, a distinction of significance in determining the amount of I-131 to be given as therapy for hyperthyroidism.

2. To correlate thyroid palpation with scintigraphic findings to determine the degree of function in a clinically-defined area or nodule (i.e., palpable).

3. To locate ectopic thyroid tissue (i.e., lingual) or determine whether a suspected "thyroglossal duct cyst" is the only functioning thyroid tissue present.

4. To assist in the evaluation of congenital hypothyroidism.

5. To evaluate a neck or substernal mass. Radionuclide scintigraphy may be helpful to confirm that the mass is functioning thyroid tissue.

6. To differentiate thyroiditis from Graves' disease and other forms of hyperthyroidism.

PROTOCOL

- *Radionuclides used:* 99mTc-pertechnetate or I-123. I-131 is not used in routine imaging of the intact gland because of high radiation exposure.
- *Dose:* For an I-123 scan, the patient ingests 300–400 µCi orally. The scan is usually acquired 4 hr later. For a 99mTc-pertechnetate scan, 3–5 mCi is administered intravenously.
- *Timing of imaging:* Iodine I-123, 4–6 hr after dose administration; 99mTc-pertechnetate, 20 minutes after radiopharmaceutical injection. Early imaging is required because Tc-99mis not organified and thus not retained within the thyroid [9].

NORMAL AND ABNORMAL THYROID SCINTIGRAPHY [10]

1. *Normal scan:* The normal scintigraphic appearance of the thyroid varies among patients. The gland has a butterfly shape, with usually thin lateral lobes extending along each side of the thyroid cartilage. The thin pyramidal lobe usually is not seen. The normal gland shows homogeneous uptake throughout. Salivary glands are routinely seen with 99mTc-pertechnetate,

imaged at 20 to 30 minutes. Esophageal activity may be seen with either radiotracer. It can usually be confirmed by having the patient swallow water to clear the esophagus.

2. *Thyroiditis:* It is the most common cause of thyrotoxicosis associated with a decreased %RAIU. Various causes include granulomatous thyroiditis (de Quervain), silent thyroiditis, and postpartum thyroiditis (occurs within a few weeks of delivery, with positive antithyroid antibodies). During the initial stage of sub-acute thyroiditis, thyrotoxicosis predominates, caused by the release of thyroid hormone as a result of inflammation and increased membrane permeability and hence suppresses TSH. As the inflammation resolves and thyroid hormone levels decrease, the scintigram may show inhomogeneity of uptake or regional or focal areas of hypofunction (Figure 21.1a and b).

3. *Toxic multinodular goiter (TMNG; aka Plummer disease):* The %RAIU is often only moderately elevated or may be in the high normal range. The thyroid scan shows high uptake within hyperfunctioning nodules but suppression of the extranodular non-autonomous tissue. A nontoxic multinodular goiter may have hot or warm nodules, but the extranodular tissue is not suppressed (Figure 21.1c and d).

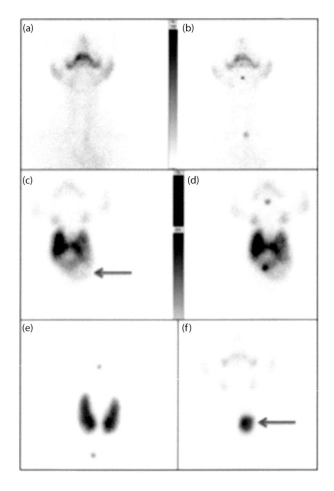

Figure 21.1   Various cases of thyroid scan: (a and b) Anterior view, and marker view; shows no tracer uptake in the thyroid bed, in a case of thyroiditis. (c and d) Anterior view and marker view; shows enlarged bilateral lobes with heterogeneous tracer uptake and presence of cold nodules in the isthmus and left lower pole—dominant nodule, features of toxic MNG. (e) Shows increased and homogenous tracer uptake in bilaterally enlarged thyroid lobes, in a case of Graves' disease. (f) Shows a single hot nodule in the left lobe with suppression of surrounding thyroid parenchyma, features of AFTN.

4. *Graves' disease (GD):* Approximately 75% of patients with thyrotoxicosis have GD as the cause. It is an autoimmune disease caused by a thyrotropin receptor stimulating antibody, which stimulates thyroid follicular cells, resulting in the production of excess thyroid hormone. A thyroid scan shows a high thyroid-to-background ratio. An elevated %RAIU confirms the diagnosis (Figure 21.1e). Thyroid scan shows increased and homogenous tracer uptake in bilaterally enlarged thyroid lobes in the case of GD.

5. *Single autonomously functioning thyroid nodule (AFTN)/toxic adenoma (TA):* Toxic nodules occur in approximately 5% of patients with a palpable nodule. Once an autonomous nodule grows to a size of 2.5–3.0 cm, it may produce the clinical manifestations of thyrotoxicosis. %RAIU may be elevated or more often remain in the normal range. The thyroid scan shows uptake in the nodule but suppression of the remainder of the gland and low background (Figure 21.1f). Thyroid scan shows a single hot nodule in the left lobe with suppression of surrounding thyroid parenchyma, features of AFTN.

6. *Ectopic thyroid:* Embryologically, the thyroglossal duct extends from the foramen cecum at the base of the tongue to the thyroid. Lingual or upper cervical thyroid tissue can present in the neonate or child as a midline mass, often accompanied by hypothyroidism. Ectopic thyroid tissue may occur in the mediastinum or even in the pelvis (struma ovarii). The typical appearance of a lingual thyroid is a focal or nodular accumulation at the base of the tongue and absence of tracer uptake in the expected cervical location. Lateral thyroid rests may be hypofunctional, functional, hyperfunctional, or be the focus of thyroid cancer. Ectopic thyroid tissue should be considered metastatic until proved otherwise (Figure 21.2a–d). Anterior and lateral views show the single focus of increased tracer uptake in the superior aspect of the neck with no evidence of tracer uptake in thyroid bed—suggestive of ectopic thyroid tissue, likely lingual thyroid.

7. *Thyroid nodules:*
   a. *Cold nodule:* Approximately 85% to 90% of thyroid nodules are cold (hypofunctional) on thyroid scans. The incidence of cancer in a cold thyroid nodule is 15% to 20%. The dominant nodule is those that are distinctly larger than the other nodules in a multinodular goiter or those that are enlarging and require further evaluation. Differentials for cold nodule apart from malignancy include benign conditions such as colloid nodule, simple cyst, hemorrhagic cyst, adenoma, and abscess.
   b. *Hot nodule:* Radioiodine uptake in a nodule denotes function. A functioning nodule is very unlikely to be malignant. Less than 1% of hot nodules are reported to harbor malignancy. RAI is the usual therapy for toxic nodules because the radiation is delivered selectively to the hyperfunctioning tissue while sparing suppressed extranodular tissues. The suppressed thyroid tissue results in a low incidence of post-therapy hypothyroidism. After successful treatment, the suppressed tissue regains function. On occasion, surgery may be performed for patients with local symptoms or cosmetic concerns.
   c. *Indeterminate nodule:* When a palpable or sonographically detected nodule >1 cm cannot be differentiated by thyroid scan as definitely "hot or cold" compared to surrounding normal thyroid, it is referred to as an indeterminate nodule. The indeterminate nodule may occur with a posterior nodule that has normal thyroid uptake superimposed anterior to it, making it appear to have normal uptake. For management purposes, an indeterminate nodule has the same significance as a cold nodule.
   d. *Discordant nodule:* Some hot or warm nodules on thyroid scans appear cold on radioiodine scans. This type of observation occurs in only 5% of patients, because some

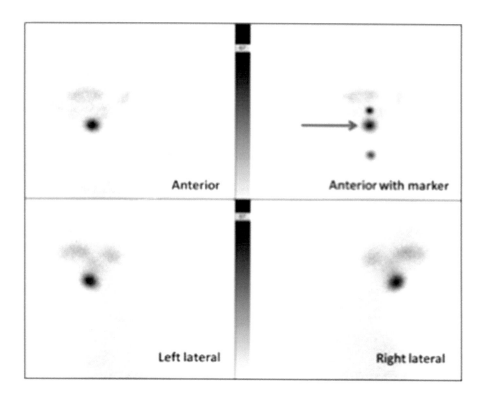

Figure 21.2 (a–d) Anterior and lateral views show a single focus of increased tracer uptake in the superior aspect of the neck with no evidence of tracer uptake in the thyroid bed—suggestive of ectopic thyroid tissue, likely lingual thyroid.

thyroid cancers maintain trapping but not organification. Of discordant nodules, 20% are malignant.

For any thyroid nodule >1 cm in any diameter, a serum TSH level should be initially obtained. If the serum TSH is subnormal, a radionuclide thyroid scan should be obtained to document whether the nodule is hyperfunctioning ("hot," i.e., tracer uptake is higher than the surrounding normal thyroid), isofunctioning ("warm," i.e., tracer uptake is equal to the surrounding thyroid), or nonfunctioning ("cold," i.e., has uptake less than the surrounding thyroid tissue). Hyperfunctioning nodules rarely harbor malignancy, and no cytologic evaluation is necessary. A higher serum TSH level, even within the upper part of the reference range, is associated with increased risk of malignancy in a thyroid nodule, as well as more advanced stage thyroid cancer [11].

131I-WHOLE BODY SCAN (WBS)

Whole body RAI imaging is used in the following situations: (1) total or near-total thyroidectomy prior to ablation of thyroid remnants and treatment of residual disease, (2) in post-therapy imaging, (3) at 6 months follow-up after ablation therapy, (4) as part of surveillance, and (5) in patients with known or suspected metastatic disease. The flowchart in Figure 21.3 depicts the management of thyroid cancer patients post-surgery.

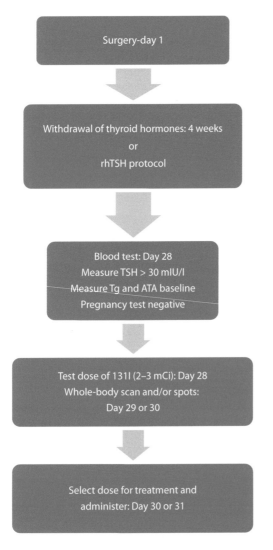

Figure 21.3   Post-surgery management of thyroid cancer patients.

Table 21.2   Drugs and foods that decrease or increase the percentage of radioactive iodine uptake

Increased uptake	Duration of effect
Iodine deficiency	
Lithium, antithyroid drugs	
Decreased uptake	
Thyroid hormones (T4)	2–4 weeks
Mineral supplements, vitamins, cough medications	2–4 weeks
Iodinated skin ointments	2–4 weeks
Iodinated drugs (Amiodarone)	Months
Radiographic contrast media (water-soluble intravascular media)	2–4 weeks
Goitrogenic foods: cabbage, turnips	
Prior radiotherapy to neck	
Antithyroid drugs	
Propylthiouracil (PTU)	3–5 days
Methimazole	5–7 days

PATIENT PREPARATION

The patients are prepared by either of these two methods: (1) withdrawal from thyroid hormone therapy (requires approximately 4–6 weeks of withdrawal from Levothyroxine (T4) replacement therapy, or lack of supplementation altogether after total or subtotal thyroidectomy) or (2) use of recombinant human TSH (rhTSH). Patients should undergo two weeks of low-iodine diet to minimize the amount of iodine in the blood that would compete with the RAI for uptake into thyroid tissue or thyroid cancer, thus increasing the diagnostic and therapeutic efficacy of RAI. Various drugs interfere with RAI uptake and should be avoided, as mentioned previously (refer Table 21.2).

rhTSH (THYROGEN)

Side effects of hypothyroidism (fatigue, depressed mood, cold intolerance, dry skin, increase in weight, constipation, hoarseness, numbness/tingling, and decreased sweating) can be debilitating for many patients, particularly those with other comorbidities. These adverse effects can be avoided with Thyrogen, a recombinant form of TSH (rhTSH), since Thyroxine therapy may be continued. The protocol differs according to centers. However, the most commonly followed protocol is shown in Figure 21.4. Blood clearance of RAI is faster in the euthyroid state favoring a higher target-to-background ratio with the use of rhTSH, since GFR is not affected. According to the recent ATA guidelines, rhTSH mediated therapy may be indicated in selected patients with underlying comorbidities making iatrogenic hypothyroidism potentially risky, in patients with a pituitary disease whose serum TSH cannot be raised, or in patients in whom a delay in therapy might be deleterious [11].

PROTOCOL

Diagnostic WBS is performed after 24–48 hr of 1–3 mCi of RAI. The post-therapy scan is performed preferably after 48–72 hr; few authors recommend scan acquisition 5–7 days after administration of therapy. The scan should extend from the head to the knees or mid-thighs, plus high-count spot views of the neck and chest, using a high-energy collimator. If metastases are suspected, imaging can be done with SPECT/CT, which allows 3D anatomic localization for documentation, future follow-up, and to guide potential surgical or external beam radiation therapy. The uptake in the neck and any other area is calculated from the counts in a region of interest (ROI) drawn over the neck, minus background activity obtained from an ROI over the thigh, divided by the total administered activity. Use of low-activity 131I (1–3 mCi) potentially reduces the negative impact of 131I WBS on RAI therapeutic efficacy for successful remnant

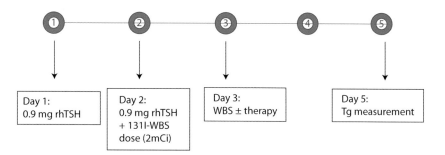

Figure 21.4   The rhTSH protocol.

ablation ("stunning"). Damle et al. concluded that the interval between diagnostic WBS and post-therapy WBS plays a critically important role in causing stunning [12].

Physiological uptake is seen in the nasal area, oropharynx, salivary glands, stomach, intestines, and urinary bladder. Uptake is commonly seen in lactating breasts and must not be confused with lung uptake. Quantification of uptake after thyroidectomy is an indicator of the adequacy of surgery, and follow-up scan uptakes allow the evaluation of therapeutic effectiveness or recurrence. According to the recent ATA guidelines, post-operative diagnostic RAI WBS may be useful when the extent of the thyroid remnant or residual disease cannot be accurately ascertained from the surgical report or neck ultrasonography, and when the results may alter the decision to treat or the activity of RAI that is to be administered. Identification and localization of uptake foci may be improved by concomitant single photon emission computed tomography-computed tomography (SPECT/CT). Also, a post-therapy WBS (with or without SPECT/CT) is recommended after RAI remnant ablation or treatment, for disease staging and document RAI avidity of any structural disease. Approximately 10% of patients show abnormal uptake on the post-therapy scan not seen on the pre-therapy scan, which may alter subsequent therapy [11].

Star artifact: The high therapeutic dose can result in intense uptake in the thyroid bed, which typically has six points of the star caused by septal penetration of the hexagonal collimator holes.

NON-RADIOACTIVE IODINE IMAGING

Non-specific tumor SPECT agents such as 201-Thallium, 123/131I-MIBG, 99mTc-sestamibi, 99mTc-DMSA (V), 111Indium-Octreotide, and PET tracers such as 18F-FDG and 68Gallium-DOTANOC are useful when poorly differentiated, tall-cell variants, or cancers composed of Hurthle cells are present, which are often less RAI avid.

a.   *18F-Fluorodeoxyglucose (FDG) PET imaging:* The recent ATA guidelines strongly recommend 18FDG PET/CT scan to be considered in high-risk DTC patients with elevated serum Tg (generally >10 ng/mL) with negative RAI imaging. 18FDG-PET/CT scanning may also be considered as a part of initial staging in poorly differentiated thyroid cancers and invasive Hurthle cell carcinomas, especially those with other evidence of disease on imaging or because of elevated serum Tg levels. This is a prognostic tool in patients with metastatic disease to identify lesions and patients at highest risk for rapid disease progression and disease-specific mortality, and evaluation of post-treatment response following systemic or local therapy of metastatic or locally invasive disease [11]. In a meta-analysis of 25 studies that included 789 patients, the sensitivity of 18FDG PET/CT

was 83%, and the specificity was 84% in non–131I-avid DTC. Factors influencing 18FDGPET/CT sensitivity included tumor dedifferentiation, larger tumor burden, and TSH stimulation. 18FDG PET/CT may prove more sensitive in picking up lesions located in retropharyngeal or retro-clavicular regions [13].

b.   *68Ga-DOTANOC PET/CT:* 68Ga-DOTANOC PET/CT has an important role in the follow-up of MTC patients, particularly those with high Calcitonin values. It also helps select potential candidates for PRRT therapy [14]. Also, a recent study has shown the correlation between 68Ga positive lesions and Calcitonin levels and between 18F-FDG positivity and CEA levels [15]. Kundu et al. conducted a prospective study evaluating 68Ga-DOTANOC PET/CT in comparison with 18F-FDG PET/CT in DTC patients with raised thyroglobulin and negative 131I-WBS. 68Ga-DOTANOC PET/CT demonstrated disease in 40/62 (65%) patients and 18F-FDG PET/CT in 45/62 (72%) patients, with no significant difference on McNemar analysis (p = 0.226). 68Ga-DOTANOC PET/CT changed management in 21/62 (34%) patients and 18F-FDG PET/CT in 17/62 (27%) patients. The authors concluded that Ga-DOTANOC PET-CT is inferior to 18F-FDG PET/CT on lesion-based but not on patient-based analysis for detection of recurrent/residual disease in DTC patients with negative WBS scan and elevated serum Tg levels, and that it can also help in selection of potential candidates for peptide receptor radionuclide therapy [16]. Another prospective study by Naswa et al. evaluated 68Ga-DOTANOC PET/CT in patients with recurrent medullary thyroid carcinoma and compared with 18F-FDG PET/CT. Their results showed a superior sensitivity for 68Ga-DOTANOC PET/CT compared to 18F-FDG PET/CT (75.61 vs. 63.4%). However, the difference was statistically not significant (p = 0.179) [17].

c.   *Radiolabeled anti-CEA monoclonal antibodies:* Because of the high prevalence of CEA antigen expression on the surface membranes of MTC, imaging with radio-labeled anti-CEA monoclonal antibodies has been investigated [18].

d.   *18F-DOPA and 124I-PET/CT* have also shown to be useful in the detection of recurrence in thyroid cancer [19].

e.   *(I-131 or I-123)-Metaiodobenzylguanidine (MIBG) and C-11 Hydroxyephedrine:* MIBG is similar in structure to norepinephrine, one of the circulating catecholamines and a sympathetic nerve neurotransmitter. Hydroxyephedrine is an analog of ephedrine, a sympathomimetic drug. MIBG and hydroxyephedrine are taken up in APUD-like neuroendocrine cells and their tumors in neurosecretory granules and have proved useful in the diagnosis of MTC. Studies have shown that the MIBG scan has a limited sensitivity of 40%–50%. However, MIBG scan helps in selecting those patients that may respond to therapy with high-dose 131I-MIBG [20–22].

f.   *111Indium-Octreotide imaging:* The overall sensitivity of 111In-octreotide is 82% sensitivity in patients who had no abnormal uptake on I-131 scintigraphy. It can be used as a predictor for the utility of therapeutic octreotide (Sandostatin), high-dose In-111 octreotide for therapy in patients refractory to I-131, or other analogs, such as Y90-labeled somatostatin analogs in octreotide positive patients [23].

g. *99mTc-DMSA (V) in MTC*: Uptake mechanism depends on the flow and phosphate groups on tumor as well as the pH of the medium. 99mTc-DMSA(V) yields a high sensitivity tumor detection rates ranging from 50%–80% in MTC [24].

h. *68Ga-PSMA-HBED-CC PET/CT*: In DTC, MTC, RAI refractory thyroid cancer, and ATC, 68Ga-PSMA-HBED-CC PET/CT is being tried and seems a potential theragnostic agent [25–27].

THERAPY

RAI therapy is most commonly indicated in GD, TMNG, TA, and thyroid cancer.

GRAVES' DISEASE (GD)

- Patients choosing RAI therapy as treatment for GD would likely place relatively higher value on definitive control of hyperthyroidism, the avoidance of surgery, and the potential side effects of ATDs, as well as a relatively lower value on the need for lifelong thyroid hormone replacement, rapid resolution of hyperthyroidism, and potential worsening or development of Graves' ophthalmopathy (GO).

- Absolute contraindications for RAI therapy include pregnancy, lactation, coexisting thyroid cancer, suspicion of thyroid cancer, and individuals unable to comply with radiation safety guidelines and used with informed caution in women planning a pregnancy within 4–6 months.

- Sufficient activity of RAI should be administered in a single application, typically a mean dose of 10–15 mCi (370–555 MBq), to render the patient with GD hypothyroid. A pregnancy test should be obtained within 48 hr before treatment in any woman with childbearing potential who is to be treated with RAI and verify a negative result before administering RAI [11]. Damle et al. evaluated the predictive role of 24 hr RAIU with respect to the outcome of radioiodine therapy in patients with diffuse toxic goiter (DTG). A total of 633 consecutive patients with DTG were given fixed-dose (185 MBq/5 mCi) of radioiodine between January 1987 and December 2006. Of these, 175 patients had an RAIU ≤50% and 458 patients had an RAIU >50%. First-dose success rate in the former group was 81.7% and in the second group 68.6% (p = 0.001). The overall first-dose success was 72%. Multivariate analysis confirmed significant role of 24 hr RAIU data to predict a successful outcome. The authors concluded that 24 hr RAIU value of ≤50% appears to be associated with a significantly better outcome compared to that of a 24 hr RAIU value of >50% in patients with DTG given as treatment a fixed dose of 185 MBq/5 mCi radioiodine [28].

- According to the recent ATA guidelines for the management of hyperthyroidism, the goal of RAI therapy in GD is to control hyperthyroidism by rendering the patient hypothyroid; this treatment is beneficial provided sufficient radiation dose is deposited in the thyroid.

- RAI can be accomplished equally well by either administering a fixed activity or by calculating the activity based on the size of the thyroid and its ability to trap RAI [11]. Jaiswal et al. conducted a prospective study to compare the results of these two approaches in a randomized patient population with 20 patients in each group. Fixed dose group patients were administered 185 MBq of 131I. Calculated dose group patients were given 131I as per the following formula: Calculated

dose = [3700 kBq/g × estimated thyroid weight(g)] ÷ 24 hr RAIU (%). Success of first dose of radioiodine was defined as clinically/biochemically euthyroid/hypothyroid status at the end of 3 months without the need for further therapy. The authors reported that there was no statistically significant difference between the success rates of the two methods at 3 months (the success rate of the first dose was 60% in the fixed group and in calculated dose group it was 65% and hence, the fixed dose approach may be used for treatment of Graves' disease as it is simple and convenient for the patient) [29].

- Follow-up within the first 1–2 months after RAI therapy for GD should include an assessment of T3, T4, and TSH. Biochemical monitoring should be continued at 4–6 week intervals for 6 months, or until the patient becomes hypothyroid and is stable on thyroid hormone replacement.

- When hyperthyroidism due to GD persists after 6 months following RAI therapy, retreatment with RAI is suggested. In selected patients with minimal response 3 months after therapy, additional RAI may be considered [11].

TMNG OR TA

- Overt hyperthyroidism due to TMNG or TA can also be treated with RAI therapy. Advanced patient age, significant comorbidity, prior surgery or scarring in the anterior neck, small goiter size, RAIU sufficient to allow therapy, and lack of access to a high-volume thyroid surgeon (the latter factor is more critical for TMNG than for TA) could be an indication for RAI therapy.

- Absolute contraindications to the use of radioactive iodine include pregnancy, lactation, coexisting thyroid cancer, and individuals unable to comply with radiation safety guidelines and should be used with caution in women planning a pregnancy within 4–6 months.

- Non-functioning nodules on radionuclide scintigraphy or nodules with suspicious ultrasound characteristics should be managed accordingly. TMNG and TA with high nodular RAI uptake and widely suppressed RAI uptake in the peri-nodular thyroid tissue are especially suitable for RAI therapy.

- The goal of therapy is the rapid and durable elimination of the hyperthyroid state. The sufficient activity of RAI should be administered in a single application to alleviate hyperthyroidism in patients with TMNG.

- The activity of RAI used to treat TMNG, calculated based on goiter size to deliver 150–200 μCi (5.55–7.4 MBq) per gram of tissue corrected for 24-hr RAIU, is usually higher than that needed to treat GD. Besides, the RAIU values for TMNG may be lower, necessitating an increase in the applied activity of RAI. Follow-up is similar to GD patients.

- For patients with TMNG who receive RAI therapy, the response is 50%–60% by 3 months, and 80% by 6 months, with an average failure rate of 15%. There is a 75% response rate by 3 months and 89% rate by 1 year following RAI therapy for TA [11].

THYROID CANCER

RAI therapy with I-131 has been a mainstay of thyroid cancer management since its first application was described by Seidlin et al. in 1946 [1]. Initial therapy of thyroid cancer consists of surgical removal of the thyroid gland and the primary tumor, along with the identification and removal of the involved lymph nodes. RAI therapy reduces the rate of cancer recurrence, extends the disease-free interval, and helps to control the inoperable disease. Most patients with metastatic disease can be managed successfully for many years with RAI therapy.

Women of childbearing age receiving RAI therapy should have a negative screening evaluation for pregnancy before RAI administration and avoid pregnancy for 6–12 months after receiving RAI. RAI should not be given to nursing women. Lactating women should have stopped breastfeeding or pumping for at least 3 months. Sperm banking should be considered in men who may receive cumulative RAI activities ≥400 mCi. Gonadal radiation exposure is reduced with proper hydration, frequent micturition to empty the bladder, and avoidance of constipation. Some specialists recommend that men wait 3 months (or one full sperm cycle) to avoid the potential for transient chromosomal abnormalities [11].

There is a wide range of therapeutic options available for the treatment of thyroid cancer—from simple observation to aggressive treatment with emerging biotechnologies—so patients should routinely undergo risk stratification analysis to determine optimal management. There are three approaches to 131I therapy: empiric fixed amounts, therapy determined by the upper limit of blood and body dosimetry, and quantitative tumor or lesional dosimetry. Dosimetric methods are often reserved for patients with distant metastases or unusual situations such as renal insufficiency, children, the elderly, and those with extensive pulmonary metastases. The efficacy of RAI therapy is related to the mean radiation dose delivered to neoplastic foci and also to the radiosensitivity of tumor tissue. The radiosensitivity is higher in patients who are younger, with small metastases from well-differentiated papillary or follicular carcinoma, and with the uptake of RAI but no or low 18FDG uptake. The maximum tolerated radiation absorbed dose (MTRD) is commonly defined as 200 rads (cGy) to the blood. The goal is to use the minimum activity necessary to achieve successful thyroid remnant ablation, particularly for low-risk patients [11].

REMNANT ABLATION

Radioiodine remnant ablation is considered a safe and effective method for eliminating residual thyroid tissue, as well as microscopic disease if at all present in the thyroid bed following thyroidectomy. The rationale is that in the absence of thyroid tissue, serum Tg measurement can be used as an excellent tumor marker. Another consideration is that the presence of significant remnant thyroid tissue makes detection and treatment of nodal or distant metastases difficult. Rarely, microscopic disease in the thyroid bed if not ablated, in the future, could be a source of anaplastic transformation [30].

Typically for remnant ablation, doses of 30 mci are administered as an outpatient procedure. Any patient receiving more than 30 mci needs to be admitted to the therapy ward, according to AERB (Atomic Energy Regulation Board). Generally, higher activities are used for ablation of thyroid remnants when there is aggressive tumor histology such as tall-cell, insular, or columnar-cell PTC variant. RAI remnant ablation is not routinely recommended after thyroidectomy for ATA low-risk DTC patients. Bal et al. conducted a randomized clinical trial to find out the smallest possible effective dose for remnant ablation in cases of DTC, between July 1995 and January 2002. A total of 565 patients were randomized into eight groups according to 131I administered activity, starting at 15 mCi and increasing activity in increments of 5 mCi until 50 mCi. The successful ablation rate in their study was statistically different in patients receiving less than 25 mCi compared with those receiving at least 25 mCi [p = 0.006]. However, there was no significant intergroup difference in outcome among patients receiving 25–50 mCi. The authors concluded that patients receiving at least 25 mCi had three times better chance of getting remnant ablation than patients receiving lesser activity of 131I, and any activity between 25 and 50 mCi appears to be adequate for remnant ablation [31,32]. RAI remnant ablation is not routinely recommended after lobectomy or total thyroidectomy for patients with unifocal papillary microcarcinoma, in the absence of other adverse features, according to the recent ATA guidelines [11]. Radioactive iodine lobar ablation (RAILA), which avoids complications associated with resurgery, is an alternative that has been recently explored in a few international centers. Santra et al. reported comparable long-term outcome in terms of recurrence rate and disease-free survival (RAILA in comparison with remnant ablation after CT) [33]. RAI remnant ablation is not routinely recommended after thyroidectomy for patients with multifocal papillary microcarcinoma in the absence of other adverse features. RAI adjuvant therapy is routinely recommended after total thyroidectomy for ATA high-risk DTC patients; however, it should be considered after total thyroidectomy in ATA intermediate-risk level DTC patients [11]. Ballal et al. conducted a two-arm retrospective cohort study with no radioiodine in Gr-I, and adjuvant RAI therapy was administered in Gr-II patients, and concluded that intermediate-risk surgically ablated patients do not need adjuvant RAI therapy and patients who failed to achieve ablation with first dose of 131I may be dynamically risk stratified as high-risk category and managed aggressively [34] (Figure 21.5).

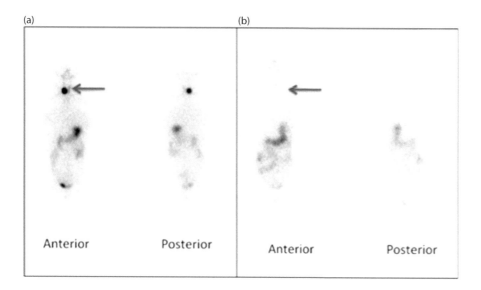

(a)   (b)

Anterior   Posterior   Anterior   Posterior

Figure 21.5   131I-WBS shows post 30 mCi 131-I therapy scan of a papillary thyroid cancer patient who underwent total thyroidectomy with the remnant in the neck (a, red arrow); with the uptake of 3.2%, the 6 months follow-up scan shows a negative WBS with successful remnant ablation (b, red arrow).

TREATMENT OF PULMONARY METASTASES

In the management of the patient with pulmonary metastases, critical criteria for therapeutic decisions include: (1) size of metastatic lesions (macronodular typically detected by chest radiography, micronodular typically detected by CT, lesions beneath the resolution of CT); (2) avidity for RAI and, if applicable, response to prior RAI therapy; and (3) stability (or lack thereof) of metastatic lesions. Pulmonary metastases should be treated with RAI therapy and be repeated every 6–12 months as long as the disease continues to concentrate RAI and respond clinically because the highest rates of complete remission are reported in these subgroups. The selection of RAI activity to administer for pulmonary metastases can be empiric (100–200 mCi, or 100–150 mCi for patients $\geq$70 years old) or estimated by dosimetry to limit whole-body retention to 80 mCi at 48 hours and 200 cGy to the bone marrow. Pulmonary pneumonitis and fibrosis are rare complications of high-dose RAI treatment. Patients with pulmonary micrometastases (<2 mm, generally not seen on anatomic imaging) that are RAI avid have the highest rates of complete remission after treatment with RAI. Significant reduction in serum Tg and the size or rate of growth of metastases or structurally apparent disease is considered a response to RAI therapy. Pulmonary function testing, including the diffusing capacity of the lungs for carbon monoxide, can be markers of pulmonary toxicity. Patients with solitary pulmonary DTC metastases may be considered for surgical resection, although the potential benefit weighed against the risk of surgery is unclear [11]. Chopra et al. suggested that patients with macro-nodular lung metastases and/or concomitant skeletal metastases have reduced odds of achieving remission. The authors also suggested that a significant number of patients recurred even after complete remission with RAI treatment, hence they recommended strict surveillance especially in patients with age >45 years and/or with follicular histology of DTC [35,36].

RAI TREATMENT OF BONE METASTASES

RAI therapy of iodine-avid bone metastases has been associated with improved survival and should be employed, although RAI is rarely curative. The RAI activity administered can be given empirically (100–200 mCi) or determined by dosimetry. Patients undergoing RAI therapy for bone metastases should also be considered for directed therapy of bone metastases that are visible on anatomical imaging. Bone metastases may include surgery, external beam radiation therapy, and other local treatment modalities [11] (Figure 21.6).

Rare sites of metastases include liver, brain, kidney, adrenal glands, breast, inguinal, and axillary lymph nodes [37–43]. Secondary malignancies are also reported in literature associated with thyroid cancer [44].

TREATMENT OF RAI REFRACTORY DISEASE

Radioiodine-refractory structurally evident DTC is classified in patients with appropriate TSH stimulation and iodine preparation in four primary ways: (1) the malignant/metastatic tissue does not ever concentrate RAI (no uptake outside the thyroid bed at the first therapeutic WBS), (2) the tumor tissue loses the ability to concentrate RAI after previous evidence of RAI-avid disease (in the absence of stable iodine contamination), (3) RAI is concentrated in some lesions but not in others; and, (4) metastatic disease progresses despite significant concentration of RAI.

When a patient with DTC is classified as refractory to RAI, there is no indication for further RAI treatment. Kinase inhibitor therapy (sorafenib, lenvatinib, vandetanib) should be considered in RAI-refractory DTC patients with metastatic, rapidly progressive, symptomatic, and/or imminently threatening disease not otherwise amenable to local control using other approaches. Patients who are candidates for kinase inhibitor therapy should be thoroughly counseled on the potential risks and benefits of this therapy as well as alternative therapeutic approaches, including best supportive care [11] (Figure 21.7).

SIDE EFFECTS AND COMPLICATIONS OF RAI THERAPY

Although generally safe, RAI therapy has some potential side effects, classified as early and late complications [45]. The early complications include gastrointestinal symptoms, radiation thyroiditis, sialadenitis/xerostomia, bone marrow

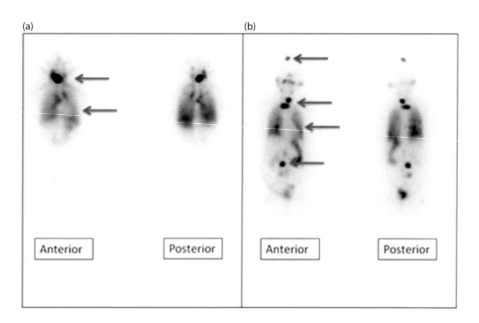

Figure 21.6 131I-WBS anterior and posterior views show increased tracer uptake in the remnant, cervical lymph nodes, and bilateral lungs (a, red arrows). 131I-WBS anterior and posterior views show increased tracer uptake in the remnant, cervical lymph nodes, bilateral lungs, and few skeletal sites (skull, thoracic and lumbar vertebrae) (b, red arrows).

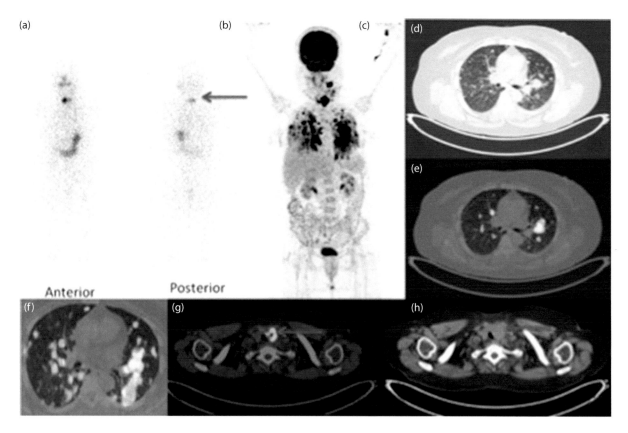

Figure 21.7 131I-WBS (anterior and posterior, a and b) shows mild tracer uptake in remnant in the thyroid bed (red arrow). However, the patient had a Tg level of 3,040 ng/mL. Hence patient was diagnosed with radioactive refractory disease, and 18FDG PET/CT was advised. Images (c–f) showed multiple soft tissue nodules with increased tracer uptake in bilateral lung fields. Images g and h (red arrows) show local recurrence in the left thyroid bed.

suppression, gonadal damage, dry eye, and nasolacrimal duct obstruction.

The late complications include secondary cancers, pulmonary fibrosis, permanent bone marrow suppression, and genetic effects. Proper hydration optimizes renal excretion of I-131, thus minimizing radiation exposure. Patients are also advised to use lemon-flavored lozenges to promote salivary flow, thus reducing exposure to the glands [46].

NON-RAI RADIOTRACER THERAPY

111In-octreotide therapy, 90Y-DOTATATE therapy, 131I-MIBG therapy, 177Lu-PRRT, and 177Lu-PSMA have also been tried in non-RAI thyroid cancer [47–50].

- TSH elevation is achieved by withdrawing Levothyroxine or injection of rhTSH.
- Residual thyroid tissues can be ablated with 131I.
- 131I is not beneficial in a patient with a T1–T2 tumor that has been thoroughly excised.
- Follow-up of patients is done with 131I-WBS and Tg measurement.
- When the radioiodine scan is negative and Tg positive, it is termed Thyroglobulin Elevated Negative Iodine Scan (TENIS); management includes use of empirical high dose therapy (100–200 mCi). Alternatively, the site of cancer can be identified by 18FDG PET/CT and treated by surgery or external radiation therapy.
- RAI is generally safe, but has a few early and late complications.

SALIENT POINTS

- RAIU study with 131-I and thyroid scan with 99mTc-pertechnetate are the two most common diagnostic investigations. The most common indications include Graves' disease, TA, TMNG, AFTN, and in the evaluation of ectopic thyroid.
- RAI therapy is most commonly indicated in GD, TMNG, TA, and thyroid cancer.
- Post-operatively 131I is used for a diagnostic whole-body scan to determine how much residual tissue or functioning metastasis is present.
- The patient should have elevated TSH (>30 μIU/mL) when a diagnostic scan or treatment with 131I is undertaken.

REFERENCES

1. Fermi E. Radioactivity induced by neutron bombardment. *Nature.* 1934;133:757.

2. Chapman E. History of the discovery and early use of radioactive iodine. *JAMA.* 1983;250:2042.

3. Hertz S, Roberts A, Evans RD. Radioactive iodine as an indicator in the study of thyroid physiology. *Proc Soc Exp Biol Med.* 1983;38:510–14.

4. Ernest LO. The medical cyclotron of the crocker radiation laboratory. *Science.* 1939;90:407.

5. Riggs DS. Iodine metabolism in man. *Pharmacol Rev.* 1952;4:285.

6. Chapman EM et al. The collection of radioactive iodine by the human fetal thyroid. *J Clin Endocrinol.* 1984;8:717.

7. Berson SA et al. The determination of thyroidal and renal plasma I-131 clearance rates as a routine diagnostic test of thyroid dysfunction. *J Clin Invest.* 1952;31:141.

8. Ballal S, Soundararajan R, Bal C. Re-establishment of normal radioactive iodine uptake reference range in the era of universal salt iodization in the Indian population. *Indian J Med Res.* 2017;145(3):358–64.

9. Balon RH et al. *Procedure guideline for Thyroid Scintigraphy V3.0.* Society of Nuclear Medicine Procedure Guidelines Manual, 2006.

10. Ziessman HA, O'Malley JP, Thrall JH. Endocrine system. In: Fahey FH (ed.) *Nuclear Medicine: The Requisites,* 4th edn. Elsevier Saunders, Philadelphia, PA, 2013, pp. 66–90.

11. Haugen BR et al. American Thyroid Association Management Guidelines for adult patients with thyroid nodules and differentiated thyroid cancer: The American Thyroid Association Guidelines Taskforce on thyroid nodules and differentiated thyroid cancer. *Thyroid.* 2016 Jan;26(1):1–133.

12. Damle NA, Bal C, Ballal S. Stunning in post (131)I therapy scans after low-dose (131)I diagnostic whole body scans with differentiated thyroid cancer in the Indian patient population: Critical importance of interval between the two scans. *Indian J Endocrinol Metab.* 2012 May;16(3):477–8.

13. Leboulleux S, Schroeder PR, Schlumberger M, Ladenson PW. The role of PET in the follow-up of patients treated for differentiated epithelial thyroid cancers. *Nat Clin Pract Endocrinol Metab.* 2007;3:112–21.

14. Couto J et al. 68 Ga DOTANOC PET CT role in the follow up of patients with medullary thyroid carcinoma. *Endocrine Abstracts.* 2013;32:P1089.

15. Souteiro P et al. 68Ga-DOTANOC and FDG PET/CT in metastatic medullary thyroid carcinoma: Novel correlations with tumoral biomarkers. *Endocrine.* 2019 May; 64(2): 322–9.

16. Kundu P, Lata S, Sharma P, Singh H, Malhotra A, Bal C. Prospective evaluation of (68) Ga-DOTANOC PET-CT in differentiated thyroid cancer patients with raised thyroglobulin and negative (131)I-whole body scan: Comparison with (18)F-FDG PET-CT. *Eur J Nucl Med Mol Imaging.* 2014 Jul;41(7):1354–62.

17. Naswa N, Sharma P, Suman Kc S, Lata S, Kumar R, Malhotra A, Bal C. Prospective evaluation of 68Ga-DOTA-NOC PET-CT in patients with recurrent medullary thyroid carcinoma: Comparison with 18F-FDG PET/CT. *Nucl Med Commun.* 2012 Jul;33(7):766–74.

18. Edington HD et al. Radioimmunoimaging of metastatic medullary carcinoma of the thyroid gland using an indium-111-labeled monoclonal antibody to CEA. *Surgery.* 1988;104:1004–11.

19. Verbeek HH et al. Clinical relevance of 18F-FDG PET and 18F-DOPA PET in recurrent medullary thyroid carcinoma. *J Nucl Med.* 2012;53:1863–71.

20. Endo K et al. Imaging of medullary thyroid cancer with I-131 MIBG. *Lancet.* 1984;2:233.

21. Hoefnagel CA et al. Radionuclide diagnosis and therapy of neural crest tumors using iodine-131 meta-iodobenzylguanidine. *J Nucl Med.* 1987;28:308–14.

22. Ohta H, Yamamoto K, Endo K. A new imaging agent for medullary carcinoma of the thyroid. *J Nucl Med.* 1984;25:323–25.

23. Krenning EP et al. Somatostatin receptor scintigraphy with In-111- DTPA-D-Phe1- and I-123-Tyr3-octreotide: The Rotterdam experience with more than 1000 patients. *Eur J Nucl Med.* 1993;20:716–31.

24. Bozkurt MF, Ugur O, Banti E, Grassetto G, Rubello D. Functional nuclear medicine imaging of medullary thyroid cancer. *Nucl Med Commun.* 2008 Nov;29(11):934–42.

25. Taywade SK, Damle NA, Bal C. PSMA expression in papillary thyroid carcinoma: Opening a new horizon in management of thyroid cancer? *Clin Nucl Med.* 2016 May;41(5):e263–5.

26. Arora S, Prabhu M, Damle NA, Bal C, Kumar P, Nalla H, Arun Raj ST. Prostate-specific membrane antigen imaging in recurrent medullary thyroid cancer: A new theranostic tracer in the offing? *Indian J Nucl Med.* 2018 Jul–Sep;33(3):261–3.

27. Damle NA, Bal C, Singh TP, Gupta R, Reddy S, Kumar R, Tripathi M. Anaplastic thyroid carcinoma on 68 Ga-PSMA PET/CT: Opening new frontiers. *Eur J Nucl Med Mol Imaging.* 2018 Apr;45(4):667–8.

28. Damle N, Bal C, Kumar P, Reddy R, Virkar D. The predictive role of 24 h RAIU with respect to the outcome of low fixed dose radioiodine therapy in patients with diffuse toxic goiter. *Hormones (Athens).* 2012 Oct–Dec;11(4):451–7.

29. Jaiswal AK, Bal C, Damle NA, Ballal S, Goswami R, Hari S, Kumar P. Comparison of clinical outcome after a fixed dose versus dosimetry-based radioiodine treatment of Graves' disease: Results of a randomized controlled trial in Indian population. *Indian J Endocrinol Metab.* 2014 Sep;18(5):648–54.

30. Bal CS, Padhy AK. Radioiodine remnant ablation: A critical review. *World J Nucl Med.* 2015 Sep–Dec;14(3):144–55.

31. Bal CS, Kumar A, Pant GS. Radioiodine dose for remnant ablation in differentiated thyroid carcinoma: A randomized clinical trial in 509 patients. *J Clin Endocrinol Metab.* 2004 Apr;89(4):1666–73.

32. Bal C, Ballal S, Soundararajan R, Chopra S, Garg A. Radioiodine remnant ablation in low-risk differentiated thyroid cancer patients who had R0 dissection is an over treatment. *Cancer Med.* 2015 Jul;4(7):1031–8.

33. Santra A, Bal S, Mahargan S, Bal C. Long-term outcome of lobar ablation versus completion thyroidectomy in differentiated thyroid cancer. *Nucl Med Commun.* 2011 Jan;32(1):52–8.

34. Ballal S, Soundararajan R, Garg A, Chopra S, Bal C. Intermediate-risk differentiated thyroid carcinoma patients who were surgically ablated do not need adjuvant radioiodine therapy: Long-term outcome study. *Clin Endocrinol (Oxf).* 2016 Mar;84(3):408–16.

35. Chopra S, Garg A, Ballal S, Bal CS. Lung metastases from differentiated thyroid carcinoma: Prognostic factors related to remission and disease-free survival. *Clin Endocrinol (Oxf).* 2015 Mar;82(3):445–52.

36. Bal CS, Kumar A, Chandra P, Dwivedi SN, Mukhopadhyaya S. Is chest x-ray or high-resolution computed tomography scan of the chest sufficient investigation to detect pulmonary metastasis in pediatric differentiated thyroid cancer? *Thyroid.* 2004 Mar;14(3):217–25.

37. Jain TK, Karunanithi S, Sharma P, Vijay MK, Ballal S, Bal C. Asymptomatic solitary cerebral metastasis from papillary carcinoma thyroid: 131I SPECT/CT for accurate staging. *Clin Nucl Med.* 2014 Nov;39(11):977–9.

38. Brient C, Mucci S, Taïeb D, Mathonnet M, Menegaux F, Mirallié E, Meyer P, Sebag F, Triponez F, Hamy A. Differentiated thyroid cancer with liver metastases: Lessons learned from managing a series of 14 patients. *Int Surg.* 2015 Mar;100(3):490–6.

39. Damle N, Singh H, Soundararajan R, Bal C, Sahoo M, Mathur S. Radioiodine avid axillary lymph node metastasis in papillary thyroid cancer: Report of a case. *Indian J Surg Oncol.* 2011 Sep;2(3):193–6.

40. Damle N, Kumar P, Maharjan S, Mathur S, Bal C. Inguinal node metastasis from follicular thyroid cancer. *Indian J Endocrinol Metab.* 2013 Mar;17(2):353–4.

41. Kumar A, Nadig M, Patra V, Srivastava DN, Verma K, Bal CS. Adrenal and renal metastases from follicular thyroid cancer. *Br J Radiol.* 2005 Nov;78(935):1038–41.

42. Biswal BM, Bal CS, Sandhu MS, Padhy AK, Rath GK. Management of intracranial metastases of differentiated carcinoma of thyroid. *J Neurooncol.* 1994;22(1):77–81.

43. Chawla M, Bal CS. Four cases of coexistent thyrotoxicosis and jaundice: Results of radioiodine treatment and a brief review. *Thyroid.* 2008 Mar;18(3):289–92.

44. Okere PC, Olusina DB, Shamim SA, Shandra V, Tushar M, Sellam K, Bal C. Pattern of second primary malignancies in thyroid cancer patients. *Niger J Clin Pract.* 2013 Jan–Mar;16(1):96–9.

45. Pant GS, Sharma SK, Bal CS, Kumar R, Rath GK. Radiation dose to family members of hyperthyroidism and thyroid cancer patients treated with 131I. *RadiatProt Dosimetry.* 2006;118(1):22–7.

46. Fard-Esfahani A, Emami-Ardekani A, Fallahi B, Fard-Esfahani P, Beiki D, Hassanzadeh-Rad A, Eftekhari M. Adverse effects of radioactive iodine-131 treatment for differentiated thyroid carcinoma. *Nucl Med Commun.* 2014 Aug;35(8):808–17.

47. Zlock DW, Greenspan FS, Clark OH, Higgins CB. Octreotide therapy in advanced thyroid cancer. *Thyroid.* 1994 Winter;4(4):427–31.

48. Stokkel MP, Verkooijen RB, Bouwsma H, Smit JW. Six-month follow-up after 111In-DTPA-octreotide therapy in patients with progressive radioiodine non-responsive thyroid cancer: A pilot study. *Nucl Med Commun.* 2004 Jul;25(7):683–90.

49. Budiawan H, Salavati A, Kulkarni HR, Baum RP. Peptide receptor radionuclide therapy of treatment-refractory metastatic thyroid cancer using (90)Yttrium and (177) Lutetium labeled somatostatin analogs: Toxicity, response, and survival analysis. *Am J Nucl Med Mol Imaging.* 2013 Dec;4(1):39–52.

50. Hoefnagel CA, Delprat CC, Valdés Olmos RA. Role of [131I] metaiodobenzylguanidine therapy in medullary thyroid carcinoma. *J NuclBiol Med.* 1991 Oct–Dec;35(4):334–6.

Chapter 22

SYSTEMIC THERAPY (TARGETED THERAPY AND IMMUNOTHERAPY) FOR THYROID CANCERS

Abhishek Vaidya and Amol Dongre

CONTENTS

Introduction 173
Molecular Pathogenesis: Genetic Changes and Altered Signaling Pathways 173
Targeted Therapy in Thyroid Cancer 174
Conclusion 176
References 176

INTRODUCTION

The incidence of thyroid cancer is increasing worldwide [1,2]. On the basis of their degree of differentiation, thyroid cancers derived from follicular cells are classified as differentiated thyroid cancers (DTC), poorly differentiated thyroid cancers (PDTC), and anaplastic thyroid cancers (ATC) [3]. DTCs account for 93% of all thyroid cancers [4]. Medullary thyroid carcinomas (MTC) are derived from parafollicular C cells, and account for about 3%–5% of thyroid cancers [5]. Most DTCs (including papillary thyroid cancers and follicular thyroid cancers) are well behaved and have an excellent survival prognosis [6]. The usual treatment for these cancers is surgery (lobectomy or total thyroidectomy), with or without radioiodine (RAI) therapy. However, a small subset (<10%) of DTCs, many MTCs and PDTCs, and most ATCs are not cured by standard treatment [7]. When grouped together, these "aggressive/advanced thyroid cancers" have a 5-year survival rate in less than 50%, in stark contrast to the >90% 20-year survival rates for DTCs [7]. ATCs account for <2% of all thyroid cancers, but are the most aggressive, accounting for about 50% of all thyroid cancer mortality [8]. It is in this subset of aggressive and advanced thyroid cancers that systemic therapy, primarily in the form of targeted therapy and immunotherapy, has a role to play.

There has been a greater understanding of molecular pathogenesis underlying thyroid cancers in recent years. Better elucidation of thyroid cancer molecular genesis has opened vistas for possible use of targeted therapy in thyroid cancers.

This chapter briefly looks at molecular pathogenesis of thyroid cancers and then focuses on targeted therapy and immunotherapy for these cancers.

MOLECULAR PATHOGENESIS: GENETIC CHANGES AND ALTERED SIGNALING PATHWAYS

A large body of research in recent years has led to the identification of specific genetic changes and putative molecular pathways involved in thyroid cancers [9]. More recently, the results from the Thyroid Cancer Genome Atlas (TCGA) gave a comprehensive analysis of papillary thyroid cancers (PTC) using next generation sequencing (NGS), which has led to the identification of specific abnormalities of founder significance in most analyzed tumors [10].

The carcinogenesis in thyroid cancers is closely associated with the activation of various tyrosine cascades and inactivation of tumor suppressor genes, including BRAF phosphatidylinositol-4,5-bisphosphate 3-kinase (PI3 K) catalytic subunit α (PIK3CA), tumor protein 53 (tp53) mutations, and telomerase reverse transcriptase (TERT) mutation [11]. These pathways may exert their effects individually or in association with each other through an extensive cross talk.

BRAF MUTATIONS AND MITOGEN-ACTIVATED PROTEIN KINASE (MAPK) PATHWAY

BRAF is the most studied and the most common gene mutation having an important role in thyroid carcinogenesis. It is a serine-threonine kinase, belonging to the family of RAF proteins, and is an intracellular mediator of the MAPK pathway. The most common BRAF mutation is $BRAF^{V600E}$ (amino acid substitution), which constitutively activates the serine-threonine kinase, thus upregulating the MAPK pathway [9]. This involves the sequential activation of MEK and ERK. The activated MAPK pathway plays a role in cell growth, proliferation, differentiation, and carcinogenesis. As stated, BRAF strongly activates this pathway. The resulting intracellular events then upregulate tumor-promoting genes and downregulate tumor-suppressing genes. Thus, BRAF mutation and activation of the MAPK pathway have an important role in thyroid cancers, especially papillary cancers [9]. $BRAF^{V600F}$ mutation is seen in about 45% of PTCs [12].

RAS MUTATIONS AND PHOSPHATIDYL INOSITOL 3 KINASE-AKT (PI3K-AKT)/MTOR PATHWAY

RAS mutations are the second most common in thyroid cancers. In its normal state, RAS is bound to GTP, and converts GTP to inactive GDP by its intrinsic GTPase activity. A mutated RAS loses its GTPase activity, thus constitutively activating GTP. RAS activates the PI3 K pathway preferentially [12]. PI3 K pathway plays a key role in cell growth, proliferation, and survival [11]. As stated, the PI3 K pathway is upregulated via RAS, and also by binding of its p85 subunit to activated tyrosine residues on activated growth factor receptors, thus showing a cross talk with the receptor tyrosine kinase (RTK) pathway. mTOR is a regulatory protein of the PI3 K/AKT/mTOR pathway and its activation results in the transcription and translation of critical growth genes [13]. The PI3K AKT pathway has a predominant role in follicular neoplasms including follicular thyroid carcinoma (FTC) [9,12].

KINASE SIGNALING ACTIVATION

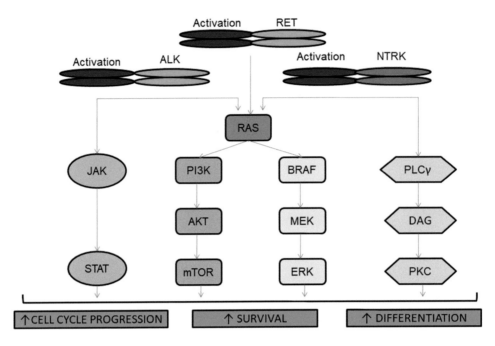

Figure 22.1   A schematic representation of molecular pathways and genetic changes underlying thyroid cancers.

RET-PTC REARRANGEMENT

RET is a proto-oncogene that encodes a cell membrane receptor tyrosine kinase (RTK). RET is highly expressed in parafollicular C cells. It is not usually expressed in follicular cells, but may be activated here by chromosomal rearrangement: the RET/PTC translocation. This translocation constitutively activates tyrosine kinase activity of RET. RET-PTC activates both the MAPK and PI3-AKT pathways [9,12]. The most common subtypes of this translocation are RET/PTC1 and RET/PTC3 [9,12,14]. RET/PTC induced carcinogenesis is mediated in part by an epidermal growth factor receptor (EGFR), and thus may be an attractive therapeutic target for tyrosine kinase inhibitors (TKI) [15].

PAX8-PPAR-γ REARRANGEMENT

Another genetic translocation involved in thyroid carcinogenesis is PAX8-PPAR-γ. This translocation leads to the fusion between the PAX8 gene and the peroxisome proliferator–activated receptor (PPAR-γ) gene. PAX8–PPAR-γ has an inactivating effect on the wild-type tumor suppressor PPAR-γ and transactivates certain PAX8-responsive genes [16]. This translocation occurs in about 40%–60% of FTC [12].

TELOMERASE REVERSE TRANSCRIPTASE (TERT) PROMOTER GENE MUTATIONS

TER promoter gene mutation is an important recent discovery in thyroid carcinogenesis. Activation of TERT promoter gene results in cells acquiring telomerase activity, thus avoiding cell death. TERT is found to be overexpressed in DTCs [7]. About 11% of FTC and 16%–40% of PTC (frequently in association to B-RAF mutations) were found to bear TERT mutations [17]. Coexistence of TERT with BRAF mutation was found to have the worst prognosis for DTC patients [18].

ANAPLASTIC LYMPHOMA KINASE (ALK)

The ALK gene may undergo either activating mutations or gene rearrangements, leading to its activation. Activating ALK, either in the form of ALK mutants and ALK fusion proteins, promote the activation of MAPK, PI3 K, and JAK/STAT downstream pathways.

ALK mutations and rearrangements are mainly found in PDTCs and ATCs, and they lead to disease progression and aggression [19,20].

The molecular pathways and genetic changes of thyroid cancer are illustrated in Figure 22.1.

TARGETED THERAPY IN THYROID CANCER

MULTI-KINASE INHIBITORS (MKI)/TYROSINE KINASE INHIBITORS (TKI)

The MAPK pathway is one of the most studied pathways in thyroid cancer. Data from TCGA has shown that PTC is MAPK driven, with the two potent activators being BRAF^{V600E} and mutated RAS.

Several tyrosine kinase inhibitors and multi-kinase inhibitors have been tried in advanced, RAI-refractory DTCs and MTCs, with promising results. For ATC, the results are varied, with a few drugs being promising. As of now, the FDA has approved four drugs targeting the MAPK pathway for treatment of advanced thyroid cancers [7,21]. These are: lenvatinib and sorafenib (for advanced, RAI-refractory, recurrent DTCs); and vandetanib and cabozantinib (for MTCs).

SORAFENIB

This MKI targets VEGFR 1–3, PDGFR, RET, RAF, and c-kit [22]. In its initial single arm phase II trial for advanced RAI-refractory thyroid cancers, sorafenib yielded a median progression free survival (PFS) of 18 months [23]. This was followed by a phase III, multicenter, randomized, placebo-controlled trial (DECISION trial). This trial enrolled 417 patients of advanced RAI-refractory thyroid cancers, and showed a significantly better PFS in the treatment group (sorafenib 400 mg orally BD) as compared to placebo controls (10.8 months vs 5.8 months; HR 0.59; p < 0.0001) [24]. However, there was no benefit in overall survival; further toxicity was seen in more than 60% of patients. Nevertheless, sorafenib received FDA approval for the treatment of advanced RAI-refractory thyroid cancers. Sorafenib has also been tried in

ATC and MTC. In ATC, in a study of 20 patients, partial response (PR) was achieved in two patients, while five had stable disease (SD) [25]. In a study of 16 advanced MCTs, sorafenib induced PR in one and SD in 14 [26].

LENVATINIB

This MKI targets and also inhibits several targets, namely VEGFR 1–3, FGFR 1–4, PDGFR, RET, and c-kit [27]. It showed promising activity in an initial phase II single arm trial of 58 treatment naïve or re-treated advanced RAI-refractory thyroid cancers [28]. This was followed by a phase III, randomized, placebo-controlled trial (SELECT trial). This trial randomized 261 patients to either receive lenvatinib (24 mg per day in 28-day cycles) or a placebo. There was significantly better PFS in the treatment arm (18.3 months vs. 3.6 months; HR 0.21; $p < 0.0001$). The response rate was promising at 64%, with four patients achieving complete response. The discontinuation rate due to toxicity was 14% [29]. Subsequently, lenvatinib was approved by the FDA for treatment of advanced RAI-refractory thyroid cancers. Owing to its better efficacy and safety profile, lenvatinib is currently regarded as the first line MKI in treatment of such thyroid cancers [30].

VANDETANIB

This MKI has been primarily researched in advanced MTCs. It targets RET, VEGFR, EGFR, and c-kit. Its efficacy was first demonstrated in a phase II trial of 30 advanced or metastatic hereditary MTCs. In this study, PR was achieved in 22 patients at a dose of vandetanib 300 mg per day [31]. This was followed by a phase III, randomized, placebo-controlled trial (ZETA trial). This trial included 331 patients with advanced MTC and showed a significantly better PFS with vandetanib as compared to the placebo group (30.5 months vs 19.3 months; HR 0.46; $p = 0.001$) [32]. The side effect profile included diarrhea, rash, nausea, and a rare but critical adverse effect in form of QT prolongation, potentially leading to *torsades de pointes* [32]. Subsequently, vandetanib became the first FDA-approved drug for treatment of unresectable, locally advanced or metastatic MTC. Although not approved for RAI-refractory DTC, vandetanib has been tested in a phase II randomized trial in this group of patients. Here it was found to have a good efficacy with an improvement in PFS in those receiving the drug over the placebo group (median PFS 11.1 months vs 5.9 months; HR 0.63; $p = 0.008$) [33]. Vandetanib is currently being studied in a phase III, randomized trial of 238 patients with advanced RAI-refractory thyroid cancers (VERIFY trial, NCT01876784). The results of this trial are being awaited at the time of writing this chapter.

CABOZANTINIB

This is a multi-inhibitor of MET, VEGF-2, and RET. The efficacy of cabozantinib was initially shown in a phase I study of 37 heavily pre-treated MTC patients [34]. This led to a phase III, randomized, placebo-controlled trial of advanced MTCs (EXAM trial), in which subjects were randomized to receive either cabozantinib (140 mg daily) or a placebo. This trial showed a significantly better PFS in the treatment arm (11.2 months vs 4 months, HR 0.28, $p < 0.001$) [35]. However, there was no benefit of overall survival between groups. In 2012, cabozantinib was approved by the FDA for treatment of advanced MTCs [36].

Cabozantinib has also been tested as a salvage therapy in RAI-resistant DTCs progressing on VEGFR inhibitors. In a phase II trial of 25 such patients, cabozantinib led to 40% overall response rate (ORR), and a 92% disease control rate [37].

Several other multi-kinase inhibitors have been evaluated in different studies for thyroid cancer. A brief synopsis of these is given in Table 22.1.

Table 22.1 A brief synopsis of MKIs (other than the four FDA approved) for thyroid cancers [7]

MKI drug	Target	Study phase	Patients	Partial response (%)	PFS (months)
Sunitinib	PDGFR, FLT3, c-kit, VEGFR, RET	II	35	31	12.8
Axitinib	VEGFR, PDGFR	II	60	30	18.1
Motesanib	VEGFR, PDGFR, c-kit	II	93	14	9.3
Pazopanib	VEGFR, PDGFR, c-kit	II	37	49	11.7
Dovitinib	FGFR, VEGFR	II	40	20.5	5.4
Imatinib	PDGFR, BCR-ABL, c-kit, RET	II	15	0	NA
Selumetinib	MEK, RAS, BRAFV600E	II	39	3	8

SINGLE/SELECTIVE INHIBITORS

MKIs form the most accepted and studied targeted therapy for advanced thyroid cancers. However, certain single target inhibitors or selective inhibitors may also be efficacious in certain cases. Several trials have investigated the role of single target inhibitors; however, without a predictive biomarker, their applicability and results are limited [11].

BRAF INHIBITOR

Vemurafenib is a selective BRAF inhibitor, which has shown encouraging efficacy in a phase II trial including 51 cases of advanced RAI-refractory PTC displaying BRAF[V600E]. The study population consisted of two as per prior treatment with an anti-VEGFR. Amongst TKI-untreated patients, 10 out of 26 (38.5%) achieved a PR, whereas nine patients (35%) achieved a SD for six months or longer, with a median PFS of 18.2 months. In the TKI-treated group, six of the 22 evaluable patients (27%) experienced a PR, while the other six had SD for at least six months, with a median PFS of 8.9 months. A further study is ongoing.

BRAF AND MEK INHIBITORS

It may be an effective strategy to combine a BRAF inhibitor (dabrafenib) with a MEK inhibitor (trametinib) in advanced thyroid cancers. A phase II trial recruiting 16 pre-treated ATC patients reported 69% ORR, including a CR. This, along with about 90% rate of ongoing responses at 12 months, represents unprecedented results for this aggressive disease. Clinical trials employing dabrafenib in combination with trametinib or lapatinib are ongoing.

SELUMETINIB

This drug targets MAP kinases MEK-1 and 2. It was found to reverse the RAI refractory state in 8 of 20 patients with metastatic thyroid cancer, as assessed by 124I-PET. Selumetinib-treated patients subsequently received RAI achieving PR (n = 5) or SD (n = 3) after the radio-metabolic treatment. Further, NRAS mutation seems to be a predictive biomarker of selumetinib efficacy. Research is underway evaluating this molecule.

ALK INHIBITORS

Owing to their role in carcinogenesis, ALK inhibitors find a role in several solid cancers. ALK inhibitors currently include first generation (crizotinib) or second-generation (ceritinib, alectinib, and brigatinib) inhibitors. There are also immunotherapeutic drugs directed against activated ALK.

Ceritinib: This is a second-generation ALK inhibitor that overcomes secondary resistance due to acquired ALK mutations or amplification or activation of alternative ALK-independent survival pathways (such as EGF, IGF, RAS/SRC, and AKT/mTOR signaling pathways). However, in a study, ceritinib had limited efficacy in ATC patients with the ALKL1198F mutation in full-length ALK or the EML4-ALK fusion protein. An additional trial is currently evaluating this drug in patients harboring ALK mutations or fusions (NCT02289144).

Crizotinib: This is a second generation TKI targeting ALK, MET, and ROS1. It has been extensively researched in ALK-fusion-positive. There is an anecdotal report of one ALK-translocated ATC patient treated with crizotinib achieving a PR. Recently, in a phase Ib study (PROFILE 1013; NCT01121588), which enrolled 44 ALK-positive metastatic patients, one patient with advanced MTC achieved a PR. However, its utility is restricted by very limited data.

PI3 K/AKT/mTOR PATHWAY INHIBITORS

Thyroid carcinogenesis has a prominent role of activation of the PI3 K/AKT/mTOR pathway. Research has shown that targeting this pathway may be an attractive proposal for patients with advanced RAIR DTCs and MTCs. Several trials have researched mTOR inhibitors in thyroid cancer.

Buparlisib: This is a class I PI3 K inhibitor. It failed to show a significant PFS benefit in 43 advanced, RAI-resistant DTCs. Though there was a reduction in tumor growth, there was no objective response, and 48.8% of patients had progressed at six months. The decrease in tumor growth may be due to an incomplete inhibition of the PI3 K oncogenic pathway.

Everolimus: This mTOR inhibitor was tested in a phase II trial of 38 patients with advanced RAI-resistant DTC. There was a median PFS of 47 weeks. Two further phase II studies analyzed everolimus safety and efficacy on seven subjects with MTC, 28 patients with metastatic or locally advanced DTC, and seven individuals with ATC. Five patients (71.4%) showed SD, and 4 (57.1%) had an SD lasting >24 weeks. A further phase II trial evaluated everolimus efficacy in patients with RAI-resistant thyroid cancer and correlated tumor mutational profiling with response. Median PFS were 12.9, 13.1, and 2.2 for DTC, MTC, and ATC cohorts, respectively, and patients with mutations in the PI3 K pathway appeared to benefit most from drug treatment.

Sirolimus: A retrospective study reported that this drug combined with cyclophosphamide generated PFS rates comparable to the standard of care for RAI-refractory DTC. One-year PFS probability was 0.45 in the sirolimus plus cyclophosphamide cohort and 0.30 in the control population.

IMMUNOTHERAPY

Many malignancies are often associated with suppression of the immune response. The malignant cells that survive the immune system surveillance may have an over-expression of programmed death-ligand 1 and 2 (PD-L1/2), which in turn binds to its receptor, programmed cell death protein 1 (PD-1), on T-cells. This causes a weakened T-cell immune response. PD-L1 is expressed in DTC and ATC and may even be a prognostic marker in ATC. Subsequent to the successful application of immunotherapy in melanoma and other solid tumors leading to FDA approval of several immunotherapies, this approach is also being tried in thyroid cancer. A phase I basket trial (NCT02054806) with pembrolizumab, an anti-PD1 drug, included a small group of DTC patients, where two of 22 (9%) patients achieved a PR to pembrolizumab monotherapy. Spartalizumab, an anti-PD1 drug, was studied in an expansion trial in ATC patients. Of 30 evaluated patients, five (17%) achieved a PR.

Studies involving combination targeted therapy with immunotherapy are underway. One study combining lenvatinib and pembrolizumab is being carried out by the International Thyroid Oncology Group (NCT02973997). Combination immunotherapy with nivolumab (anti-PD-1) plus ipilimumab (inhibitor of cytotoxic T lymphocyte A4, CTLA4) for all types of thyroid cancer is currently under investigation (NCT03246958).

Another phase II study is enrolling ATC and PDTC patients to various targeted therapies in combination with atezolizumab, an anti-PD-L1 drug (NCT03181100). The type of targeted therapy is selected on the basis of the driver mutation present in the tumor. Further trials are also investigating the combination of EBRT given to a metastatic site (SBRT) in combination with immunotherapy in thyroid cancers (NCT02239900, NCT03122496).

CONCLUSION

A small subset of DTCs, larger proportion of MTCs, and most of ATCs will be amenable to cure by standard therapy of surgery with RAI therapy. Systemic therapy has a role to play in such scenarios. The elucidation of genetic and epigenetic changes involved in thyroid carcinogenesis has allowed newer drugs against specific targets to be explored in such advanced thyroid cancers. Amongst the various targeted therapies studied, only four drugs have undergone phase III trials with significant results to qualify them for FDA approval. Lenvatinib is the first line therapy for RAI-refractory advanced thyroid cancers; sorafenib being the other approved drug in this scenario. For MTCs, vandetanib and cabozantinib are approved for metastatic and recurrent advanced cancers. The advent of immunotherapy has thrown open attractive prospects in systemic therapy of advanced thyroid cancers, especially when combined with multi-kinase inhibitors. Results of several such combination trials are awaited in the near future.

REFERENCES

1. Pellegriti G, Frasca F, Regalbuto C, Squatrito S, Vigneri R. Worldwide increasing incidence of thyroid cancer: Update on epidemiology and risk factors. *J Cancer Epidemiol.* 2013;2013:965212.

2. Vaccarella S, Franceschi S, Bray F, Wild CP, Plummer M, Dal Maso L. Worldwide thyroid-cancer epidemic? the increasing impact of overdiagnosis. *N Engl J Med.* 2016;375(7):614–7.

3. O'Neill JP, Shaha AR. Anaplastic thyroid cancer. *Oral Oncol.* 2013;49(7):702–6.

4. Liska J, Altanerova V, Galbavy S, Stvrtina S, Brtko J. Thyroid tumors: Histological classification and genetic factors involved in the development of thyroid cancer. *Endocr Regul.* 2005;39(3):73–83.

5. Nikiforov YE, Nikiforova MN. Molecular genetics and diagnosis of thyroid cancer. *Nat Rev Endocrinol.* 2011;7(10):569–80.

6. Davies L, Welch HG. Current thyroid cancer trends in the United States. *JAMA Otolaryngol Head Neck Surg.* 2014;140(4):317–22.

7. Naoum GE, Morkos M, Kim B, Arafat W. Novel targeted therapies and immunotherapy for advanced thyroid cancers. *Mol Cancer*. 2018;17(1):51.

8. Smallridge RC et al. American Thyroid Association guidelines for management of patients with anaplastic thyroid cancer. *Thyroid*. 2012;22(11):1104–39.

9. D'Cruz AK et al. Molecular markers in well-differentiated thyroid cancer. *Eur Arch Oto-Rhino-Laryngol*. 2018; 275(6):1375–84.

10. Cancer Genome Atlas Research N. Integrated genomic characterization of papillary thyroid carcinoma. *Cell*. 2014;159(3):676–90.

11. Li Z, Zhang Y, Wang R, Zou K, Zou L. Genetic alterations in anaplastic thyroid carcinoma and targeted therapies. *Exp Ther Med*. 2019;18(4):2369–77.

12. Xing M. Molecular pathogenesis and mechanisms of thyroid cancer. *Nat Rev Cancer*. 2013;13(3):184–99.

13. Saji M, Ringel MD. The PI3K-Akt-mTOR pathway in initiation and progression of thyroid tumors. *Mol Cell Endocrinol*. 2010;321(1):20–8.

14. Tallini G, Asa SL. RET oncogene activation in papillary thyroid carcinoma. *Adv Anat Pathol*. 2001;8(6):345–54.

15. Croyle M et al. RET/PTC-induced cell growth is mediated in part by epidermal growth factor receptor (EGFR) activation: Evidence for molecular and functional interactions between RET and EGFR. *Cancer Res*. 2008;68(11):4183–91.

16. Kroll TG et al. PAX8-PPARgamma1 fusion oncogene in human thyroid carcinoma [corrected]. *Science*. 2000;289(5483):1357–60.

17. Liu R, Xing M. TERT promoter mutations in thyroid cancer. *Endocr Relat Cancer*. 2016;23(3):R143–55.

18. Landa I et al. Frequent somatic TERT promoter mutations in thyroid cancer: Higher prevalence in advanced forms of the disease. *J Clin Endocrinol Metab*. 2013;98(9):E1562–6.

19. Landa I et al. Genomic and transcriptomic hallmarks of poorly differentiated and anaplastic thyroid cancers. *J Clin Invest*. 2016;126(3):1052–66.

20. Tirro E et al. Molecular alterations in thyroid cancer: From bench to clinical practice. *Genes*. 2019;10(9).

21. Haugen BR et al. 2015 American Thyroid Association Management Guidelines for adult patients with thyroid nodules and differentiated thyroid cancer: The American Thyroid Association Guidelines task force on thyroid nodules and differentiated thyroid cancer. *Thyroid*. 2016;26(1):1–133.

22. Wilhelm SM et al. BAY 43-9006 exhibits broad spectrum oral antitumor activity and targets the RAF/MEK/ERK pathway and receptor tyrosine kinases involved in tumor progression and angiogenesis. *Cancer Res*. 2004;64(19):7099–109.

23. Schneider TC, Abdulrahman RM, Corssmit EP, Morreau H, Smit JW, Kapiteijn E. Long-term analysis of the efficacy and tolerability of sorafenib in advanced radio-iodine refractory differentiated thyroid carcinoma: Final results of a phase II trial. *Eur J Endocrinol*. 2012;167(5):643–50.

24. Brose MS et al. Sorafenib in radioactive iodine-refractory, locally advanced or metastatic differentiated thyroid cancer: A randomised, double-blind, phase 3 trial. *Lancet*. 2014;384(9940):319–28.

25. Savvides P et al. Phase II trial of sorafenib in patients with advanced anaplastic carcinoma of the thyroid. *Thyroid*. 2013;23(5):600–4.

26. Lam ET et al. Phase II clinical trial of sorafenib in metastatic medullary thyroid cancer. *J Clin Oncol*. 2010;28(14):2323–30.

27. Okamoto K et al. Antitumor activities of the targeted multi-tyrosine kinase inhibitor lenvatinib (E7080) against RET gene fusion-driven tumor models. *Cancer Lett*. 2013; 340(1):97–103.

28. Cabanillas ME et al. A phase 2 trial of lenvatinib (E7080) in advanced, progressive, radioiodine-refractory, differentiated thyroid cancer: A clinical outcomes and biomarker assessment. *Cancer*. 2015;121(16):2749–56.

29. Schlumberger M et al. A Phase II Trial of the Multitargeted Tyrosine Kinase Inhibitor Lenvatinib (E7080) in Advanced Medullary Thyroid Cancer. *Clin Cancer Res*. 2016;22(1):44–53.

30. Haddad RI et al. NCCN guidelines insights: Thyroid carcinoma, version 2.2018. *J Natl Compr Canc Netw*. 2018;16(12):1429–40.

31. Wells SA Jr et al. Vandetanib for the treatment of patients with locally advanced or metastatic hereditary medullary thyroid cancer. *J Clin Oncol*. 2010;28(5):767–72.

32. Wells SA Jr et al. Vandetanib in patients with locally advanced or metastatic medullary thyroid cancer: A randomized, double-blind phase III trial. *J Clin Oncol*. 2012;30(2):134–41.

33. Leboulleux S et al. Vandetanib in locally advanced or metastatic differentiated thyroid cancer: A randomised, double-blind, phase 2 trial. *Lancet Oncol*. 2012;13(9):897–905.

34. Kurzrock R et al. Activity of XL184 (Cabozantinib), an oral tyrosine kinase inhibitor, in patients with medullary thyroid cancer. *J Clin Oncol*. 2011;29(19):2660–6.

35. Elisei R et al. Cabozantinib in progressive medullary thyroid cancer. *J Clin Oncol*. 2013;31(29):3639–46.

36. Traynor K. Cabozantinib approved for advanced medullary thyroid cancer. *Am J Health-Syst Pharm*. 2013;70(2):88.

37. Cabanillas ME et al. Cabozantinib as salvage therapy for patients with tyrosine kinase inhibitor-refractory differentiated thyroid cancer: Results of a multicenter phase II International Thyroid Oncology Group Trial. *J Clin Oncol*. 2017;35(29):3315–21.

Chapter 23

SURGICAL MANAGEMENT OF PARATHYROID DISORDERS

Neeti Kapre Gupta, Gregory W. Randolph, and Dipti Kamani

CONTENTS

Introduction 179
Clinical Profile 179
Diagnosis 179
Minimally Invasive Parathyroidectomy 181
Pathology 183
Conclusions 184
References 184

INTRODUCTION

In the early 1900s, physicians considered enlargement of the parathyroid glands to be caused by deficiency or hypoparathyroidism, and it was treated with parathyroid extract transplantation. It was only when the first parathyroidectomy, performed by Dr. Felix Mandl in Vienna in 1925, yielded prompt initial successful outcomes that the real treatment for hyperparathyroidism was determined. Subsequently, the famous yet unfortunate story of marine Captain Charles Martell at Massachusetts General Hospital in Boston provided probably the first real lesson in parathyroid surgery. Captain Martell, so troubled by his bone and renal conditions subsequent to parathyroid disease, would spend hours researching gland anatomy and surgical principles at the Harvard library. He persuaded Dr. Cope and Dr. Churchill [1] to perform a mediastinal exploration to identify and successfully resect an ectopic adenoma. This team of doctors went on to perform a series of successful parathyroid surgeries and established the technique at the endocrinology department in the hospital.

Hyperparathyroidism (HPT) can be divided into primary, secondary, or tertiary. Primary HPT (PHPT) is a result of increased production of parathyroid hormone (PTH) due to hyperplasia or neoplastic pathology of one or multiple parathyroid glands. Secondary hyperparathyroidism (SHPT) refers to a compensatory increase in PTH secretion in response to low serum calcium levels and is most commonly seen in chronic renal diseases, less commonly with long-term lithium therapy, and rarely with gastrointestinal absorption disorders and pseudohypoparathyroidism. Tertiary HPT (THPT) occurs after longstanding SHPT in which there is severe parathyroid hyperplasia, with autonomous PTH secretion that is no longer effectively responsive to the serum calcium levels. THPT is seen in post renal transplant patients who have developed resistance to PTH receptors.

PHPT could be a result of single adenoma (85%–90%), multiglandular disease, double adenoma, and rarely parathyroid carcinoma (1%) [2]. Primary HPT is known to occur in syndromic and non-syndromic situations. MEN1, MEN2A, and hyperparathyroidism with jaw tumor syndrome are the more significant ones. Table 23.1 illustrates syndromes commonly associated with hyperparathyroidism. Primary hyperparathyroidism characterized by hypercalcemia and increased parathyroid hormone levels was classically described as the clinical presentation of groans, moans, and stones! However, with increased awareness and better diagnostic tools such as the advent of an automated serum chemistry analyzer, the detection of asymptomatic primary hyperparathyroidism has become fairly common. Therefore, on one hand where there were no doubts regarding indications for surgery in the earlier scenario, indications for incidentally detected asymptomatic hyperparathyroid patients have to be stringent. The revised guidelines, therefore, serve as a very important reference for making surgical decisions [3].

Parathyroidectomy should be recommended for the following asymptomatic hyperparathyroidism patients: (1) those <50 years of age, (2) those who cannot participate in appropriate follow-up, (3) those with a serum calcium level >1.0 mg/dL above the normal range, (4) those with creatinine clearance <60 mL/min, or (5) those with T-score lower than 2.5 SD at any site or any previous fracture fragility [3].

CLINICAL PROFILE

Women are affected more than men in a ratio of approximately 3:1 and generally in the fifth and sixth decades of life. Syndromic hyperparathyroidism patients generally manifest symptoms in the second or third decade of life. Constitutional complaints, such as weakness, easy fatigability, depression, and intellectual weariness are frequently reported. Diseases epidemiologically (although not etiologically) linked with primary hyperparathyroidism, such as hypertension and peptic ulcer disease, are also seen commonly. Kidney stones and fractures, although uncommon, continue to be seen in some neglected population sets. Both general examination and local neck examination may not yield any significant findings and the diagnosis is primarily biochemical.

DIAGNOSIS

Diagnosis is purely biochemical. Elevated serum PTH and calcium are hallmarks of HPT. Concomitant presence of renal dysfunction, vitamin D deficiency, and phosphate metabolism need to be evaluated to differentiate the type and cause of HPT. A close differential diagnosis of HPT is familial hypocalcuric hypercalcemia (FHH) [4].

Table 23.1 Syndromic associations with hyperparathyroidism

Syndrome	Incidence of HPT	Co-existent features	Genetic mutation	Surgical management
Multiple Endocrine Neoplasia 1 (MEN 1)	High (90%–100%)	Pancreatic tumors, gastrinomas, stomach ulcers (Zollinger-Ellison syndrome)	MEN 1 (11q13)	Multigland excision
Multiple Endocrine Neoplasia 2A (MEN 2A)	Low (15%–30%)	MTC and pheochromocytoma	RET (10q21)	Excision of hypertrophic glands only
Hyperparathyroidism with Jaw Tumor Syndrome (HPTJT)	High (80%) Increased risk of parathyroid carcinoma	Fibro-osseous tumors of maxilla or mandible, increased risk of renal tumors (nephroblastomas, hamartomas, or Wilms' tumors), and uterine tumors	HRPT2	Multigland excision
Familial Hypocalciuric Hypocalcemia (FHH)	High	Asymptomatic mild hypercalcemia with relative hypocalciuria, hypermagnesemia in half of the patients, low calcium/creatinine ratio with total calcium/24-hour urine collection <100 mg	CASR (3q 21–24)	Treatment only if symptomatic
Familial Isolated Hyperparathyroidism (FIHPT)	Low (12%–14%)	Very rare	MEN 1, CASR, HRPT2	Multigland excision

This can be determined by measuring the urinary calcium excretion and urinary calcium-creatinine ratio.

Several physicians consider that pre-operative localization studies are not necessary for first time explorations. However, in the wake of minimal access parathyroid surgeries, they have a definite role. These studies become further relevant with re-exploration parathyroid surgeries. Non-invasive as well as invasive, and structural as well as functional imaging studies are available. As a first line, ultrasonography (USG) and sestamibi scans are useful diagnostic tools [5] (Figure 23.1). When performed by experienced radiologists, accuracy rates are very high for detection as well as localization of the concerned parathyroid gland harboring the adenoma. Studies show that a combination of USG and multiplexed ion beam imaging (MIBI) scan has an accuracy of approximately 92% for single adenomas [6]. However, sestamibi scan lacks sensitivity for multi-gland disease. Imaging studies are concordant in up to 65% of patients with primary HPT. When results from these tests are discordant, SPECT-CT, 4D-CT, and MRI may be employed [7,8]. The fourth dimension implying timing of contrast perfusion provides the added advantage of both anatomical and physiological details about the parathyroid gland in question. The parathyroid adenomas have rapid uptake and early washout of intravenous contrast compared to the thyroid. F-fluorocholine (FCH) PET/CT imaging has been proven superior for accurate pre-operative localization of

parathyroid adenomas, especially for ectopic or small parathyroid lesions [9]. For discordant studies or re-explorations, rarely invasive test such as selective venous sampling for PTH may be required [10]. An ultrasound or CT guided FNAC can also be performed along with PTH measurements from the washout to further clinch the diagnosis [11]. During surgery, intra-operative ultrasound proves to be a surgeon's friend to aid in localization.

MANAGEMENT

Surgery remains the mainstay of treatment. Medical management can be employed for patients who are not suitable candidates for surgery. Oral bisphosphonates, calcimimetic agents, and selective estrogen receptor modulators (especially for post-menopausal women) have been tried with reasonable success.

It is aptly said that appropriate surgery performed at the first time stands the best chance for cure. A thorough knowledge of anatomy is paramount to assure good surgical outcomes.

SURGICAL ANATOMY

A large autopsy study identified four parathyroid glands in 84% of human cadavers, five or more glands in 13%, and only three parathyroid glands in 3% [12]. Normal parathyroid glands are approximately 5–6 mm in greatest dimension, weigh 15–35 mg, and can be inconspicuous with their orange-tan color embedded

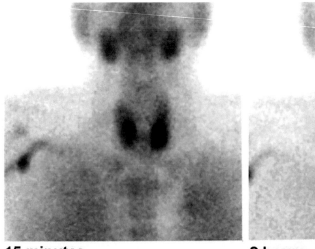 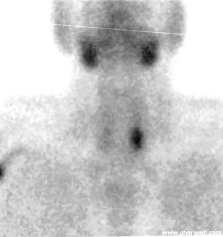

15 minutes   **2 hours**

Figure 23.1 Left-sided inferior parathyroid adenoma visualized on functional imaging.

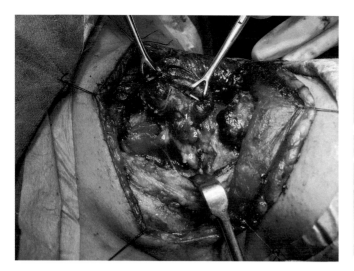

Figure 23.2 Parathyroids with their supplying vasculature and central compartment nodes seen separately (1- Thyroid, 2- Parathyroid, 3- Central compartment lymph node, 4- Fat).

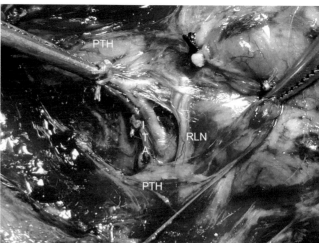

Figure 23.3 Superior and inferior parathyroid glands separated by the plane of the recurrent laryngeal nerve.

or flattened within a surrounding yellow fatty tissue envelope. Parathyroid glands are often confused with central compartment lymph nodes, fat globules, or rarely thyroid nodules (Figure 23.2). Several characteristics will help to differentiate between the four structures (Table 23.2).

The superior parathyroid glands arise from the fourth pharyngeal pouch and descend along with the thyroid gland. They are generally seen in a 1 cm area around the intersection of the recurrent laryngeal nerve and inferior thyroid artery roughly near the entry point at the crico-thyroid joint. The inferior parathyroid glands arise from the third pharyngeal pouch and descend down along with the thymus. They are generally seen within 1 cm area from the lower pole of the thyroid gland. Although these are the standard locations for these glands, they are notorious for ectopic presence. Therefore, one must be aware of the various anatomically variant locations as follows:

1. Dorsum of the superior pole of the thyroid gland
2. Retro-esophageal
3. Parapharyngeal
4. Within the carotid sheath
5. Thyrothymic tract
6. Mediastinal
7. Aorto-pulmonary window

Table 23.2 Differentiating characteristics for identification of parathyroid glands

Characteristic	Parathyroid	Fat	Lymph node	Thyroid
Color	Orange tan	Yellow	Pinkish white	Reddish brown
Hilar vessel	Present, can be traced up to inferior thyroid artery	Absent	May or may not be present	Absent
Roving sign[a]	Positive	Negative	Negative	Negative
Consistency	Soft to firm	Soft mushy	Firm to hard	Nodular
Shape	Bean shaped	Globular	Oval to round	Nodular

[a] Roving sign: The parathyroid gland housed in its capsule glides over the thyroid in a roving motion.

The surest method of differentiating superior and inferior parathyroid glands is following the plane of recurrent laryngeal nerve (Figure 23.3). Glands that are dorsal to it are superior and those which are ventral to it are inferior. Intra-thyroidal parathyroid glands are seen in approximately 1% of cases and contrary to embryological theories, inferior glands are more often intra-thyroidal according to autopsy studies.

The following types of surgical procedures exist for the management of hyperparathyroidism:

1. Minimally invasive parathyroidectomy
2. Bilateral neck exploration

There is abundant literature including some meticulously conducted meta-analysis to determine superiority between the approaches [13]. Jinih et al. conclude that compared with bilateral exploration, focused exploration has similar recurrence, persistence, and reoperation rates but significantly lower overall complication rates and shorter operative time [14]. The failures of focused exploration are often blamed on presence of double adenomas or misdiagnosed multiple gland disease. However, chances of these remaining undetected before the end of surgery are significantly decreased by routine implementation of intra-operative serum PTH estimations. The decision rests on results of localization studies, history of previous interventions, disease status, and often on surgeon/institution preference [15,16]. With stringent selection criteria, surgeons have reported some success with minimal parathyroid surgery for negative localization studies as well [17]. Cost effective studies show a superiority of open minimally invasive over video-assisted parathyroidectomy [18]. Also, it is pertinent to note that scar satisfaction rates were no different between the open and minimally invasive or remote access approaches [19]. Therefore, it is necessary to strike a balance between maximizing cosmesis and ensuring quality and cost-effectiveness of care.

MINIMALLY INVASIVE PARATHYROIDECTOMY

This implies limited neck exploration to selectively target and excise the parathyroid gland in question. Localization studies are a pre-requisite for this procedure and results are most promising for single adenomas. This can further be of the following types:

a. *Open minimally invasive parathyroidectomy*: A small incision (3–3.5 cm) is placed either in the midline midway between the cricoid cartilage and suprasternal notch, preferably in a natural skin crease. This allows bilateral exploration if required.

b. *Endoscopic assisted minimally invasive parathyroidectomy*: A mini skin incision (1–1.5 cm) is placed horizontally in the midline or along the anterior border of the sternocleidomastoid muscle. Earlier requirements of CO_2 insufflation are no longer deemed essential. The endoscopic assistance provides magnification and therefore aids in better identification of the vasculature and the recurrent laryngeal nerve.

c. *Radio-guided parathyroidectomy*: 20 mCi of 99mTc-sestamibi is administered half an hour prior to surgery. Intra-operatively, a gamma camera evaluates the functioning parathyroid glands. In vivo counts are documented. After excision or ex-vivo counts more than 20 as compared to the remnant, background activity is considered as successful excision of the concerned parathyroid gland.

BILATERAL NECK EXPLORATION

Before the advent of advanced localization studies and intra-operative PTH measurements, bilateral neck exploration was the norm. The dictum was: "Do not remove anything until you have seen everything." This is still preferred by many surgeons. All four glands are examined and the morphologically abnormal glands or those identified on localization studies are resected. Bilateral explorations are essential for the treatment of multiglandular hyperplasia, syndromic primary HPT, and secondary and tertiary HPT. Summarized below are indications for bilateral neck exploration:

- Multiple endocrine neoplasia syndromes
- Secondary and tertiary hyperparathyroidism
- Intra-operative PTH does not fall by >50% even 20 minutes after resection of suspected single gland
- Failure to locate suspected gland prompted by localization studies or detection of more than one suspicious gland on intra-operative examination
- Localization studies fail to identify abnormal gland
- Indication for simultaneous thyroid surgery (co-existent goiter or thyroid cancer)
- Surgeons often prefer to perform bilateral exploration for discordant pre-operative imaging studies (Table 23.3)

EXTENT OF SURGERY

For primary hyperparathyroidism caused by single adenoma, resection of the involved gland is considered adequate surgery. Intra-operative PTH monitoring criteria (mentioned in detail below) guide the surgeon toward successful removal of the gland in question. For multiglandular hyperplasia and syndromic HPT, the choice remains between three to three and a half gland resection, that is subtotal parathyroidectomy versus total parathyroidectomy with auto-graft. Since subsequent neck surgery for medullary carcinoma thyroid is suspected in MEN 2 syndromes, the remnant parathyroid should preferably be transplanted in the forearm muscle brachioradialis.

For other scenarios, the sternocleidomastoid muscle is a suitable alternative. The auto-graft should be marked with titanium clips or non-absorbable sutures for ease of identification in case of re-operative parathyroid or thyroid surgery.

For secondary and tertiary hyperparathyroidism, the management is primarily medical. However, patients whose HPT is not controlled or who are symptomatic in spite of maximum medical management are surgical candidates. K/DOQI guidelines from the U.S. Kidney Foundation have proposed that parathyroidectomy should be recommended in patients with severe SHPT (persistent serum levels of intact PTH >800 pg/mL), associated with hypercalcemia or hyperphosphatemia, which is refractory to medical therapy. Both subtotal parathyroidectomy and total parathyroidectomy with auto-graft are recommended options (Table 23.4).

There is considerable debate between subtotal versus total parathyroidectomy as surgery of choice for patients with MEN 1 disorders, secondary, and tertiary hyperparathyroidism [20,21]. The effects on post-operative serum calcium and PTH measurements, the chances of recurrence/persistence, and re-operations are similar for both the approaches. It is recommended that anything less than a subtotal parathyroidectomy is unacceptable on account of high percentage of failures and recurrences for MEN 1 and secondary hyperparathyroidism [22]. In an interesting study by Pitt et al. in 2009, the scope for less than subtotal resection of parathyroid glands for tertiary hyperparathyroidism was explored [23].

The morphologically smallest gland without nodularity should be chosen as the remnant. Inferior parathyroid glands are easier to preserve due to their more ventral location. However, they should be marked with metallic clips to ease identification later. Also the remaining glandular tissue must be confirmed as normal preferably by frozen section in order to prevent re-explorations. Even 1–2 mm tissue is sufficient for an experienced pathologist to report on frozen section examination.

OPERATIVE ADJUNCTS

Intra-operative PTH (IOPTH) monitoring with turn-back times as low as 10–15 minutes has truly revolutionized the technique of minimally invasive parathyroidectomy [24,25]. It works on the premise that the half-life of PTH is 3–5 minutes. Therefore, a substantial fall of >50% in PTH values 10–20 minutes post resection is routinely practiced criterion for performance of

Table 23.4   Surgical indications for secondary hyperparathyroidism

Surgical Indications for Secondary Hyperparathyroidism Modified by Japanese Society for Dialysis Therapy (JSDT) Guideline
Essential Components
1. Persistent high serum level of intact PTH level >500 pg/mL 2. Hyperphosphatemia (serum P >6 mg/dL) or hypercalcemia (serum Ca >10 mg/dL), which is refractory to medical therapy 3. To detect estimated volume of the largest gland >300–500 mm³ or long axis >1 cm
Clinical Findings
If patients have one of the following factors mentioned, parathyroidectomy should be absolutely recommended: 1. Severe osteitis fibrosa, high bone turnover 2. Progressive ectopic calcification 3. Subjective symptoms (bone and joint pain, arthralgia, muscle weakness, irritability, pruritus, depression) 4. Calciphylaxis 5. Progressive reduction in bone mineral content 6. Anemia resistant to erythropoietin stimulating agent (ESA) 7. Dilated cardiomyopathy/cardiac failure

Table 23.3   Advantages and drawbacks of both these approaches

	Minimally invasive thyroidectomy	Bilateral neck exploration
Overall morbidity	Less	More
Hypocalcemia	Less pronounced	More pronounced
Risk of recurrence/ persistence	More	Less
Risk of overall failure	More	Less

adequate parathyroidectomy [26]. Some surgeons prefer taking a pre-incision sample, pre-excision samples (ligation of feeder vessel to the parathyroid adenoma), and 10 minutes post-excision samples. Evidence also indicates that IOPTH to ≤40 pg/mL are associated with the lowest persistence rates after parathyroidectomy for primary hyperparathyroidism, and patients with values between 41–65 pg/mL will require a careful follow-up [27,28].

One can also perform PTH estimation on the aspirate from the excised parathyroid tissue. Values above 2,500 pg/mL are considered confirmatory. IOPTH improves the success rate of minimally invasive procedures significantly. In a large prospective study at the University of Wisconsin, the cure rate for initial unilateral exploration guided by IOPTH is 98.5% versus a predicted rate of 87% when decision-making is based on ipsilateral parathyroid gland appearance alone [29].

Low pre-incision values and co-existing renal disease can sometimes make IOPTH interpretations less reliable. However, similar criteria of >50% decline in pre-operative values were still a reliable indicator of success [30].

There has also been some critique toward the cost effectiveness of IOPTH monitoring since it is not routinely available in all institutions [31]. The CaPTHUS [32] (pre-operative calcium, parathyroid hormone, ultrasound, sestamibi, concordance imaging) scoring model was introduced first in 2006 to predict presence of single parathyroid adenoma and consequently predict long-term success after focused neck explorations for hyperparathyroidism. Although it was a very reliable formula to estimate chances of cure after focused or unilateral parathyroid explorations, it was not acceptable to substitute or replace IOPTH estimations completely [33] (Table 23.5).

PARATHYROID AUTOFLUORESCENCE (PTAF) AND INTRA-OPERATIVE PARATHYROID GLAND DETECTION

Parathyroid glands can be differentiated from surrounding tissue by virtue of their ability to emit autofluorescence when stimulated by near-infrared light. The utilization of PTAF for thyroid and parathyroid surgeries is a very recent advancement and is still in early stages. Some initial studies have found its utility in the identification of parathyroid glands in surgery for primary hyperparathyroidism [34,35]. DiMarco et al. found that routine use of PTAF in parathyroid surgery is presently not justified [36]. With further enhancements in this technology, PTAF's role in parathyroid surgery may expand.

POST-OPERATIVE MONITORING

Several centers are promoting outpatient/same-day discharge surgeries for parathyroid pathologies. However, the authors propose a period of a minimum 24–48 hours stay in hospital. Serum PTH and calcium estimations should ideally be conducted approximately 24 and 48 hours post-surgery. Severe hypocalcemia may precipitate in certain patients, especially those with very high PTH levels or severe bone demineralization pre-operatively (hungry bone syndrome).

REVISION SURGERY

Failure of PTH values to normalize 6 months after primary surgery and persistence or appearance of symptoms suggestive of hyperparathyroidism should prompt work-up for re-exploration surgery. The following precautions can help to ensure optimal results for revision surgeries:

1. Re-confirm diagnosis.
2. Review all previous imaging, biochemical, and histology reports.
3. Review prior operative notes.
4. Perform localization studies.
5. Utilization of intra-operative adjuncts such as IOPTH, Intra-operative nerve monitoring, and loop magnification.
6. Some surgeons prefer the back-door technique, where the parathyroid glands are approached laterally from underneath the strap muscles. This helps to avoid scar tissue in the central compartment from previous surgical intervention.
7. Usual anatomical variations such as thymic, retro-esophageal, etc., should be verified before resorting to severe measures such as thyroid lobectomy.

PARATHYROID CARCINOMA

Parathyroid carcinoma contributes to approximately 1% of all cases of HPT [33]. Previous head and neck radiation, chronic stimulation from renal failure, or familial syndromes are likely etiological factors. This may be a phenotypic variant of HPT-JT syndrome.

Hallmarks of this disease are significantly elevated serum calcium (3.75–3.97 mmol/L) and PTH (5–10 times the normal range) and suspicious ultrasound or CT features [38]. Clinically, a hard mass can be palpated in the neck. There may be signs of local invasion such as recurrent laryngeal nerve palsies. There may be presence of features of end organ involvement such as renal disease or skeletal manifestations.

Staging can be broadly classified as:

1. Disease localized to the parathyroid gland
2. Local infiltration into surrounding structures
3. Distant metastases

Adequate surgery should include ipsilateral thyroid lobectomy, central compartment nodal clearance, and removal of all fibrofatty tissue from level VI [37]. There is no recommendation of lateral compartment neck dissection in the absence of proven or suspected disease. Recommendations for adjuvant radiation include R+ resection, the post-operative lack of normalization of parathyroid hormone, as well as multifocal recurrence or soft tissue deposits in recurrent patients.

PATHOLOGY

Morphologically there are meager differentiating features between adenoma and hyperplasia. On microscopic examination, the percentage of fat cells is an important criterion. Hypercellularity that exceeds 50:50 ratio of oxyphil cells over fat cells implies the diagnosis of adenoma. A differentiation of parathyroid carcinoma over benign tumor may be challenging on an intra-operative frozen section. However, the triad of high mitotic rate (>5 per 50 high power fields), macro nucleoli, and necrosis are predictors of recurrent or metastatic disease. Immunohistochemical staining

Table 23.5 CaPTHUS scoring model

Predictive factor	Points
Pre-operative total serum Ca level ≥3 mmol/L or ≥12 mg/dL	1
Intact PTH level ≥2 times upper limit of normal PTH levels	1
Sestamibi scan results positive for 1 enlarged parathyroid gland	1
Neck ultrasound results positive for 1 enlarged thyroid gland	1
Concordant sestamibi and neck ultrasound study results (identifying 1 enlarged gland on the same side of the neck)	1
Total	0–5

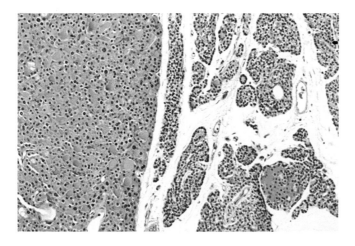

Figure 23.4 Photomicrograph of the histological appearance of parathyroid adenoma.

with the monoclonal MIB-1 antibody, which detects the cell cycle–associated marker, Ki 67 antigen, and cell aneuploidy are also important pathological features (Figure 23.4).

CONCLUSIONS

The norm for parathyroid surgery remains that the first chance is the best chance. Rational surgical decision-making, adequate pre-operative diagnostic workup, and surgical expertise including utilization of appropriate intra-operative adjuncts are the keys to ensure success rates of treatment. The consensus statement of the European Society of Endocrine Surgeons (ESES) assumed that even if bilateral neck exploration has excellent results and is always an option for the surgical treatment of primary HPT, minimally invasive parathyroidectomy is a safe and cost-effective procedure to treat selected patients with sporadic primary HPT, especially in cases of positive pre-operative localization tests. Minimally invasive procedures have certain distinct advantages, especially in terms of less post-operative hypocalcemia, shorter operative time, earlier discharge, better cosmetic result, and reduced post-operative pain.

REFERENCES

1. Organ CH Jr. The history of parathyroid surgery, 1850–1996: The Excelsior Surgical Society 1998 Edward D Churchill Lecture. *J Am Coll Surg*. 2000 Sep;191(3):284–99.

2. Callender GG, Udelsman R. Surgery for hyperparathyroidism. *Cancer*. 2014 Dec 1;120(23):3602–16.

3. Bilezikian JP, Khan AA, Potts JT Jr. Guidelines for the management of asymptomatic primary hyperparathyroidism: Summary statement from the third international workshop. *J Clin Endocrinol Metab*. 2009 Feb;94(2):335–9.

4. Christensen SE, Nissen PH, Vestergaard P. Familial hypocalciuric hypercalcaemia: A review. *Curr Opin Endocrinol Diabetes Obes*. 2011 Dec;18(6):359–70.

5. Moghadam RN, Amlelshahbaz AP, Namiranian N, Sobhan-Ardekani M, Emami-Meybodi M, Dehghan A, Rahmanian M, Razavi-Ratki SK. Comparative diagnostic performance of ultrasonography and 99mTc-Sestamibi scintigraphy for parathyroid adenoma in primary hyperparathyroidism; Systematic review and meta-analysis. *Asian Pac J Cancer Prev*. 2017 Dec 28;18(12):3195–200.

6. Ibrahim EAG, Elsadawy ME. Combined Tc-99 m sesta MIBI scintigraphy and ultrasonography in preoperative detection and localization of parathyroid adenoma. *Egypt J Radiol Nucl Med*. 2015;46:937–41.

7. Cheung K, Wang TS, Farrokhyar F, Roman SA, Sosa JA. A meta-analysis of preoperative localization techniques for patients with primary hyperparathyroidism. *Ann Surg Oncol*. 2012 Feb;19(2):577–83.

8. Treglia G, Sadeghi R, Schalin-Jäntti C, Caldarella C, Ceriani L, Giovanella L, Eisele DW. Detection rate of (99 m) Tc-MIBI single photon emission computed tomography (SPECT)/CT in preoperative planning for patients with primary hyperparathyroidism: A meta-analysis. *Head Neck*. 2016 Apr;38(Suppl 1):E2159–72.

9. Thanseer N et al. Comparative effectiveness of ultrasonography, 99mTc-Sestamibi, and 18F-Fluorocholine PET/CT in detecting parathyroid adenomas in patients with primary hyperparathyroidism. *Clin Nucl Med*. 2017 Dec;42(12):e491–7.

10. Ibraheem K, Toraih EA, Haddad AB, Farag M, Randolph GW, Kandil E. Selective parathyroid venous sampling in primary hyperparathyroidism: A systematic review and meta-analysis. *Laryngoscope*. 2018 Nov;128(11):2662–7.

11. Aydın C, Polat SB, Dellal FD, Kaya C, Dogan HT, Turkolmez S, Kılıç M, Ersoy R, Çakır B. The diagnostic value of parathyroid hormone washout in primary hyperparathyroidism patients with negative or equivocal 99 m Tc-MIBI results. *Diagn Cytopathol*. 2019 Feb;47(2):94–9.

12. Akerström G, Malmaeus J, Bergström R. Surgical anatomy of human parathyroid glands. *Surgery*. 1984 Jan;95(1):14–21.

13. Singh Ospina NM et al. Outcomes of parathyroidectomy in patients with primary hyperparathyroidism: A systematic review and meta-analysis. *World J Surg*. 2016 Oct;40(10):2359–77.

14. Jinih M, O'Connell E, O'Leary DP, Liew A, Redmond HP. Focused versus bilateral parathyroid exploration for primary hyperparathyroidism: A systematic review and meta-analysis. *Ann Surg Oncol*. 2017 Jul;24(7):1924–34.

15. Reeve TS, Babidge WJ, Parkyn RF, Edis AJ, Delbridge LW, Devitt PG, Maddern GJ. Minimally invasive surgery for primary hyperparathyroidism: Systematic review. *Arch Surg*. 2000 Apr;135(4):481–7.

16. Kiernan CM, Wang T, Perrier ND, Grubbs EG, Solórzano CC. Bilateral neck exploration for sporadic primary hyperparathyroidism: Use patterns in 5,597 patients undergoing parathyroidectomy in the collaborative endocrine surgery quality improvement program. *J Am Coll Surg*. 2019 Apr;228(4):652–9.

17. Scott-Coombes DM, Rees J, Jones G, Stechman MJ. Is unilateral neck surgery feasible in patients with sporadic primary hyperparathyroidism and double negative localisation? *World J Surg*. 2017 Jun;41(6):1494–9.

18. Barczyński M, Cichoń S, Konturek A, Cichoń W. Minimally invasive video-assisted parathyroidectomy versus open minimally invasive parathyroidectomy for a solitary parathyroid adenoma: A prospective, randomized, blinded trial. *World J Surg*. 2006 May;30(5):721–31.

19. Linos D, Economopoulos KP, Kiriakopoulos A, Linos E, Petralias A. Scar perceptions after thyroid and parathyroid surgery: Comparison of minimal and conventional approaches. *Surgery.* 2013 Mar;153(3):400–7.

20. Yuan Q, Liao Y, Zhou R, Liu J, Tang J, Wu G. Subtotal parathyroidectomy versus total parathyroidectomy with autotransplantation for secondary hyperparathyroidism: An updated systematic review and meta-analysis. *Langenbecks Arch Surg.* 2019 Aug;404:669–79.

21. Chen J, Jia X, Kong X, Wang Z, Cui M, Xu D. Total parathyroidectomy with autotransplantation versus subtotal parathyroidectomy for renal hyperparathyroidism: A systematic review and meta-analysis. *Nephrology (Carlton).* 2017 May;22(5):388–96.

22. Schreinemakers JM, Pieterman CR, Scholten A, Vriens MR, Valk GD, Rinkes IH. The optimal surgical treatment for primary hyperparathyroidism in MEN1 patients: A systematic review. *World J Surg.* 2011 Sep;35(9):1993–2005.

23. Pitt SC, Panneerselvan R, Chen H, Sippel RS. Tertiary hyperparathyroidism: Is less than a subtotal resection ever appropriate? A study of long-term outcomes. *Surgery.* 2009 Dec;146(6):1130–7.

24. Sebag F, Shen W, Brunaud L, Kebebew E, Duh QY, Clark OH. Intraoperative parathyroid hormone assay and parathyroid reoperations. *Surgery.* 2003 Dec;134(6):1049–55.

25. Dobrinja C, Santandrea G, Giacca M, Stenner E, Ruscio M, de Manzini N. Effectiveness of intraoperative parathyroid monitoring (ioPTH) in predicting a multiglandular or malignant parathyroid disease. *Int J Surg.* 2017 May;41(Suppl 1):S26–33.

26. Carneiro-Pla DM, Solorzano CC, Lew JI, Irvin GL 3rd. Long-term outcome of patients with intraoperative parathyroid level remaining above the normal range during parathyroidectomy. *Surgery.* 2008 Dec;144(6):989–93.

27. Claflin J, Dhir A, Espinosa NM, Antunez AG, Cohen MS, Gauger PG, Miller BS, Hughes DT. Intraoperative parathyroid hormone levels ≤40 pg/mL are associated with the lowest persistence rates after parathyroidectomy for primary hyperparathyroidism. *Surgery.* 2019 Jul;166(1):50–4.

28. Wharry LI, Yip L, Armstrong MJ, Virji MA, Stang MT, Carty SE, McCoy KL. The final intraoperative parathyroid hormone level: How low should it go? *World J Surg.* 2014 Mar;38(3):558–63.

29. Rajaei MH, Oltmann SC, Adkisson CD, Elfenbein DM, Chen H, Carty SE, McCoy KL. Is intraoperative parathyroid hormone monitoring necessary with ipsilateral parathyroid gland visualization during anticipated unilateral exploration for primary hyperparathyroidism: A two-institution analysis of more than 2,000 patients. *Surgery.* 2014 Oct;156(4):760–6.

30. Trinh G, Noureldine SI, Russell JO, Agrawal N, Lopez M, Prescott JD, Zeiger MA, Tufano RP. Characterizing the operative findings and utility of intraoperative parathyroid hormone (IOPTH) monitoring in patients with normal baseline IOPTH and normohormonal primary hyperparathyroidism. *Surgery.* 2017 Jan;161(1):78–86.

31. Badii B, Staderini F, Foppa C, Tofani L, Skalamera I, Fiorenza G, Qirici E, Cianchi F, Perigli G. Cost-benefit analysis of the intraoperative parathyroid hormone assay in primary hyperparathyroidism. *Head Neck.* 2017 Feb;39(2):241–6.

32. Kebebew E, Hwang J, Reiff E, Duh QY, Clark OH. Predictors of single-gland vs multigland parathyroid disease in primary hyperparathyroidism: A simple and accurate scoring model. *Arch Surg.* 2006 Aug;141(8):777–82; discussion 782.

33. Elfenbein DM, Weber S, Schneider DF, Sippel RS, Chen H. CaPTHUS scoring model in primary hyperparathyroidism: Can it eliminate the need for ioPTH testing? *Ann Surg Oncol.* 2015 Apr;22(4):1191–5.

34. Serra C, Silveira L, Canudo A, Lemos MC. Parathyroid identification by autofluorescence - preliminary report on five cases of surgery for primary hyperparathyroidism. *BMC Surg.* 2019 Aug 28;19(1):120.

35. Falco J, Dip F, Quadri P, de la Fuente M, Rosenthal R. Cutting edge in thyroid surgery: Autofluorescence of parathyroid glands. *J Am Coll Surg.* 2016 Aug;223(2):374–80.

36. DiMarco A, Chotalia R, Bloxham R, McIntyre C, Tolley N, Palazzo FF. Autofluorescence in parathyroidectomy: Signal intensity correlates with serum calcium and parathyroid hormone but routine clinical use is not justified. *World J Surg.* 2019 Jun;43(6):1532–7.

37. Goswamy J, Lei M, Simo R. Parathyroid carcinoma. *Curr Opin Otolaryngol Head Neck Surg.* 2016 Apr;24(2):155–62.

38. Wächter S, Holzer K, Manoharan J, Brehm C, Mintziras I, Bartsch DK, Maurer E. Surgical treatment of parathyroid carcinoma: Does the initial en bloc resection improve the prognosis? *Chirurg.* 2019 Jul; 90:90–912.

Chapter 24

PEDIATRIC THYROID SURGERY

Rajendra Saoji

CONTENTS

Introductions   187
Benign Conditions Warranting Surgical Management   187
Thyroid Malignant Lesions   188
Who Should Be Operating on Children?   189
Thyroid Pain and Abscess   189
Ectopic Thyroid Gland   189
References   189

INTRODUCTIONS

Thyroid pathologies for children treat a varied mix of benign and malignant conditions. Functionality of the gland may vary physiologically and pathologically. Surgical problems are often a manifestation of the embryological remnant variations, and therefore thorough anatomical knowledge is a must for due planning, e.g., thyroid cyst or resultant abscess due to infection prone remnants of otherwise uncommon third and fourth branchial arches or thyroglossal duct cyst containing entire thyroid tissue and likewise. Since these are majorly indolent conditions, it is essential to minimize or avoid iatrogenic morbidity. Pediatric thyroid cancers are a distinct entity with a different biological behavior than the adult counterpart. They are much more aggressive with higher chances of nodal and distant metastases. Many of these require adjuvant treatment in view of higher stages. However, prognosis is excellent with more than 95% 10-year survival outcomes in a major series [1].

Types of thyroid swellings which need surgical attention:

Goiters	Graves' disease Toxic nodule Congenital
Cysts	Simple cyst Cyst of remnant of third or fourth pharyngeal pouch
Abscess	Infections of uncommon branchial pouches in close proximity of thyroid lobe.
Neoplastic	Adenoma Differentiated thyroid cancer (DTC) Medullary thyroid cancer (MTC) and associated familial syndromes
Others	Ectopic thyroid tissue

BENIGN CONDITIONS WARRANTING SURGICAL MANAGEMENT

AUTOIMMUNE THYROIDITIS OR GRAVES' DISEASE

Graves' disease is an autoimmune condition which causes hyperthyroidism or thyrotoxicosis secondary to the production of autoantibodies to the thyroid-stimulating hormone (TSH) receptor. The incidence of Graves' disease in the pediatric population is approximately 1 per 100,000 per year. This represents 0.1 per 100,000 in the child and 3 per 100,000 in the adolescent population [2]. Children with Graves' disease should be managed with antithyroid drugs (ATD), viz. Methimazole and Propylthiouracil (PTU). To counter cardiovascular sequelae of the disease process, beta blockers are commonly added to the medical management of thyrotoxicosis. Such medications need to be given over long periods of time and then discontinued or reduced gradually. Very careful monitoring is needed for side effects such as agranulocytosis, joint pain, fever, skin rash, and the like, resulting from Methimazole. The dose should be adjusted until the patient is rendered biochemically euthyroid and the symptoms of Graves' disease are relieved. The other frequently employed drug PTU has the very serious side effect of liver failure and has been banned for use in the pediatric population in many countries. The role of surgery, as a definitive therapy, comes in when patients either cannot be managed with Methimazole due to severely troublesome side effects or fail to undergo lasting remission. The non-surgical alternative of radioactive iodine is again not suitable for the pediatric population because of risk of radiation exposure. A potential association between parathyroid hyperplasia and hyperparathyroidism after radio-iodine therapy has also been reported.

Therefore, surgery is an acceptable form of therapy for pediatric Graves' disease. Thyroid surgery should be chosen when definitive therapy for Graves' disease is indicated and the child is too young for I-131 or the required dose of I-131 is too high.

The operation of choice is total or near-total thyroidectomy, performed with the intent of rendering the patient hypothyroid. Subtotal thyroidectomy should be avoided due to an unacceptably high incidence of recurrence. In order to avoid the possibility of hemodynamic instability or thyroid storm in the operating room, children with Graves' disease undergoing thyroidectomy should be euthyroid prior to surgery, and Methimazole with/out beta-blockers given as necessary. Methimazole is typically given for one to two months in preparation for thyroidectomy. Potassium iodide should be given in the immediate pre-operative period.

Potassium iodide (50 mg iodide/drop) can be given as 3–7 drops three times daily for 10 days prior to surgery. Beta-blockers also may be needed in patients with persistent tachycardia or allergy to Methimazole.

Graves' patients who undergo thyroidectomy are more likely to suffer from hypocalcemic complications compared to patients who undergo thyroidectomy for other indications [3]. There are several hypotheses for this finding, including hungry bone syndrome, increased secretion of calcitonin as a result of thyroid manipulation, and increased vascularity and inflammation of the gland which may cause bleeding that can obscure the operative field or result in direct adhesions to the parathyroid glands. At some centers, calcitriol (25–50 μg twice per day) is started three days pre-operatively as prophylaxis for post-operative hypocalcemia.

According to the largest published series of 78 thyroidectomies in children from the Mayo clinic over 17 years, the most common risks of thyroidectomy include recurrent laryngeal or superior laryngeal nerve injury and permanent hypoparathyroidism (0%–6%) [4]. Other less common risks include bleeding, which can occur up to 72 hours after the time of surgery, and wound infection.

TOXIC NODULE

Toxic adenomas are autonomously functioning benign tumors that cause symptomatic hyperthyroidism. The true incidence of toxic adenomas in children is too low for accurate epidemiologic estimates. In the case of children with solitary or unilobar toxic adenomas, thyroid lobectomy is the recommended procedure (or rarely, isthmusectomy, if the toxic nodule is in the isthmus). Subtotal lobectomy and nodulectomy are inadequate resections and increase the risk of recurrence. As in the case of Graves' disease, these patients should be rendered biochemically and clinically euthyroid prior to surgery. The risk of lobectomy includes bleeding and recurrent laryngeal nerve injury.

CONGENITAL GOITER

Another benign thyroid disease that can require surgical intervention is congenital goiter. Congenital goiters can be solitary or multinodular. The true incidence of these pathologies is low enough to preclude epidemiologic estimates. Large goiters can be symptomatic. If a patient develops symptoms of compression related to mass effect, such as discomfort or pain ("globus sensation"), dysphagia, dysphonia, or difficulty in breathing particularly when lying flat, surgery should be considered. Uninodular goiters are amenable to lobectomy, while multinodular goiters require near-total or total thyroidectomy.

THYROID MALIGNANT LESIONS

Thyroid nodules occur rarely in children but require investigation because the incidence of malignancy is higher in the pediatric population than in adults. Evaluation of a thyroid nodule should begin with a history and physical examination, along with a biochemical evaluation. This is typically followed by an ultrasound. In patients who are hyperthyroid, ultrasound should be followed by a nuclear medicine ("uptake") scan in order to determine if the pathology is a "warm" or "hot" nodule (that is, a toxic adenoma). Suspicious nodules should undergo interrogation with an ultrasound-guided fine-needle aspiration biopsy (FNAB). If the evaluation of a thyroid nodule reveals an FNAB with cytology that is consistent with follicular or Hurthle cell neoplasia, surgical excision is warranted for definitive histologic diagnosis; cytology cannot identify vascular or capsular invasion and discriminate adenomas from carcinomas. There are no specific professional society guidelines addressing the approach to follicular or Hurthle cell neoplasms in children. In these cases, the general recommendation is thyroid lobectomy with completion thyroidectomy if the pathology demonstrates vascular

and/or capsular invasion, except in the case of bilateral nodularity, where a total thyroidectomy is warranted initially.

Incidence of DTC is 0.49 per 100,000 per year, but is rising steeply, largely because of the rapid expansion of papillary thyroid cancer that has been observed around the world. Compared to adults, pediatric patients with DTC present with more extensive disease; lymph node involvement at the time of diagnosis is seen in 40%–80% of children compared to 20%–50% of adults. Distant metastases at presentation is seen in 20%–30% of cases. Nevertheless, prognosis is favorable, with an associated 5-year survival rate of 95%–99%, and a 20-year survival rate of 90% documented in literature. Owing to the relative rarity of DTC in children, there have been no prospective randomized clinical trials to determine optimal management. When thorough lymphadenectomy was performed in conjunction with total thyroidectomy, patients with clinically or radiographically positive lymph nodes achieved survival rates that were similar to those of patients who presented with node-negative diseases. In this particular case, the authors defined lymph node management as "complete" if it included a modified radical neck dissection [5]. Moreover, PTC is frequently multifocal and bilateral within the thyroid gland; therefore, near-total or total thyroidectomy is usually indicated. This operative approach further facilitates the administration of radioactive iodine post-operatively and long term surveillance with thyroglobulin (Tgb) levels. Data also show that risk of recurrence and even survival are enhanced statistically with near-total or total thyroidectomy compared to lobectomy in adults. Consequently, there is growing consensus that children with DTC should undergo total or near total thyroidectomy with central compartment lymph node dissection for clinically or radiographically positive lymph node disease.

MTC arises from the calcitonin-producing parafollicular C cells of the thyroid gland. It has an incidence in children of 0.03 per 100,000 population per year. MTC can occur sporadically or as part of a spectrum of familial MTC syndromes. In adults, sporadic MTC accounts for 65%–75% of MTC, but in the pediatric population, sporadic carcinomas are exceedingly rare; the vast majority of MTC diagnosed in childhood is hereditary. Hereditary MTC can occur independently as familial MTC (FMTC). It can also occur as part of a triad in the multiple endocrine neoplasia (MEN) syndromes with pheochromocytoma and primary hyperparathyroidism in MEN 2A, or with pheochromocytoma, marfanoid habitus, and mucosal neuromas with MEN 2B. As such, it is nearly always the first component of the MEN 2 phenotypes. Both syndromes are related to selected mutations of the RET proto oncogene. The MTC related to MEN 2B is the most virulent, followed by that of MEN 2A and FMTC, respectively. Patients (e.g., parents and parents-to-be) with MTC should be informed about the possibility of inheritable cancer syndromes and offered genetic testing and counseling as appropriate.

After genetic counseling and RET testing of all first degree relatives, risk categories and recommendations for prophylactic thyroidectomy have been made by the American Thyroid Association [7] (Table 24.1).

Post-operatively, patients require diligent surveillance for disease recurrence. Biochemical evidence of disease recurrence includes new calcitonin elevation or rapid calcitonin or carcinoembryonic antigen (CEA) doubling time. Palpable disease in the surgical bed or draining nodes is also indicative of recurrent disease. In cases of suspected recurrence, imaging with ultrasound is indicated, with the diagnosis confirmed by FNA. If extra-cervical disease is suspected, computed tomography (and magnetic resonance imaging for the liver, in particular) can facilitate confirmation.

Table 24.1 Risk categories and recommendations for prophylactic thyroidectomy

Codon mutation	Syndrome	Risk category	Timing for prophylactic thyroidectomy
918	MEN 2B	Highest	As early as possible within the first year or first month of life
883	MEN 2B	High	Within first 5 years of life
634	MEN 2A	High	Within first 5 years of life

WHO SHOULD BE OPERATING ON CHILDREN?

In a literature review examining more than 20 case series reports on a total of 1,800 pediatric patients, rates of permanent recurrent laryngeal nerve injury and permanent hypoparathyroidism were lowest in operations by high-volume thyroid surgeons [6]. The reported range of complication rates was considerable:

- Nerve injury rates ranged from 0% to 40%
- Hypoparathyroidism rates varied from 0% to 32%

The authors go on to note, "all surgery should be performed by high-volume, experienced endocrine, pediatric, and head and neck surgeons." A multidisciplinary approach that involves pediatric endocrinologists, pediatricians, surgeons, nuclear medicine physicians, anesthesiologists, and pathologists is an essential part of the pre-operative, post-operative, and long-term management of children with thyroid disease and especially those who are undergoing thyroidectomy.

THYROID PAIN AND ABSCESS

It is a rare benign condition known for its recurrence and curiously more common on the left side at the mid- and upper pole of the thyroid gland. As such it is due to infection in the remnant of third or fourth branchial pouch. Because of complex course, due to their embryological origin, presentation appears as an abscess of the thyroid gland. These remnants can also present as a cold nodule in the thyroid gland before any infective episode or after clearance of infection and need to be considered in differential diagnosis with other nodules of the thyroid gland. Anatomical familiarity and knowledge is essential to avoid recurrence and injury to vital neurovascular structures.

This pathology essentially needs complete excision of the remnant tissue after initial drainage of the abscess. Surgical therapy of third and fourth arch anomalies is similar to that of the more common second arch anomaly with the following exceptions. Endoscopy should be used to identify pyriform sinus entry point. This identification helps in settling diagnosis of the infected branchial remnant as cause and also allows cannulation or injection of dye in the tract to aid with dissection. Fourth arch anomaly resections require ipsilateral hemithyroidectomy to complete excision of the tract and sometimes partial resection of thyroid cartilage to provide adequate exposure of pyriform fossa sinus.

ECTOPIC THYROID GLAND

In thyroid dysgenesis, nearly 66% of remnants thyroid gland are found in an ectopic location, anywhere from base of the tongue (lingual thyroid) to the normal position in the neck (hypoplasia). It may present as an asymptomatic or symptomatic (breathing or feeding difficulty) mass at the base of the tongue or in the midline of the neck at supra- or infrahyoid position. Sometimes it can get infected if located in the thyroglossal duct cyst. Clinical importance lies in the fact that ectopically located thyroid tissue could be the only functioning thyroid tissue available in the body. Should it need to be removed, then a post-operative hypothyroid state is expected. Therefore, these patients will need lifelong thyroid hormone supplements or transplantation of ectopically located thyroid tissue to other suitable locations and long term surveillance for hypothyroidism.

REFERENCES

1. Bilimoria KY, Bentrem DJ, Ko CY, Stewart AK, Winchester DP, Talamonti MS, Sturgeon C. Extent of surgery affects survival for papillary thyroid cancer. *Ann Surg.* 2007;246:375–84.

2. Birrell G, Cheetham T. Juvenile thyrotoxicosis; can we do better? *Arch Dis Child.* 2004;89:745–50.

3. Pesce CE, Shiue Z, Tsai HL, Umbricht CB, Tufano RP, Dackiw AP, Kowalski J, Zeiger MA. Postoperative hypocalcemia after thyroidectomy for Graves' disease. *Thyroid.* 2010;20:1279–83. Epub 2010 Oct 18.

4. American Thyroid Association (ATA) Guidelines Taskforce on Thyroid Nodules and Differentiated Thyroid Cancer, Cooper DS et al. Revised American Thyroid Association management guidelines for patients with thyroid nodules and differentiated thyroid cancer. *Thyroid.* 2009;19:1167–214.

5. Handkiewicz-Junak D, Wloch J, Roskosz J, Krajewska J, Kropinska A, Pomorski L, Kukulska A, Prokurat A, Wygoda Z, Jarzab B. Total thyroidectomy and adjuvant radioiodine treatment independently decrease locoregional recurrence risk in childhood and adolescent differentiated thyroid cancer. *J Nucl Med.* 2007;48:879–88.

6. Scholz S, Smith JR, Chaignaud B, Shamberger RC, Huang SA. Thyroid surgery at Children's Hospital Boston: A 35-year single institution experience. *J Pediatr Surg.* 2011;46:437–42.

7. Wu LS, Roman SA, Sosa JA. Medullary thyroid cancer: An update of new guidelines and recent developments. *Curr Opin Oncol.* 2011;23:22–7.

INDEX

A

ABBA, *see* Axillo-bilateral breast approach
Active surveillance, as alternative to surgery, 105–106
Adena Pipe, 1, 2
Aerodigestive injury, thyroid surgery and, 120
Aerodigestive tract, invasion of, 127–129
    intra-laryngotracheal luminal invasions, 129
    larynx invasion, 128
    respiratory tract invasion, 128
    tracheal invasion, 128–129
Agranulocytosis, 51
Airway concerns, in thyroid surgery, 120–123
    difficult intubation, 120
    hypoparathyroidism, 121–122
    hypothyroidism, 122
    injury to EBSLN, 120–121
    thyroid storm, 122–123
AIT, *see* Amiodarone induced thyrotoxicosis
ALK, *see* Anaplastic lymphoma kinase
ALK inhibitors, 175–176
Amiodarone, 53
Amiodarone induced thyrotoxicosis (AIT), 53
Anaplastic lymphoma kinase (ALK), 174
Anaplastic thyroid cancers (ATC)
    clinical presentation, 147–148
        clinical evaluation, 147–148
        clinical findings, 147
        diagnosis, 147
        staging, 148
    imaging of, 31–40
        lymphadenopathy, 37, 40, 41
        primary thyroid lymphoma, 33
        ultrasound elastography, 33, 37, 39, 40
    neoadjuvant chemotherapy, role of, 149
    neoadjuvant pre-operative radiotherapy, 148
    overview, 147
    pathology, 49
    post-operative external beam radiotherapy, 148
    treatment of, 148–149
Anesthesia, for thyroid surgery, 3
    awake intubation, 61
    cervical epidura, *see* Cervical epidural anesthesia, for thyroid surgery
    general, 61
    induction of, 61–62
    maintenance of, 61–62
    recovery from, 62
    regional, 63
Ansa cervicalis, surgical anatomy of, 8, 9
Anterior jugular veins, surgical anatomy of, 7–8
Anti-thyroglobulin antibodies (Anti-TG AB), 152
Asepsis, 3
ATC, *see* Anaplastic thyroid cancers
Autoimmune thyroiditis, 24–25
Autonomously functioning thyroid nodule (AFTN), 163
Axillo-bilateral breast approach (ABBA), 83

B

BABA, *see* Bilateral axillo-breast approach
Babcock, William Wayne, 4
Babcock forceps, 4
Beahr's triangle, 12, 13
Berry's ligament, 13, 71, 72
Bethesda system for reporting of thyroid cytopathology (BSRTC), 45
Bigelow, Henry Jacob, 3, 5
Bilateral axillo-breast approach (BABA), 83, 84, 86
Bilroth, Theodor, 4
Blood supply, of thyroid gland, 10–12
    inferior thyroid artery, 10
    pyramidal artery, 10–11
    superior thyroid artery, 10
    thyroid ima artery, 10
    thyroid veins, 11–12
Bovie, William T., 4
BRAF inhibitor, 175
B-RAF mutations, 155, 173
BSRTC, *see* Bethesda system for reporting of thyroid cytopathology
Buparlisib, 176

C

Cabozantinib, 175
Capsule, of thyroid gland, 9
CCND, *see* Central compartment neck dissection
Central compartment neck dissection (CCND), 113–115
Ceritinib, 176
Cervical epidural anesthesia, for thyroid surgery, 63–66
    indications, 64
    intra-operative management, 65
    method for, 64–65
    post-operative management, 65–66
    pre-medication, 64
Colloid goiter, 46
Colloid nodules, 28
Cricothyroid joint, 13
Crizotinib, 176
Cushing, Harvey, 4

D

Decompressive craniotomy, 3
De humani corporis fabrica, 97
De Quervain's (sub-acute) thyroiditis, management of, 52–53
Differentiated thyroid cancers (DTC)
    completion thyroidectomy, 106–107
    extent of surgery, 106
    hemi-thyroidectomy vs total thyroidectomy, 107–108
    low risk thyroid cancer *vs.* high risk thyroid cancer, 106
    metastases neck nodes in, surgery of, 113–116
    nodal recurrence in, risk of, 116
    surgery for, 105–106
    surgical tips and tricks, 108–109
Drug-induced thyroiditis, management of, 52
DTC, *see* Differentiated thyroid cancers

E

Ectopic thyroid, 163
EFVPTC, *see* Encapsulated Follicular Variant of Papillary Thyroid Carcinoma
Embryology, of thyroid gland, 7–8
Encapsulated Follicular Variant of Papillary Thyroid Carcinoma (EFVPTC), 47
Eustachius, Bartholomew, 1
Everolimus, 176
External branch of the superior laryngeal nerve (EBSLN), 12, 109

F

Fine needle aspiration cytology (FNAC), 45
FNAC, *see* Fine needle aspiration cytology
Follicular neoplasia, pathology of, 47

G

Gillette, King Camp, 4
Globus hystericus, 17
Goiter
    earliest artistic depictions, 1, 2
    history of, 1–2
Graves' disease, 24, 25, 163
    beta adrenergic blockers for, 52
    management of, 51–52
    potassium iodide therapy, 52
    radioiodine therapy, 52
    RAI therapy for, 166
Gross, Jack, 2
Gross, Samuel David, 4

H

Halsted, William Steward, 4
Harington, Charles, 2
Hashimoto's thyroiditis, 25–26
Hematoma, thyroid surgery and, 119–120
Hemi-thyroidectomy, 42
Hultl, Humer, 4
Hurthle cell neoplasm, 46
    ultrasound of, 29, 31
Hyperparathyroidism (HPT), 179
    minimally invasive parathyroidectomy, 181–183
        bilateral neck exploration, 182
        extent of surgery, 182
        intraoperative parathyroid gland detection, 183
        operative adjuncts, 182–183
        parathyroid autofluorescence, 183
        parathyroid carcinoma, 183
    syndromic associations with, 180
Hypertrophic or keloid scar, thyroid surgery and, 120
Hypoparathyroidism, 121–122

Hypothyroidism, 122
    management of, 53–54
        central hypothyroidism, 53
        primary hypothyroidism, 53–54

I

Infections, thyroid surgery and, 119
Inferior thyroid artery, 10
Insular carcinoma, pathology of, 49–50
Intra-operative neural monitoring (IONM), 97,
        106
    continuous vagal monitoring, 102
    intra-operative setup, 100
    laryngeal examination, importance of,
        97–98
    loss of signal during, 100, 101
    neural injury prevention, 102
    neural mapping using, 98
    non-recurrent laryngeal nerve, intra-
        operative identification of, 102
    passive EMG activity during, 100
    routine use of, 101
    safety, 100
    setup, 99–100
    and staged thyroidectomy in thyroid cancer
        surgery, 100–101
    standards for, 98–100
    superior laryngeal nerve monitoring, 102
    technique, 98–99
    utility and applications, 98
IONM, *see* Intra-operative neural monitoring
Ipsilateral vocal cord paralysis, 97
Isthmus
    discovery of, 1
    relations of, 9
131I-whole body scan, 164–165

K

Kendall, Edward C., 2
Kocher, Emil Theodor, 4, 5

L

Laryngeal nerve palsy, recurrent, 82
LATC, *see* Locally advanced thyroid cancer
Lenvatinib, 175
Levator glandulae thyroidae, 13
Linea alba cervicalis, 94
Lister, Joseph, 3, 5
List of Essential Medicines, 1
Liston, Robert, 4
Locally advanced thyroid cancer (LATC),
        127–133
    aerodigestive tract, invasion of, 127–129
        intra-laryngotracheal luminal invasions,
            129
        larynx invasion, 128
        respiratory tract invasion, 128
        tracheal invasion, 128–129
    overview, 127
    pharyngeal and esophageal involvement,
        132
    strap muscles, invasion of, 127
    surgical management, 129–132
    vascular invasion, 132
Lore's triangle, 12
LOS, *see* Loss of signal
Loss of signal (LOS), 98
    during IONM, 100, 101
Lugol, Jean Guillaume Auguste, 1
Lugol's Solution (aqueous iodine), 1

M

Malampatti grading, 60
MAPK pathway, *see* Mitogen-activated protein
        kinase pathway
Maryland dissector, 93
Medullary thyroid cancer (MTC)
    external beam radiotherapy, adjuvant, 142
    features of, 135
    imaging of, 30–31, 38
    immunohistochemical features of, 137
    metastasis, 142
    oncocytic variant of, histological features
        of, 137
    pathology of, 48, 49
    pre-operative evaluation, 135–138
    prophylactic cancer surgery, 142–143
    recurrence, 142
    residual, 142
    TNM classification AJCC (8th edition) for,
        138–142
        palliative surgery, 138
        surgical steps, 139–142
        surgical treatment, 138–139
        unresectability criteria, 138
MEK inhibitor, 175
Metastasis to thyroid, imaging of, 40–42
    computed tomography, 41–42
    contrast-enhanced ultrasound, 41
    hemi-thyroidectomy, 42
    magnetic resonance imaging, 41–42
    positron emission tomography-computed
        tomography, 41–42
    post-thyroidectomy, 42
Midline tuberculous abscess, 16
Minimally invasive parathyroidectomy, 181–183
Minimally invasive video-assisted thyroidectomy
        (MIVAT) technique, 83
Mitogen-activated protein kinase (MAPK)
        pathway, 173
MIVAT technique, *see* Minimally invasive
        video-assisted thyroidectomy
        technique
Molecular pathogenesis, 173–174
mTOR pathway, 173
Muco-epidermoid carcinoma, 50
Multi-kinase inhibitors (MKI), 174–175
Multinodular goiter, surgery of, 75–77
    evolution of, 75
    follow-up strategy, 76–77
    genesis of thyroid nodule, 75–76
    indications for surgery, 75–76
    optimizing surgical treatment, 76
    overview, 75
    structural issues, 76
Murphy, John, 3–4
Myxedema coma, 62

N

Natural orifice transluminal endoscopic surgery
        (NOTES), 83
Neoplastic lesions, pathology of, 47–50
    follicular neoplasia, 47
    insular carcinoma, 49–50
    medullary carcinoma, 48, 49
    papillary carcinoma, 47, 48
    poorly differentiated carcinoma, 49–50
Nerves, of thyroid gland, 12–13
Nerve supply, of thyroid, 11–12
Next generation sequencing (NGS), 173
NIFTP, *see* Non-invasive follicular thyroid
        neoplasm with papillary nuclear
        features

Nodal metastasis in thyroid cancer
    diagnosis, 113
    lateral compartment, 115–116
    metastases neck nodes, in DTC, 113–114
    quantification of problem, 113
    surgical tips, 114–115
    therapeutic CCND, 113–115
Nodule of Zuckerkandl, 12, 13
Non-Hodgkin's lymphoma (NHL), 49
Non-invasive follicular thyroid neoplasm with
        papillary nuclear features (NIFTP)
    histology, 47
    nuclear inclusions in, 47
Non-neoplastic lesions, 46
Non-radioactive iodine imaging, 165–169
Non-RAI radiotracer therapy, 169
Non-recurrent laryngeal nerve (NRLN), 13, 102
NOTES, *see* Natural orifice transluminal
        endoscopic surgery
NRLN, *see* Non-recurrent laryngeal nerve

P

Papanicolaou stain, 46
Papillary thyroid carcinoma, imaging of, 29–30,
        32–36
Papillary thyroid microcarcinoma (PTMC), 105
    imaging of, 30, 37
Parathyroid disorders, surgical management of
    clinical profile, 179
    diagnosis, 179–181
        management, 180
        surgical anatomy, 180–181
    minimally invasive parathyroidectomy,
        181–183
        bilateral neck exploration, 182
        extent of surgery, 182
        intraoperative parathyroid gland
            detection, 183
        operative adjuncts, 182–183
        parathyroid autofluorescence, 183
        parathyroid carcinoma, 183
    overview, 179
    pathology, 183–184
Parathyroid (PT) glands, 12
Parathyroid hormone (PTH), history of, 2–3
Parathyroid insufficiency, 82
Parker, Morgan, 4
PAX8-PPARγ rearrangement, 174
Pediatric thyroid surgery, 187–189
    autoimmune thyroiditis, 187–188
    benign conditions warranting surgical
        management, 187–188
    congenital goiter, 188
    ectopic thyroid gland, 189
    Graves' disease, 187–188
    malignant lesions, 188
    overview, 187
    right surgeons for, 189
    thyroid pain and abscess, 189
    toxic adenomas, 188
Petz, Aladar, 4
Phosphatidyl inositol 3 kinase-AKT
        (PI3K-AKT), 173
Pitt-Rivers, Rosalind, 2
Platysma muscle, surgical anatomy of, 7
Poorly differentiated carcinoma, pathology of,
        49–50
Postpartum thyroiditis, management of, 52
Potts, John Thomas, 2
Primary hypothyroidism, 53–54
Processus posterior glandulae thyroidea, 12
Prograsp forceps, 93
Prophylactic cancer surgery, 142–143

Propylthiouracil (PTU), 51
PTMC, *see* Papillary thyroid microcarcinoma
PTU, *see* Propylthiouracil
Pyramidal artery, 10–11

R

Radiation-induced thyroiditis, management of, 53
Radioiodine (RAI)
　imaging with, molecular basis of, 161–165
　　131I-whole body scan, 164–165
　　normal and abnormal thyroid scintigraphy,
　　　162–164
　　thyroid scan, 162
　　thyroid uptake study, 161
RAI refractory disease, treatment of, 168
RAI therapy
　of bone metastases, 168
　for Graves' disease, 166
　pulmonary metastases, treatment of, 168–169
　remnant ablation, 167
　side effects and complications of, 168–169
　of thyroid cancer, 166–167
　TMNG or TA, 166
RAS mutations, 155, 173
Recurrent laryngeal nerve (RLN), 12–13, 16
　management of, 71
　with preoperative vocal cord paralysis, 101
　robotic thyroidectomy, 92, 93
RET-PTC rearrangement, 174
Retrosternal goiter (RSG)
　chest X-ray, 80
　classification, 80–81
　clinical manifestations, 79
　CT scan, 80
　investigation for, 79–80
　overview, 79
　sternotomy approach for, 82
　treatment, 81–82
rhTSH (thyrogen), 164
RLN, *see* Recurrent laryngeal nerve
RLN paralysis, 97
Robotic or endoscopic thyroidectomy, remote
　　access
　advantages and limitations of, 84–86
　axillo-bilateral breast approach, 83
　bilateral axillo-breast approach, 83, 84, 86
　classification, 83–86
　　operative procedures, 83–84
　comparison of, 88
　experience of, 86–87
　gasless postauricular facelift approach, 84
　gasless unilateral axillary approach, 83–84,
　　85
　history of, 83
　postauricular facelift approach, 87
　transoral vestibular approach, 84
　　with carbon dioxide insufflation, 88
Robotic thyroidectomy, 91–95
　indications and contraindications for,
　　91–95
　outcomes, 94–95
　overview, 91
　techniques, 91–94
　　axillo-breast approach, 93
　　retroauricular approach, 93–94
　　trans-axillary approach, 91–93
　　transoral approach, 94
RSG, *see* Retrosternal goiter

S

Sanzio, Raffaello, 1
Schreger, C. H. T., 1

Selumetinib, 175
Seroma, thyroid surgery and, 119
Sirolimus, 176
Skull trephining, 3
Solitary thyroid nodule (STN), 45
Sorafenib, 174–175
Strap muscles, surgical anatomy of, 8
Superior thyroid artery, 10
Suppurative infection, 16
Surgery, history of, 3–4
Surgical anatomy, of thyroid gland, 7–9
　ansa cervicalis, 8, 9
　anterior jugular veins, 7–8
　platysma muscle, 7
　strap muscles, 8
Surgical instruments, history of, 3–4
Surveillance, post-treatment, of thyroid cancer
　dynamic risk stratification, 155–157
　initial risk stratification, 153–155
　　molecular markers, profiling of, 155
　　thyroid cancer mortality risk, 153–154
　　thyroid cancer recurrence risk, 154–155
　overview, 151
　strategies for, 157–158
　　according to risk and response to
　　　treatment, 158
　　high-risk patients, 158
　　low-risk or intermediate-risk patients,
　　　157–158
　surveillance tools for DTC, 151–153
　　anti-thyroglobulin antibodies, 152
　　computed tomography scans, 153
　　positron emission tomography scans, 153
　　serum thyroglobulin, 151–152
　　ultrasonography of neck, 152
　　whole body RAI scans, 152–153
System of Surgery, A, 4

T

TA, *see* Toxic adenoma
Targeted therapy, in thyroid cancer, 174–176
　AKT pathway inhibitor, 176
　ALK inhibitors, 175–176
　immunotherapy, 176
　mTOR pathway inhibitor, 176
　multi-kinase inhibitors, 174–175
　PI3 K pathway inhibitor, 176
　tyrosine kinase inhibitors, 174–175
Teratoma, 50
TERT promoter gene mutation, 174
TERT promoter mutations, 155
Thyroglobulin (Tg), 151–152
Thyroglossal cyst, 16
Thyroidectomy, 67–73
　anesthesia for, 68, 69
　appliances and technology for, 68–69
　incision planning, 69
　injuries in, identifying, 73
　overview, 67
　parathyroid injuries, 73
　patients at risk, identification of, 67
　position for, 69
　RLN injuries, 73
　safety steps for, 69–72
　size of thyroid masses, 67–68
Thyroid gland
　anatomical understanding of, historical
　　perspective, 1–2
　capsule of, 9
　embryology of, 7–8
　enlargement of, *see* Goiter
　hormones, history of, 2–3
　relations of, 10

surgical anatomy, *see* Surgical anatomy, of
　　thyroid gland
　venous drainage of, 11
Thyroid ima artery, 10
Thyroid Imaging, Reporting, and Data System
　　(TIRADS), 26
Thyroiditis, 162
　autoimmune, imaging of, 24–25
　Hashimoto's, imaging of, 25–26
　management of, 52–53
　　De Quervain's (sub-acute) thyroiditis,
　　　52–53
　　drug-induced thyroiditis, 52
　　infectious or post-infectious thyroiditis, 52
　　postpartum thyroiditis, 52
　　radiation-induced thyroiditis, 53
　pathology of, 46, 47
Thyroid nodule, clinical assessment of, 15–18
　clinical questionnaire for functionality, 18
　patient clinical history, gathering, 15–17
　physical examination, 17–18
　thyroid swellings, clinical questionnaire
　　for, 18
Thyroid nodules, 163–164
Thyroid nodules, imaging of, 26–29, 30
　benign, 28
　colloid nodules, 28
　evaluation for size, 26
　malignant, 28–29
　TIRADS risk category, 26–28
Thyroid-stimulating hormone (TSH), 151
Thyroid storm, 122–123
Thyroid surgery
　airway examination, 60
　airway management, preparation of, 61
　anesthesia for
　　cervical epidural, 63–66
　　induction of, 61–62
　　regional, 63
　complications of, 119–123; *see also* specific
　　complications
　history of, 4
　medical history of patient, 59–60
　post-operative complication, 62–63
　pre-operative assessment, 57–59
　pre-operative preparation, 60–61
　radiological assessment, 60
Thyroid swellings, clinical questionnaire for, 18
Thyroid veins, 11–12
Thyrotoxicosis, 25
Thyrotoxic state, 15
Thyrotoxic storm, 62–63
Thyroxine (T4), 2
TIRADS, *see* Thyroid Imaging, Reporting, and
　　Data System
TMNG, *see* Toxic multinodular goiter
TOETVA, *see* Transoral endoscopic thyroidectomy
　　through a vestibular approach
Toxic adenoma (TA), 163
Toxic multinodular goiter (TMNG), 162
Transfiguration, The, 1, 3
Transoral endoscopic thyroidectomy through a
　　vestibular approach (TOETVA), 94
3,5,3′-Triiodothyronine (T3), 2
Tyrosine kinase inhibitors (TKI), 174–175
Tyrosine kinase inhibitors, for drug-induced
　　thyroiditis, 53

U

Ultrasound, of thyroid gland, 21–26
　in diffuse thyroid disorders, 24–26
　　autoimmune thyroiditis, 24–25
　　Hashimoto's thyroiditis, 25–26

Ultrasound, of thyroid gland (*Continued*)
    embryology and ectopic thyroid glands, 24
    of follicular neoplasm, 29, 31
    history and evolution, 21
    Hurthle cell neoplasm, 29, 31
    principle and physics of, 21–22
    technique and patient position, 24
    thyroid anatomy, 22–24

V

Vandetanib, 175
VANS, *see* Video-assisted neck surgery
VCP, *see* Vocal cord palsy
Vertical hemilaryngectomy, 129
Vesalius, Andreas, 1
Video-assisted neck surgery (VANS), 83

Vocal cord palsy (VCP), 101
von Haller, Albrecht, 2
von Luschka, Herbert, 1

W

Whole body RAI imaging, 164–165
Whole body RAI scans (WBS), 152–153